T0263064

Neurocritical Care

Editors

DEEPA MALAIYANDI
LORI SHUTTER

CRITICAL CARE CLINICS

www.criticalcare.theclinics.com

Consulting Editor
GREGORY S. MARTIN

January 2023 • Volume 39 • Number 1

ELSEVIER

1600 John F. Kennedy Boulevard • Suite 1800 • Philadelphia, Pennsylvania, 19103-2899

http://www.theclinics.com

CRITICAL CARE CLINICS Volume 39, Number 1
January 2023 ISSN 0749-0704, ISBN-13: 978-0-323-89732-7

Editor: Joanna Collett
Developmental Editor: Hannah Almira Lopez

Critical Care Clinics (ISSN: 0749-0704) is published quarterly by Elsevier Inc., 360 Park Avenue South, New York, NY 10010-1710. Months of issue are January, April, July, and October. Business and Editorial Offices: 1600 John F. Kennedy Blvd., Suite 1800, Philadelphia, PA 19103-2899. Customer Service Office: 6277 Sea Harbor Drive, Orlando, FL 32887-4800. Periodicals postage paid at New York, NY and additional mailing offices. Subscription prices are $274.00 per year for US individuals, $779 per year for US institutions, $100.00 per year for US students and residents, $305.00 per year for Canadian individuals, $976.00 per year for Canadian institutions, $348.00 per year for international individuals, $976.00 per year for international institutions, $100.00 per year for Canadian students/residents, and $150.00 per year for foreign students/residents. To receive student/resident rate, orders must be accompanied by name of affiliated institution, date of term, and the signature of program/residency coordinator on institution letterhead. Orders will be billed at individual rate until proof of status is received. Foreign air speed delivery is included in all *Clinics* subscription prices. All prices are subject to change without notice. POSTMASTER: Send address changes to *Critical Care Clinics*, Elsevier Periodicals Customer Service, 11830 Westline Industrial Drive, St. Louis, MO 63146. **Customer Service: 1-800-654-2452 (US). From outside of the US, call 1-314-447-8871. Fax: 1-314-447-8029. E-mail: journalscustomerservice-usa@elsevier.com (for print support) or journalsonlinesupport-usa@elsevier.com (for online support).**

Reprints. For copies of 100 or more of articles in this publication, please contact the Commercial Reprints Department, Elsevier Inc., 360 Park Avenue South, New York, NY 10010-1710. Tel.: 212-633-3874; Fax: 212-633-3820; E-mail: reprints@elsevier.com.

Critical Care Clinics is also published in Spanish by Editorial Inter-Medica, Junin 917, 1er A, 1113, Buenos Aires, Argentina.

Critical Care Clinics is covered in *MEDLINE/PubMed (Index Medicus), EMBASE/Excerpta Medica, Current Concepts/Clinical Medicine, ISI/BIOMED*, and *Chemical Abstracts*.

Contributors

CONSULTING EDITOR

GREGORY S. MARTIN, MD, MSC
Professor, Division of Pulmonary, Allergy, Critical Care and Sleep Medicine, Research Director, Emory Critical Care Center, Director, Emory/Georgia Tech Predictive Health Institute, Co-Director, Atlanta Center for Microsystems Engineered Point-of-Care Technologies (ACME POCT), President, Society of Critical Care Medicine, Atlanta, Georgia, USA

EDITORS

DEEPA MALAIYANDI, MD, FNCS
Assistant Professor and Division Director of Neurocritical Care, Department of Neurology, University of Toledo College of Medicine, Neurointensivist, Department of Neurology, ProMedica Toledo Hospital and Neurosciences Center, Toledo, Ohio, USA

LORI SHUTTER, MD, FNCS, FCCM
Professor of Critical Care Medicine, Neurology, and Neurosurgery, Vice Chair for Education, Division Director of Neurocritical Care, Director of Multidisciplinary Critical Care and Neurocritical Care Training Programs, Department of Critical Care Medicine, UPMC/University of Pittsburgh School of Medicine, Pittsburgh, Pennsylvania, USA

AUTHORS

FIRAS ABDULMAJEED, MD
Assistant Professor of Critical Care Medicine and Neurology, Department of Critical Care Medicine, University of Pittsburgh School of Medicine, Pittsburgh, Pennsylvania, USA

ABDALLA AMMAR, PharmD, FCCM, BCCCP, BCPS
Clinical Pharmacist-Neurocritical Care, NewYork-Presbyterian/Weill Cornell Medical Center, New York, New York, USA

MAHMOUD A. AMMAR, PharmD, FCCM, BCCCP, BCPS
Critical Care Pharmacist-Trauma-Surgical Critical Care, Yale New Haven Hospital, New Haven, Connecticut, USA

FRANCIS BERNARD, MD, FRCPC, FNCS
Consultant, Critical Care, Professor, Department of Medicine, Hôpital du Sacré-Cœur de Montréal, University of Montréal, Director of CENA (Center of Excellence for Advance Neuromonitoring), Montréal, Québec, Canada

CHERYLEE W.J. CHANG, MD, FACP, FCCM, FNCS
Division Chief, Neurocritical Care, Professor, Department of Neurology, Duke University, Durham, North Carolina, USA

TIFFANY R. CHANG, MD
Associate Professor, Departments of Neurosurgery and Neurology, University of Texas Health Science Center at Houston, Houston, Texas, USA

PATRICK J. COPPLER, PA-C
Department of Emergency Medicine, University of Pittsburgh, Pittsburgh, Pennsylvania, USA

SALVATORE A. D'AMATO, MD
Neurocritical Care Fellowship Program, Department of Neurosurgery, University of Texas Health Science Center at Houston, Houston, Texas, USA

JONATHAN ELMER, MD, MS
Departments of Emergency Medicine, Critical Care Medicine, and Neurology, University of Pittsburgh, Pittsburgh, Pennsylvania, USA

TRACEY H. FAN, DO
Department of Neurology, Division of Neurocritical Care, Massachusetts General Hospital, Department of Neurology, Division of Neurocritical Care, Brigham and Women's Hospital, Boston, Massachusetts, USA

VICTORIA FLEMING, BA
Departments of Neurology, University of Massachusetts Chan Medical School, Worcester, Massachusetts, USA

DIANA GREENE-CHANDOS, MD, FNCS
Associate Professor of Neurology, Program Director, Neurocritical Care Fellowship, School of Medicine Block Director, Neurointensivist and Vascular Neurologist, Department of Neurology, University of New Mexico, Albuquerque, New Mexico, USA

MOHANAD HAMANDI, MD
Medicine Resident, Department of Medicine, University of Pittsburgh School of Medicine, Pittsburgh, Pennsylvania, USA

ELYSIA JAMES, MD
Assistant Professor of Neurology, Division of Neurocritical Care, Assistant Dean of Diversity, University of Toledo College of Medicine, Toledo, Ohio, USA

SHRADDHA MAINALI, MD
Department of Neurology, Virginia Commonwealth University, Richmond, Virginia, USA

DEEPA MALAIYANDI, MD, FNCS
Assistant Professor and Division Director of Neurocritical Care, Department of Neurology, University of Toledo College of Medicine, Neurointensivist, Department of Neurology, ProMedica Toledo Hospital and Neurosciences Center, Toledo, Ohio, USA

ASMA M. MOHEET, MD, MHDS, FNCS
Medical Director, Neurocritical Care, OhioHealth Riverside Methodist Hospital, Columbus, Ohio, USA

SUSANNE MUEHLSCHLEGEL, MD, MPH, FNCS, FCCM, FAAN
Departments of Neurology, Anesthesiology/Critical Care, and Surgery, University of Massachusetts Chan Medical School, Worcester, Massachusetts, USA

CASEY OLM-SHIPMAN, MD, MS
Assistant Professor of Neurology and Neurosurgery, University of North Carolina School of Medicine, Chapel Hill, North Carolina, USA

SOOJIN PARK, MD
Department of Neurology, Department of Biomedical Informatics, Columbia University, New York, New York, USA

JOSE JAVIER PROVENCIO, MD
Louis Nerancy Professor in Neurology, Department of Neurology, University of Virginia, Charlottesville, Virginia, USA

DANIA QARYOUTI, MD
Department of Neurology, Neurology Resident Physician, University of New Mexico, Albuquerque, New Mexico, USA

ERIC S. ROSENTHAL, MD
Department of Neurology, Division of Neurocritical Care, Division of Clinical Neurophysiology, Massachusetts General Hospital, Boston, Massachusetts, USA

ANGELA HAYS SHAPSHAK, MD, FNCS
Associate Professor of Neurology and Anesthesiology, Director, Neurocritical Care Fellowship, Associate Director, Neurology Residency, The University of Alabama at Birmingham, Birmingham, Alabama, USA

LORI SHUTTER, MD, FNCS, FCCM
Professor of Critical Care Medicine, Neurology, and Neurosurgery, Vice Chair for Education, Division Director of Neurocritical Care, Director of Multidisciplinary Critical Care and Neurocritical Care Training Programs, Department of Critical Care Medicine, UPMC/University of Pittsburgh School of Medicine, Pittsburgh, Pennsylvania, USA

GENE SUNG, MD, MPH
Director, Neurocritical Care and Stroke, University of Southern California, LAC+USC Medical Center, Los Angeles, California, USA

KRISTI TEMPRO, MD
Fellow, Department of Neurology, Neurocritical Care, Duke University, Durham, North Carolina, USA

ELJIM P. TESORO, PharmD, FNCS, FCCM, BCCCP
Department of Pharmacy Practice, College of Pharmacy, University of Illinois at Chicago, Chicago, Illinois, USA

Contents

The History of Neurocritical Care as a Subspecialty   1

Kristi Tempro and Cherylee W.J. Chang

> The role of the neurointensivist as a subspecialist has been cemented in modern medicine globally. It was forged through the collaboration of neurologists, neurosurgeons, internists, anesthesiologists, general surgeons, emergency medicine physicians, and pediatricians. As with all critical care areas, it requires a multiprofessional environment. Neurocritical care harnesses knowledge, technology, resources, and research opportunities to embrace a multisystem approach to care for the neurologically critically ill. Although recently formally recognized, its crucial role to serve patients with acute, life-threatening neurologic insults has been well established.

Quality Improvement in Neurocritical Care   17

Casey Olm-Shipman and Asma M. Moheet

> Quality improvement is key to advancing outcomes for neurocritically ill patients. Variation in neurocritical care practice can lead to differences in health outcomes and contribute to health disparities. The implementation of evidence-based best practice standards represents a major opportunity to improve their care. Neurocritical care performance measures have recently been developed and may be used to target high priority areas for improvement. In addition, neurocritical care clinicians should be aware of the heavily weighted pay-for-performance and publicly reported performance measures that are directly relevant to neurocritical care practice.

Neurocritical Care Education in the United States   29

Angela Hays Shapshak and Lori Shutter

> Neurocritical care is a relatively young subspecialty that is rapidly coming into its own. As the neurocritical care community has expanded, the process of training and credentialing physicians in this growing field has undergone a rapid evolution. This article will review the history and current state of neurocritical care training and education, physician certification, and program accreditation in the United States within the larger context of critical care training across subspecialties.

Neurocritical Care Research: Collaborations for Curing Coma   47

Jose Javier Provencio

> One of the most common questions asked by family members of patients with brain injuries who are in a coma is "will my loved one wake up?".

Despite substantial improvements in the care of patients with neurological diseases, the medical and scientific community struggles to answer this simple question. More importantly, the technology and treatment strategies to improve the trajectory of patients with impaired consciousness in the acute setting are limited. The Curing Coma Campaign was developed by the Neurocritical Care Society as a multispecialty, multi-interest community of researchers and caretakers who are focused on patients with disorders of consciousness (DoC) in the acute phase of care. Over the first few years of the group, several publications have focused on identifying the gaps in our knowledge to encourage research in the area. In this review, the current understanding of DoC is reviewed. The work of the Curing Coma Campaign to identify gaps in our knowledge is highlighted.

This article reviews the care of patients with ischemic stroke in the intensive care unit, including early general critical care interventions for airway control blood pressure goals according to the type of acute stroke treatment, poststroke cerebral edema management, hemorrhagic conversion in ischemic stroke, fibrinolytic reversal, and management of carotid endarterectomy and infective endocarditis. The importance of preventing common intensive care complications is discussed, including aspiration pneumonia, deep venous thrombosis, urinary tract infections, cardiac arrhythmias, and hyperglycemia.

Aneurysmal subarachnoid hemorrhage and intracerebral hemorrhage are devastating injuries causing significant morbidity and mortality. However, advancements made over decades have improved outcomes. This review summarizes a systematic approach to stabilize and treat these patient populations.

In this review, we discuss treatment and considerations for status epilepticus in general intensive care unit patients, acquired brain injury, autoimmune conditions, toxidromes, pediatrics, and pregnancy.

(▶) Video content accompanies this article at http://www.criticalcare. theclinics.com.

Although intracranial pressure (ICP) monitoring has been the mainstay of traumatic brain injury (TBI) management for decades, new understanding of TBI physiopathology calls for paradigm shifts. The complexity of TBI management precludes ICP being taken as an isolated value with a specific threshold. Multimodality monitoring is crucial to expanding our comprehension of individualized pathophysiology, allowing for a precise and tailored treatment approach. This article will review keys concepts to interpret and apply published ICP management guidelines and statements.

CRITICAL CARE CLINICS

SERIES OF RELATED INTEREST

Emergency Medicine Clinics
https://www.emed.theclinics.com/
Clinics in Chest Medicine
https://www.chestmed.theclinics.com/

THE CLINICS ARE AVAILABLE ONLINE!
Access your subscription at:
www.theclinics.com

Preface

Neurocritical Care Past, Present, and Future

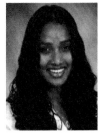 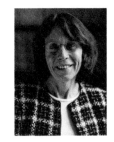

Deepa Malaiyandi, MD, FNCS   Lori Shutter, MD, FNCS, FCCM
Editors

In this issue, we have attempted to portray the evolution of both the science and the field of Neurocritical Care from its organic origins out of the polio epidemic to its ree-mergence as one of the burgeoning subspecialities in the landscape of modern critical care. Despite the remarkable growth in number of board-certified neurointensivists, specialty trained advanced practice providers, pharmacists, nurses, respiratory thera-pists, and other allied health care professionals, there continues to be a severe shortage of neurocritical care programs throughout the world. As such, patients with neurologic failure or who are at high risk for neurologic failure continue to be cared for by nonneurointensivists in a variety of general and other specialty intensive care units (ICUs). These units and their providers play a crucial role in the ability of these pa-tients to achieve their best possible functional outcome. The validation of neurocritical care-specific quality metrics is much anticipated to provide support and guide practice as well as fund allocation efforts.

The recognition of neurocritical care as an Accreditation Council for Graduate Medical Education (ACGME) -accredited subspecialty in 2021 marked a crowning moment for the many pioneers and visionaries who have deliberately persevered to-ward this status. A glimpse into the development of neurocritical care education is included as many institutions seek to add ACGME accreditation to their existing programs.

Neurocritical Care research is a rapidly expanding area that focuses on crucial clin-ical issues and the need to understand gaps in our current knowledge. The Curing Coma Campaign underway by the Neurocritical Care Society is one example of the vast international and multidisciplinary research collaborations in the field.

With respect to the practice of neurocritical care, we review fundamentals for bedside management as well as the state of the science for acute ischemic stroke, subarachnoid and intracerebral hemorrhage, status epilepticus, neurotrauma and

Crit Care Clin 39 (2023) xiii–xiv
https://doi.org/10.1016/j.ccc.2022.08.004
0749-0704/23/© 2022 Published by Elsevier Inc.

elevated intracranial pressure, death by neurologic criteria, neuromuscular weakness, neuroprognostication, neurocritical care in the general ICU, neuropharmacology, multimodal monitoring, and the emerging field of big data science and artificial intelligence in neurocritical care. Technology and advanced diagnostics are opening new avenues of investigation and patient care. In summary, the future of the field is bright with ongoing rapid scientific discovery in all areas. We are both honored and excited for this opportunity to provide a review of our specialty, updates in clinical care of critically ill neurologic patients, and a glimpse into some of the advances in our field with the readers.

Deepa Malaiyandi, MD, FNCS
Division of Neurocritical Care, Department of Neurology, University of Toledo College of Medicine, UT/PPG Neuroscience Center, 2130 West Central Avenue, Suite 201, Room 2355, Toledo, OH 43606, USA

Lori Shutter, MD, FNCS, FCCM
Department of Critical Care Medicine
UPMC/University of Pittsburgh School of Medicine
3550 Terrace Street
Scaife Hall, Room 646
Pittsburgh, PA 15261, USA

E-mail addresses:
deepa.malaiyandi@utoledo.edu (D. Malaiyandi)
shutter@upmc.edu (L. Shutter)

The History of Neurocritical Care as a Subspecialty

Kristi Tempro, MD, Cherylee W.J. Chang, MD,*

KEYWORDS

- History • Neurointensive care • Neurocritical care
- Subspecialty critical care medicine • Subspecialty certification

KEY POINTS

- The practice of intensive care has been integral to the treatment and recovery of critically ill patients since the nineteenth century.
- Neurologists established their role as intensivists during the poliomyelitis epidemic. Fueled by neurovascular and epilepsy advances, neurocritical care continues to evolve particularly for those with disorders of consciousness and traumatic injury.
- Neurocritical care embraces physicians from multiple primary specialties and includes multiprofessional teams proven to better patient outcomes.
- Recent ABMS subspecialty recognition, ACGME accreditation, efforts toward global collaboration, and guideline standardization will continue to refine the role of neurointensivists in modern health care.

INTRODUCTION

The early impetus for the development of the modern intensive care unit has been driven in part by neurologic conditions and their impact on other body systems. Yet the journey to recognition of neurocritical care (NCC) as a subspecialty has been long (**Fig. 1**). One major driver was the development of a postoperative neurosurgery area at the Johns Hopkins Hospital in 1923, under the aegis of neurosurgeon Walter Dandy. Moreover, the polio epidemics in the early 1900s resulted in vast numbers of patients with neuromuscular respiratory failure, which spurred technological advances in mechanical ventilation, tracheostomy, and endotracheal intubation. In the ensuing years, the bedside critical care clinician has become increasingly aware of the need to interweave growing knowledge of the nervous system, its pathobiological states, and pharmacologic and technological advances into their practice and research. In the United States, the coming of age of NCC has included being formally

Department of Neurology, Neurocritical Care, Duke University, 40 Duke Medicine Circle, Box 3824, Durham, NC 27710, USA
* Corresponding author.
E-mail address: Cherylee.chang@duke.edu
Twitter: @changc808 (C.W.J.C.)

Crit Care Clin 39 (2023) 1–15
https://doi.org/10.1016/j.ccc.2022.06.001
0749-0704/23/© 2022 Elsevier Inc. All rights reserved.

criticalcare.theclinics.com

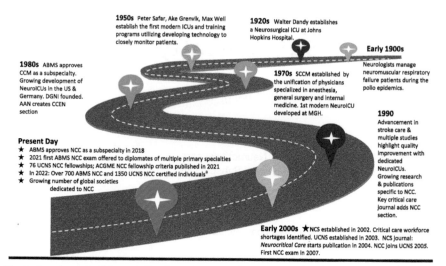

Fig. 1. Roadmap to Subspecialization—Journey of Neurocritical Care. Legend: ABMS, American Board of Medical Subspecialties; ACGME, Accreditation Council for Graduate Medical Education; CCM, Critical Care Medicine; DGNI, German Neurological Society of Neurological Intensive Care and Emergency Medicine; MGH, Massachusetts General Hospital; NCC, Neurocritical care; NCS, Neurocritical Care Society; NeuroICU, Neurocritical care unit; SCCM, Society of Critical Care Medicine; UCNS, United Council for Neurologic Subspecialties. [a]Some individuals with overlapping (UCNS and ABMS) certification.

recognized as a subspecialty of medicine by the American Board of Medical Specialties (ABMS) in 2018, the international growth of NCC societies, integration of NCC into larger critical care societies, and inclusion into their journals. This article delves into the history of NCC, its evolving presence among critical care subspecialties, and steps toward certification of individuals. A separate article will focus on education of neurointensivists and accreditation of training programs.

HISTORICAL REVIEW
The Development of Intensive Care Medicine as a Specialty

Historically, famine and vector-borne pathogens, such as plague, were the major cause of premature death. However, by the mid-1850s, waterborne infectious diseases became a major cause of death and a subject of intense study for the prevention and treatment through improved sanitation.[1] During this Victorian era, medicine began transforming its paradigm from tradition-based to science-based practice. It was during this time of scientific evolution that critical care medicine (CCM) was born.

From its inception, critical care has been a multiprofessional and multidisciplinary field. Its practice was forged in the 1850s by Florence Nightingale in British Military camps during the Crimean War.[2] She developed Nightingale Rose diagrams, which demonstrated that mortality predominantly involved preventable deaths rather than traumatic war injury. Improved sanitation and hygiene, and a novel practice of triaging more severely injured soldiers to beds closest to nursing stations for closer monitoring decreased mortality. Similar to Nightingale's practice, Dr Walter Dandy established a 4-bed neurosurgical intensive care unit in 1923 at the Johns Hopkins Hospital in Baltimore where continuous specialized postcraniotomy nursing care took place close to operating rooms.[3]

The polio epidemic of the early 1900s brought neurologists to the forefront of critical care teams. Their involvement was integral to providing the impetus to improve techniques for large-scale ventilatory care, standardization of frequent intensive monitoring, and skilled nursing care.[4,5] In the 1920s, the first effective negative pressure ventilator, the Drinker-Shaw iron lung, was tested on a poliomyelitis patient.[6] By the 1930s, endotracheal and tracheostomy tubes advanced from rigid metal tubes and positive pressure ventilators were developed. Intensive care was focused on airway management, optimization of ventilation, pulmonary toileting, and maintenance of hemodynamic stability. Additionally, nursing care addressed pressure relief by frequent repositioning, an issue highlighting another contribution to critical care by a neurologist. Jean-Martin Charcot described the progression of *Decubitus ominosus* in bed-bound patients with severe neurologic disease and inadequate nutrition in 1877.[7]

With the development of the polio vaccine, fewer patients with primary neurologic disease required ventilatory support. The military conflicts of World War II, Korean and Vietnam Wars, led to advances in resuscitation and postsurgical care. Specialized areas of intensive care were focused on postoperative patients led by surgeons and anesthesiologists. Because further technological advances occurred with greater understanding of pulmonary and cardiac pathophysiology, internists, chiefly pulmonologists, became involved in the care of patients in intensive care areas. Neurologists distanced themselves from the intensive care arena until the 1970s. During this interim, due in part to the "space race" and biotechnological needs for aerospace medicine,[8] advances in computers and telemetry with cardiac and respiratory monitoring led to further specialization. These changes supported the development of a care team with specialty training including nurses and respiratory therapists, and eventually pharmacologists, dieticians, occupational, physical, and speech therapists.

To advance the growth of this new specialty, there was a great need to develop and harmonize training, standards of practice, units' physical requirements, organizational structure, and specific roles of each member of the multiprofessional critical care team. Forward-thinking individuals including Drs Max Harry Weil, Peter Safar, William Shoemaker, and Ake Grenvik pioneered this study.[9–13] Together, with 30 other physicians, they founded the Society of Critical Care Medicine (SCCM) in 1971. The challenge at the time, and as it remains today, was to define the role of CCM because it relates to other specialties.

Throughout the next decade, in the United States, specialties continued to debate whether to create a new specialty board of CCM through the ABMS to certify individuals. The effort was not successful, and the American Board of Anesthesiology (ABA), American Board of Internal Medicine (ABIM), American Board of Pediatrics, and American Board of Surgery (ABS) moved forward separately to create independent processes for critical care subspecialty certification.[13,14] Neurology and emergency medicine did not pursue CCM as a subspecialty area at that time. In 2013, diplomates of the American Board of Emergency Medicine (ABEM) were able to obtain formal critical care certification through the ABA.[14] Involvement of the American Board of Neurosurgery (ABNS) will be discussed in a later discussion.

Neurologists Reemerge in the Field of Critical Care Medicine

In the United States, a small number of neurologists reentered the arena of critical care in the early 1970s. These individuals typically were dually trained in internal medicine or anesthesiology.[15] Neurologic surgeons remained involved in the intensive care unit (ICU) through postoperative management of their patients, including patients with aneurysmal subarachnoid hemorrhage (aSAH), traumatic brain (TBI), and spinal cord injuries (SCI). Early Neurointensive care units (NeuroICUs) started with combined expertise of specialists. The Massachusetts General Hospital established a neuroICU in 1969 under the direction of 2 neurosurgeons, Robert Ojemann and Nicholas Zervas, MD, in close collaboration with neurologist, J. Phillip Kistler. A dedicated training program was established there in 1978.[16] Subsequent NeuroICUs and training programs emerged during the next decades (**Table 1**).

With the approval of intravenous recombinant tissue plasminogen activator for acute ischemic stroke (AIS) in 1996[17] and early studies in endovascular techniques,[18] neurologists regained primary roles as intensivists. The detachable Guglielmi coil began revolutionizing the endovascular treatment of aneurysms.[19] Patients with AIS and aSAH required intensive monitoring and specialized bedside neuroscience nursing. The hourly nursing neurologic examination became recognized as an essential tool in the critical care arsenal for the early detection of potentially reversible neurologic injury. The neuroscience nurse has been pivotal in creating a safe neuroICU. An intensivist in a neuroICU not only had clinical duties but also had the added responsibilities of providing education regarding the nuances of the neurologic examination and emphasizing the implications of neglecting seemingly subtle signs and symptoms.

Demonstrating improvement in patient outcomes was essential to validate the neuroICU model and secure resources to establish additional units and training programs. Administrators needed to see the value of specially trained NCC physicians, nurses, advanced practice providers (APPs), pharmacists, rehabilitation therapists, respiratory therapists, and dieticians. A robust body of literature has emerged in the United States and internationally (eg, Japan, Korea, Saudi Arabia, Switzerland, and the United Kingdom) to make the case. The establishment of dedicated neuroICUs is associated with decreased ICU and hospital lengths of stay, cost, and mortality, as well as improved discharge disposition for patients with cerebrovascular disease, TBI and SCI.[20–35]

Table 1			
Early neurocritical care units/training programs in the United States			
Program	Year Established	Founders	Background
MGH NeuroICU	1969	Robert Ojemann, MD	Neurosurgery
MGH training	1978	Nicholas Zervas, MD	Neurosurgery
		J. Phillip Kistler, MD	Neurology
		Allan Roper, MD	Neurology/Internal Medicine
		Sean Kennedy	Anesthesiology
Johns Hopkins Hospital	1984	Daniel Hanley, MD	Neurology/Internal Medicine
		Cecil Borel, MD	Neuroanesthesiology
Columbia U	1984	Matthew Fink, MD	Neurology/Internal Medicine
UVA	1989	E. Clark Haley, MD	Neurology/Internal Medicine
		Thomas Bleck, MD	Neurology/Internal Medicine
Wash U	1992	Michael Diringer, MD	Neurology
Duke U	1993	Cecil Borel, MD	Neuroanesthesiology
		Joanne Hickey, PhD, ACNP	Neuroscience Nursing
UCSF	1994	Darryl Gress, MD	Neurology

Abbreviations: MGH, Massachusetts general hospital; NeuroICU, Neurointensive Care Unit—all programs but MGH established training programs concomitant with the development of the critical care unit; U, University; UCSF, University of California, San Francisco; UVA, University of Virginia; Wash U, Washington, University at St. louis.

Early Beginnings: Formal Organization of Neurocritical Care Professionals

In Germany, the first independent neuroICUs emerged in the 1960s in Giessen, Chemnitz, and the University of Hamburg. The acute management of cerebrovascular disease was also the impetus for the development of more specialized units throughout Germany including the University of Heidelberg in 1986, Leipzig in 1991, and 1997 in Munich, Frankfurt, Dresden, Wuerzburg, and others. Leaders such as Werner Hacke and Karl Einhäul have been inspirational in the international field of NCC. The German Neurological Society of Neurological Intensive Care and Emergency Medicine (DGNI) were founded in 1984. In 2009, the DGNI merged with the section of Neurocritical Care of the German Society for Neurosurgery.[36,37]

In the United States during the mid-1980s, neurologists interested in CCM helped create a Critical Care and Emergency Neurology (CCEN) section within the American Academy of Neurology (AAN). However, to embrace the unique qualities of NCC as an international, multidisciplinary, multiprofessional field, leaders in NCC created an independent organization that would be inclusive of all care team members. The Neurocritical Care Society (NCS) was established in 2002 as an international organization to improve outcomes for patients with life-threatening neurologic illness. The first meeting in 2003 had nearly 100% of its 70 members in attendance. The NCS has now grown to more than 2800 national and international members including physicians, nurses, pharmacists, APPs, trainees, and other critical care professionals. Subsequently, established critical care societies have become inclusive of NCC expertise and other international societies have been founded specifically to address the neurologically critically ill.

Neurointensivists and the Critical Care Workforce Shortage

In 1998, the American College of Chest Physicians, the American Thoracic Society and SCCM formed a Committee on Manpower for Pulmonary and Critical Care Societies. They were tasked with assessing the critical care workforce supply, based on the current workforce and training estimates, compared with the demand, accounting for population growth and aging. In 2000, this group projected that by 2020 there would be a 22% shortfall in intensive care specialist hours. This shortfall was expected to increase to 35% by 2035.[38,39]

The recognition that a trained intensivist adds quality and improved patient outcomes threatened to increase this workforce gap.[40] In 2000, the National Quality Forum together with the Leapfrog Group, set out to improve the quality, equity, and availability of health care by proposing specific regulatory guidelines to improve hospital safety, quality, and cost containment. They hoped to leverage hospital compliance by showcasing compliant hospitals to payors and consumers. In the critical care area, hospitals were evaluated on whether critical care certified physicians were present within 5-minutes, on-site or by telemedicine, to staff their ICUs.[41]

Four years into this initiative, it was evident the health-care system fell short, as 63% to 90% of the estimated 4.4 million ICU admissions were still being cared for without recommended ICU physician staffing measures. Barriers included inadequate supply of critical care physicians and perceived increased hospital costs.[42–44] A 2003 survey found that many hospitals lacked an identified ICU director. Resistance to implementing full-time intensive care presence included fear of loss of income and control by those currently providing that care without requisite training.[45]

Critical care-trained neurologists could help fill this workforce gap. Discussed in later discussion, United Council for Neurologic Subspecialty (UCNS)-certified neurointensivists was recognized in 2008 by the Leapfrog Group. This lent support to the role of a neurologically trained intensivist.[46] However, the initial proposal limited neurointensivists to fulfilling physician staffing requirements in a "neuroICU" because a formalized route to prove adequate training and competency on par with other intensivists was lacking.[47] This nuance furthered the impetus to seek an ABMS subspecialty designation for NCC through the Accreditation Council for Graduate Medical Education (ACGME). The Leapfrog language also compelled neurosurgery to address NCC as a subspecialty.

Given their limited workforce, NCC physicians were not the only solution. The early 2000s saw a surging interest in NCC APPs.[48,49] These nonphysician providers have significantly increased immediate bedside presence of advanced neuroscience expertise. Timely bedside evaluation, alongside implementation of evidence-based protocols, is key contributor to mortality benefit of an intensivist and ICU-focused teams.

Neurocritical Care Subspecialty Recognition and Certification

The first dedicated neurointensivists were trained in both neurology and internal medicine or were neuroanesthesiologists or neurosurgeons with embedded critical care training. By1985, the only path to critical care certification was through an ABMS primary Board certification from the ABIM, ABS, and ABA; and in 2013, ABEM.[14] In the late 1980s, an increasing number of hospital administrators, academicians, and clinicians recognized the need for neurologically trained intensivists to manage post-thrombolysis or neuroendovascular patients, support and educate specialized neuroscience nurses and APPs, and provide administrative guidance for a NeuroICU.

Expansion of the field also led to increasing literature related to the specialty of NCC. SCCM's official journal, *Critical Care Medicine*, added a permanent section dedicated to NCC in 1993,[15] and the official journal of NCS, *Neurocritical Care* started publication in 2004 with Eelco Widjicks at the helm as Editor-in-Chief.

To create a pathway for accreditation of NCC programs and certification of individuals, in 2005, the NCS, with joint sponsorship from the AAN, CCEN section, and Society for Neuroscience in Anesthesiology and Critical Care (SNACC), petitioned and received recognition as a subspecialty by the UCNS. The first subspecialty NCC certification examination was offered in 2007.

As neurointensivists integrated into nonneurological ICUs, alongside their critical care colleagues, it became apparent that they would be better supported in privileging and credentialing if the NCC training programs had the same rigorous standards, milestones, and certification of competency as those with ACGME oversight. Additionally, the perceived training limitations of NCC physicians potentially preventing them from working outside a NeuroICU had been raised by Leapfrog and others.[46,47] However, when compared with other critical care training programs, NCC was similar in many ways.[50] In 2016, NCS leadership sought support from the AAN to assist its petition to the American Board of Psychiatry and Neurology (ABPN) for recognition of NCC as an ABMS subspecialty.

Supporting letters were provided by the AAN, American Neurological Association, Association of University Professors of Neurology, Child Neurology Society, Professors of Child Neurology, and SNACC. Information was provided on the maturation of NCC to support recognition as an ABMS subspecialty, including an adequate number of providers, training programs, and unique subspecialty focused literature. At the time of the petition in 2016, there were 1241 UCNS Diplomates certified in NCC and 60 UCNS accredited NCC fellowships. From the training standpoint, all 149 neurology and 106 neurosurgery ACGME-accredited residency programs included a NCC core curriculum component to comply with the Review and Recognition Committee requirements.

Other evidence to support the petition included the fact that international critical care professional societies such as the SCCM and European Society of Intensive Care Medicine (ESICM) created neuroscience sections within their societies to allow dialog and opportunities for collaboration for members with an interest in this area. Additionally, in 2016 SCCM designated a seat for a neuroscience representative on their governing Council. Specialty-focused conferences, the development of specialty-specific guidelines, and the national and global popularity of the NCS-sponsored Emergency Neurological Life Support enhanced the awareness of the importance of this critical care subspecialty.

Furthermore, in 2016, the National Uniform Claim Committee (NUCC) approved a NCC taxonomy code (2084A2900X).[51] NUCC is an organization chaired by the American Medical Association and Centers for Medicare and Medicaid Services charged with developing a standardized data set to transmit claim and encounter information between institutions and third-party payers. The taxonomy code designates a provider's classification and specialization. By achieving its own taxonomy code, NCC was validated and supported as a "medical subspecialty devoted to the comprehensive multisystem care of the critically ill neurological patient." This helped differentiate critical care neurologists from other neurologists. Additionally, it clarified that "like other intensivists, the neurointensivist generally assumes the primary role for coordinating the care of his or her patients in the ICU, both the neurologic and medical management of the patient."[51]

In 2017, the ABPN agreed to sponsor NCC as an ABMS subspecialty and requested cosponsors of other member Boards to maintain multidisciplinary collaboration. In May 2018, 38 years after the first ABMS recognition of CCM as a subspecialty, the ABMS approved the ABPN application for NCC with the initial cosponsoring boards including the ABA, ABEM, and ABNS. In 2020, the ABIM joined as a cosponsor. Representation from these cosponsoring member boards developed the content outline and examination. In 2021, the ABA offered to sponsor certification for ABS diplomates.

The first ABMS NCC certification examination was administered in October 2021. More than 1000 candidates took the examination, reflecting the growth and coming of age of NCC as a subspecialty.

Neurosurgeons and Neurocritical Care Certification

Historically, neurologic surgery training programs have been inclusive of all areas in which a neurosurgeon may need to practice in their community, including the critical care management of their patients. Therefore, the ABNS does not offer subspecialty board certification. In 1985, the ABNS applied and was endorsed by ABMS to provide certification of special competence in CCM but chose not to develop training programs or an examination process at that time.[13] Diplomates of neurosurgery have been eligible to complete CCM training and take the written examination in an ABS or ABA critical care program. CCM certification is awarded after the candidate also passes the ABNS oral examination.[52,53]

To address the emergence of fellowship training programs in neurosurgery, the Society of Neurologic Surgeons (SNS) created the Committee for Accreditation of Subspecialty Training (CAST) in 1999.[54] CAST became involved in NCC after UCNS began issuing NCC certification to individuals, including neurosurgeons, and the Leapfrog initiative recognized that the quality of care in hospital ICUs were impacted favorably by trained intensivists. In 2013, CAST was renamed the Committee on Advanced Subspecialty Training and formalized fellowship review committees and began issuing individual certificates in NCC.[54]

In addition, the concept of a recognized focused practice (RFP) designation was approved by ABMS in March 2017. This designation recognizes the value of the board-certified individual who chooses to focus within a specific setting, population, condition, or specialized procedures, Examples include hospital medicine (ie, hospitalists) within the ABIM or American Board of Family Medicine or bariatric surgery within the ABS. Focused practice is an added designation to a primary board certification. The designation is maintained by meeting clinical practice requirements for the specified area, and as of September 2019, the ABNS has taken the RFP route for NCC certification.[55,56]

Challenges Along the Way

Challenges offer opportunities. In 2005, the Brain Attack Coalition's recommendations for Comprehensive Stroke Centers managing stroke patients requiring "high intensity medical and surgical care," did not include the essential element of NCC expertise.[57] This was based on the premise that there were too few neurointensivists available. However, there was an opposing opinion that centers wishing to provide care to the most complex stroke patients should provide the most advanced high quality of care.[58] Because the availability of neurointensivists increased and further literature emerged demonstrating quality improvement, recommendations were adjusted.

Simultaneously, as noted above, concern for critical care workforce shortages arose. In 2008, some proposed that subspecialty units and neurointensivists with limited general and other subspecialty critical care exposure during training would fragment and threaten the quality of critical care.[47,59] This concern pushed for a high level of comprehensive critical care training in UCNS NCC fellowships and pursuit of ABMS certification and ACGME training accreditation for NCC. Harmonizing critical care training across specialties has been a long-standing issue, and there is ongoing interest in revisiting the concept of a common comprehensive core critical care curriculum in training programs across all specialties.[60]

Efforts to standardize and improve the quality of NeuroICUs led to NCS publishing standards for NeuroICUs regarding organizational structure and processes, physical structure, personnel, equipment, and collaborative relationships to guide hospital administrators and directors charged with establishing a successful and sustainable NeuroICU.[61] This emphasized the importance of teamwork and collaborative relationships between critical care units and colleagues to ensure best practice.[62]

International Neurocritical Care Certification

The Competency Based Training in Intensive Care Medicine in Europe (CoBaTrICE) was formed to evaluate the general critical care certification.[63] A CoBaTrICE survey regarding the certification process within its 41 affiliated countries revealed a lack of standardized training and certification and demonstrated that critical care is not a monolithic specialty but instead, quite a complex one.[64] Its goal was to produce guidelines, a comprehensive core syllabus and educational resources to ensure standardized critical care within its participating organizations/countries.[65,66]

The efforts of CoBaTrICE and the Multidisciplinary Joint Commission in Intensive Care Medicine resulted in the first international critical care certification, the European Diploma In Critical Care (EDIC). Currently, ESICM is the sole official provider of the EDIC.[65] There are routes to critical care certification in other countries such as the Royal College of Physicians and Surgeons of Canada and the College of Intensive Care Medicine of Australia and New Zealand. However, to date, there is no international NCC certification. Of note, the UCNS provides an eligibility pathway for NCC

Table 2
Global partners of the neurocritical care society

Asian/Oceanian Chapter	Middle East/South African Chapter	North/Central American Chapter	South American Chapter	European Partners[a]
College of Intensive Care Medicine of Australia and New Zealand (2017)	International Pan Arab Critical Care Society (2011)	Canadian Neurocritical Care Society (2018)	Sociedad Argentina de Terapia Intensiva (2013) Neurointensive Care	German Society for Neurointensive and Emergency Medicine (2016)
Indian Society of Neuroanaesthesiology (2015)	Ethiopian Neurological Association (2022)	Neurocritical Care Society, Guatemalan Chapter (2011)	Brazilian Association (2015)	Swedish Acute Neurology Society (2012)
Indian Society of Critical Care Medicine (2015)		Colegio Mexicano de Medicina Critica A.C (2015)	Sociedad Chilean de Medicina Intensiva (2016)	
Society of Neurocritical Care, India (2018)		Panama Chapter of the Caribbean and Centro-American Societies of Critical Care (2012)	Colombian Association of Intensive and Critical Care (2016)	
Neurocritical Care Society of India (2020)				
The Japan Society of Neurologic Emergencies and Critical Care (2013)				
Korean Neurocritical Care Society (2011)				
Philippine Neurocritical Care Society (2017)				
Brain R.E.S.C.U.E[b] (2017)				
Society of Intensive Care Medicine, Singapore (2018)				
Nepalese Society of Critical Care Medicine (2015)				

( ) Year Partnership Established.
[a] Not an official NCS regional chapter.
[b] R.E.S.C.U.E: Responders and Educators to Strengthen Care for Neurologic Critical-Emergency Patients.

certification for internationally trained candidates who are faculty in a UCNS-accredited NCC training program.[67]

Global Recognition of Neurocritical Care as a Subspecialty

Despite a focus on recognition of NCC as a subspecialty in the United States, Germany was well ahead in the creation of NeuroICUs and DGNI. In 2019, the European Academy of Neurology recognized NCC as a new medical subspecialty and the importance of a multidisciplinary "neuroscience team" in managing the spectrum of neurologic conditions. A diverse Scientific Panel on NCC was created to provide support for related research and education in European countries.[68]

With the global growth of NCC, the NCS created 4 regional chapters (Asia/Oceania, Middle East/Africa, North/Central America, and South America), each with a designated seat on the NCS Board of Directors. As of March 2022, NCS has 23 global NCC /critical care partners (**Table 2**).

NCC's global growth and recognition during the last century created opportunities for collaborative research and knowledge sharing. In 2020, 257 sites from 47 countries participated in a point prevalence study to gather data on organization and care patterns of NCC.[69,70] Similar collaboration will continue to advance NCC because it moves through practitioner certification, training program accreditation, better understanding of disease processes, and development of diagnostic and prognostic indicators to benefit the neurocritically ill.

SUMMARY

Since its inception in the 1920s, NCC has evolved into a unique and integral field within CCM. With continued advancements in the field, the role of neurointensivists is crucial. NCC teams are multiprofessional and multidisciplinary collaborations that include physicians from multiple specialties, APPs, nurses, pharmacists, respiratory therapists, dieticians, and rehabilitation services. These collaborations have shifted the paradigm for critical care. The recent pandemic highlighted the importance of collaboration across critical care units and providers. This awareness has had global impact and resulted in significant international growth within the field. Improvement of the neurologic patient's morbidity and mortality following consistent care by neurointensivists has now been data proven. Although this is paramount, the practice of NCC also requires an ever-present and equally important ethical and sociocultural mindfulness. This is due to pathophysiologic states unique to this field such as coma, unresponsive wakefulness syndrome, and death by neurologic criteria. These and other clinical conditions with emerging biotechnology can elucidate diagnostic, therapeutic, and prognostic advances and create opportunities for further research and expansion of NCC. With the springboard of established subspecialty recognition, growing global presence and societal collaboration, the future of NCC is promising.

CLINICS CARE POINTS

- Dedicated neurointensive care units, staffed by those specially trained in NCC, can decrease ICU and hospital lengths of stay, cost, and mortality; and improve the discharge disposition of patients with TBI, SCI and cerebrovascular disease.
- Timely bedside (on-site or remote) evaluations by critical care-trained physicians and APPs are directly linked to improved quality of care and outcomes for critically ill patients.

- Critical care workforce shortages were anticipated decades ago and are a reality in the present day especially in the face of the current pandemic. An additional labor force founded through the subspecialty of NCC has expanded the availability of critical care expertise.
- Through collaboration of multiple specialty Boards, there exist multiple pathways to obtain individual certification for NCC dependent on ones' primary board certification.

DISCLOSURE

The authors have nothing to disclose.

REFERENCES

1. Shaw-Taylor L. An introduction to the history of infectious diseases,epidemics and the early phases of the long-run decline in mortality. Econ Hist Rev 2020; 73:E1–19.
2. Nightingale F. Notes on matters affecting the health, efficiency, and hospital administration of the British Army. Founded chiefly on the experience of the late War. Presented by request to the Secretary of state for war. Privately printed for Miss Nightingale. London: Harrison and Sons; 1858.
3. Sherman IJ, Kretzer RM, Tamargo RJ. Personal recollections of Walter E. Dandy and his brain team. J Neurosurg 2006;105:487–93.
4. Hardy AD. Poliomyelitis and the neurologists: the View from England, 1896- 1966. Bull Hist Med 1997;71:249–72.
5. Ropper AH. Neurological intensive care. Ann Neurol 1992;32:564–9.
6. Drinker P, McKhann CF. The use of a new apparatus for the prolonged administration of artificial respiration: a fatal case of poliomyelitis. JAMA 1929;92: 1658–60.
7. Levine JM. Historical perspective on pressure ulcers. J Am Geriatr Soc 2005;53: 1248–51.
8. Pitt JA. The human factor in long-duration manned spaceflight. In: the Human Factor- Biomedicine in the manned space program to 1980. The NASA History Series. Washington DC: National Aeronautics and Space Administration; 1985. p. 52–72.
9. Weil MH, Tang W. From Intensive care to critical care medicine- a historical perspective. Am J Respir Crit Care Med 2011;183:1451–3.
10. Weil MH. The society of critical care medicine, its history and its destiny. Crit Care Med 1973;1:1–4.
11. [No Authors Listed]. Guidelines for organization of critical care units. JAMA 1972; 222:1532–5.
12. Grenvik A, Leonard JJ, Arens JF, et al. Critical care medicine certification as a multidisciplinary subspecialty. Crit Care Med 1981;9:117–25.
13. Grenvik A. Subspecialty certification in critical care medicine by American specialty boards 1985;13:1001–3.
14. American Board of Medical Specialties. ABMS Board certification report 2020-2021. Available at: https://www.abms.org/wp-content/uploads/2022/01/ABMS-Board-Certification-Report-2020-2021.pdf. Accessed March 13, 2022.
15. Bleck TP. Historical aspects of critical care and the nervous system. Crit Care Clin 2009;25:153–64.

16. History of neurocritical care at Mass general. Available at: https://www. massgeneral.org/neurology/neurocritical-care/about/history. Accessed March 25, 2022.
17. National Institute of Neurological Disorders and Stroke rt-PA Stroke Study Group. Tissue plasminogen activator for acute ischemic stroke. N Engl J Med 1995;333: 1581–7.
18. del Zoppo GJ, Higashida RT, Furlan AJ, et al. PROACT: a phase II randomized trial of recombinant pro-urokinase by direct arterial delivery in acute middle cerebral artery stroke. PROACT Investigators Prolyse Acute Cereb Thromboembolism. Stroke. 1998;29:4–11.
19. Viñuela F, Duckwiler G, Mawad M. Guglielmi detachable coil embolization of acute intracranial aneurysm: perioperative anatomical and clinical outcome in 403 patients. J Neurosurg 1997;86:475–82.
20. Mirski MA, Chang CWJ, Cowan R. Impact of a neuroscience intensive care unit on neurosurgical patient outcomes and cost of care: evidence-based support for an intensivist-directed specialty ICU model of care. J Neurosurg Anesthesiol 2001;13:83–92.
21. Diringer MN, Edwards DF. Admission to a neurologic/neurosurgical intensive care unit is associated with reduced mortality rate after intracerebral hemorrhage. Crit Care Med 2001;29:635–40.
22. Suarez JI, Zaidat OO, Suri MF, et al. Length of stay and mortality in neurocritically ill patients: impact of a specialized neurocritical care team. Crit Care Med 2004; 32:2311–7.
23. Lerch C, Yonekawa Y, Muroa C, et al. Specialized neurocritical care, severity grade, and outcome of patients with aneurysmal subarachnoid hemorrhage. Neurocrit Care 2006;05:85–92.
24. Varelas PN, Eastwood HJY, Spanaki MV, et al. Impact of a neurointensivist on outcomes in patients with head trauma treated in a neurosciences intensive care unit. J Neurosurg 2006;104:713–9.
25. Bershad EM, Feen ES, Hernandez OH, et al. Impact of a specialized neurointensive care team on outcomes of critically ill acute ischemic stroke patients. Neurocrit Care 2008;9:287–92.
26. Varelas PN, Schultz L, Conti M, et al. The impact of a neuro-intensivist on patients with stroke admitted to a neurosciences intensive care unit. Neurocrit Care 2008; 9:293–9.
27. Josephson SA, Douglas VC, Lawton MT, et al. Improvement in intensive care unit outcomes in patients with subarachnoid hemorrhage after initiation of neurointensivist co-management. J Neurosurg 2010;112:626–30.
28. Samuels O, Webb A, Culler S, et al. Impact of a dedicated neurocritical care team in treating patients with aneurysmal subarachnoid hemorrhage. Neurocrit Care 2011;14:334–40.
29. Knopf L, Staff I, Gomes J, et al. Impact of a neurointensivist on outcomes in critically ill stroke patients. Neurocrit Care 2012;166:63–71.
30. Damian MS, Ben-Shlomo Y, Howard R, et al. The effect of secular trends and specialist neurocritical care on mortality for patients with intracerebral haemorrhage, myasthenia gravis and Guillain-Barré syndrome admitted to critical care : an analysis of the Intensive Care National Audit & Research Centre (ICNARC) national United Kingdom database. Intensive Care Med 2013;39:1405–12.
31. Egawa S, Hifumi T, Kawakita K, et al. Impact of neurointensivist-managed intensive care unit implementation on patient outcomes after aneurysmal subarachnoid hemorrhage. J Crit Care 2016;32:52–5.

32. Ryu JA, Yang JH, Chung CR, et al. Impact of neurointensivst co-management on the clinical outcomes of patients admitted to the neurosurgical intensive care unit. J Korean Med Sci 2017;32:1024–30.

33. Soliman I, Aletreby WT, Faqihi F, et al. Improved outcomes following the establishment of a neurocritical care unit in Saudi Arabia. Crit Care Res Pract 2018;2764907.

34. Jeong JH, Bang JS, Jeong WJ, et al. A dedicated neurological intensive care unit offers improved outcomes for patients with brain and spine injuries. J Intensive Care Med 2019;34:104–8.

35. Kim TJ, Lee JS, Yoon JS, et al. Impact of the dedicated neurointensivists on the outcome in patients with ischemic stroke based on the linked big data for stroke in Korea. J Korean Med Sci 2020;35:e135–43.

36. Wartenberg KE. Neurointensive care Units in Germany. ICU management & practice ICU Volume 10, Issue 2. 2010. Available at: https://healthmanagement.org/c/icu/issuearticle/neurointensive-care-units-in-germany. Accessed March 25, 2022.

37. Kunze K. Neurologische Intensivmedizin in Deutschland. Spec Edition Neurologische Intensivmedizin aktuell 2006;1435–2966. ISSN.

38. Angus D, Kelley MA, Schmitz RJ, et al. Committee on Manpower for Pulmonary and Critical Care Societies (COMPACCS): Caring for the critically ill patient. Current and projected workforce requirements for care of the critically ill and patients with pulmonary disease: can we meet the requirements of an aging population? JAMA 2000;284:2762–70.

39. Health Resources and Services Administration (HRSA). Report to Congress—The critical care workforce: a study of the supply and demand for critical care physicians, 2006. Requested by: Senate Report 108 – 81.

40. Kelley MA, Angus D, Chalfin DB, et al. The critical care crisis in the United States: a report from the profession. Chest 2004;125:1514–7.

41. Gasperino J. The Leapfrog initiative for intensive care unit physician staffing and its impact on intensive care unit performance: a narrative review. Health Policy 2011;102:223–8.

42. Pronovost P, Needham D, Waters H, et al. Intensive care unit physician staffing: financial modeling of the Leapfrog standard. Crit Care Med 2004;32:247–53.

43. National Quality Forum (NQF). Safe practice 11: intensive care Unit care. In: Safe practices for better healthcare–2010 Update: a Consensus Report. Washington, DC: NQF; 2010. p. 169–74.

44. Halpern NA, Pastores SM, Oropello JM, et al. Critical care medicine in the United States: addressing the intensivist shortage and image of the specialty. Crit Care Med 2013;41:2754–61.

45. Kahn JM, Matthews FA, Angus DC, et al. Barriers to implementing the Leapfrog Group recommendations for intensivist physician staffing: a survey of intensive care unit directors. J Crit Care 2007;22:97–103.

46. The Leapfrog group. Hospital survey: Factsheet: ICU physician staffing. Available at: https://preview2021.ratings.leapfroggroup.org/sites/default/files/inline-files/2021%20IPS%20Fact%20Sheet_3.pdf. Accessed March 22, 2022.

47. Krell K. Critical care workforce. Crit Care Med 2008;36:1350–3.

48. Caserta FM, Depew M, Moran J. Acute care nurse practitioners: the role in neuroscience critical care. J Neurol Sci 2007;261:167–71.

49. Yeager S. The neuroscience acute care nurse practitioner: role development, implementation, and improvement. Crit Care Nurs Clin North Am 2009;21:561–93.

50. Marcolini E, Seder D, Bonomo J, et al. The present state of neurointensivist training in the United States: a Comparison to other critical care training programs. Crit Care Med 2018;46:307–15.
51. National Uniform Claim Committee. Available at: https://www.nucc.org/index.php/21-provider-taxonomy/229-new-7-1-2016. Accessed March 22, 2022.
52. American College for Graduate Medical Education. ACGME program requirements for Graduate medical education in surgical critical care. Available at: https://www.acgme.org/globalassets/PFAssets/ProgramRequirements/442_SurgicalCriticalCare_2020.pdf?ver=2020-06-22-090711-273&ver=2020-06-22-090711-273. Accessed March 27, 2022.
53. American College for Graduate Medical Education. ACGME program requirements for Graduate medical education in Anesthesia critical care. Available at: https://www.acgme.org/globalassets/pfassets/programrequirements/045_anesthesiologycriticalcare_2021.pdf. Accessed March 27, 2022.
54. Society of Neurological Surgeons. CAST history. Available at: https://sns-cast.org/history/. Accessed March 26, 2022.
55. American Board of Medical Specialties. Focused practice designation. Available at: https://www.abms.org/board-certification/board-certification-requirements/focused-practice-designation/. Accessed March 26, 2022.
56. Society of Neurological Surgeons. CAST: structure. Available at: https://sns-cast.org/structure/. Accessed March 25, 2022.
57. Alberts MJ, Latchaw RE, Selman WR, et al. Recommendations for comprehensive stroke centers. A consensus statement from the brain Attack Coalition. Stroke 2005;36:1597–616.
58. Hemphill JC, Bleck T, Carhuapoma JR, et al. Is neurointensive care really optional for comprehensive stroke care. Stroke 2005;36:2344–5.
59. Chang CW, Torbey MT, Diringer MN, et al. Neurointensivists: Part of the problem or part of the solution? Crit Care Med 2008;36:2963–4.
60. Tisherman S, Spevetz A, Blosser S, et al. A case for change in adult critical care training for physicians in the United States: a white Paper developed by the critical care as a specialty Task Force of the society of critical care medicine. Crit Care Med 2018;46:1577–84.
61. Moheet AM, Livesay SL, Abdelhak T, et al. Standards for neurologic critical care Units: a statement for healthcare professionals from the neurocritical care society. Neurocrit Care 2018;29:145–60.
62. Kaplan L, Moheet AM, Livesay SL, et al. A perspective from the neurocritical care society and the society of critical care medicine: team-based care for neurological critical illness. Neurocrit Care 2020;32:369–72.
63. De Lange S, Van Aken H, Burchardi H. European society of intensive care medicine statement: intensive care medicine in Europe—structure, organisation and training guidelines of the multidisciplinary joint committee of intensive care medicine (MJCICM) of the European union of medical specialists (UEMS). Intensive Care Med 2002;28:1505–11.
64. Barrett H, Bion JF. An international survey of training in adult intensive care medicine. Intensive Care Med 2005;31:553–61.
65. CoBaTrCE Collaboration The. Development of core competencies for an international training programme in intensive care medicine. Intensive Care Med 2006;32:1371–83.
66. European Society of Intensive Care Medicine. European diploma in intensive care Medicine. Available at: https://www.esicm.org/education/edic2-2/. Accessed March 25, 2022.

67. United Council of Neurologic Subspecialties. Neurocritical care certification examination eligibility criteria. Available at: https://www.ucns.org/Online/Online/Certification/Neurocritical_Cert.aspx. Accessed March 22, 2022.
68. European Academy of Neurology. Neurocritical care. Available at: https://www.ean.org/home/organisation/scientific-panels/neurocritical-care. Accessed March 23, 2022.
69. Suarez JI, Martin RH, Bauza C, et al. Worldwide organization of neurocritical care: Results from the PRINCE study Part 1. Neurocrit Care 2020;32:172–9.
70. Venkatasubba Rao CP, Suarez JI, Martin RH, et al. Global survey of outcomes of neurocritical care patients: analysis of the PRINCE study Part 2. Neurocrit Care 2020;32:88–103.

Quality Improvement in Neurocritical Care

Casey Olm-Shipman, MD, MS[a],*, Asma M. Moheet, MD, MHDS, FNCS[b]

KEYWORDS

- Quality improvement • Value-based care • Benchmarking • Performance measures
- Neurocritical care

KEY POINTS

- Measurement is core to quality improvement in neurocritical care.
- Variation in the delivery of neurocritical care impacts patient outcomes and may worsen health disparities.
- Neurocritical care performance measures represent evidence-based "best practices" and are targets for quality improvement initiatives.
- External benchmarking and pay-for-performance programs are designed to incentivize high-value care; several measures used in these programs are directly relevant to neurocritical care practice.
- Opportunities exist for improved patient outcomes through the development of neurocritical care quality improvement collaboratives and disease/condition-specific registries.

INTRODUCTION

Quality improvement is an iterative process integral to neurocritical care delivery that is rooted in patient safety and advocacy. Measurement of health care quality indicators gained significant traction in the 1990s to 2000s, fueled by the "To Err is Human" and "Crossing the Quality Chasm" reports.[1,2] These reports brought to light the following deficiencies in care delivery and patient safety:

- Widespread, unexplained variation in practice
- Overutilization of resources driven by supply-led demand (eg, more physicians who perform a specific procedure may lead to more of these procedures being performed, resulting in higher costs of care without necessarily improving patient health outcomes)

[a] University of North Carolina School of Medicine, 101 Manning Drive, Physicians Office Building, Chapel Hill, NC 27516, USA; [b] Neurocritical Care, OhioHealth Riverside Methodist Hospital, 3535 Olentangy River Road, Columbus, OH 43214, USA
* Corresponding author. University of North Carolina School of Medicine, Department of Neurology Physicians, Office Building 170 Manning Ddrive, Chapel Hill, NC 27599
E-mail address: caseyo@neurology.unc.edu

Crit Care Clin 39 (2023) 17–28
https://doi.org/10.1016/j.ccc.2022.06.002
0749-0704/23/© 2022 Elsevier Inc. All rights reserved.
criticalcare.theclinics.com

- Unacceptably high rates of medical errors resulting in morbidity and mortality

This work laid the foundation for the "Quadruple Aim" to improve patient outcomes, population health, cost-effective (high value) care delivery, and the clinician experience of providing care.[3]

Measurement is core to quality improvement and enables the assessment of interventions to determine effectiveness.[4] In addition, quality measures are used to identify gaps in practice and unwarranted variation that may contribute to health disparities and inappropriate service utilization. There is a significant opportunity to impact the quality of care delivered to neurocritically ill patients given their high risk for hospital-acquired infections and other complications.[5] It is therefore important for neurocritical care clinicians to understand the basics of quality improvement measurement and how to apply these in clinical practice to achieve better health outcomes for patients, reduce health disparities, and navigate complex benchmarking and pay-for-performance programs which significantly impact a hospital's reputation and financial bottomline.

There is growing recognition of the need for quality measurement to assess gaps in care delivery. In neurocritical care, regional and hospital-based variation in care delivery contributes to differences in mortality rates for several neurocritical care patient populations, including traumatic brain injury, ischemic stroke, and hemorrhagic stroke.[6–10] The PRINCE study, which included 31 countries and 257 sites, demonstrated significant geographic variation in resource availability, care access, use of clinical practice protocols, and the delivery of neurocritical care across hospitals and intensive care units. Additional research is needed to better understand this variation and its impact on health outcomes. Standardizing high value care delivery and implementing evidence-based best practices are key drivers in reducing unwarranted variation and improving outcomes for neurocritically ill patients.[11,12] This has been exemplified in the field of acute stroke, where longitudinal outcomes data from the Get With the Guidelines (GWTG) registry indicate that quality improvement efforts to standardize care delivery have resulted in better patient outcomes.[13]

In 2020, the Neurocritical Care Society (NCS) published a survey assessing neurocritical care clinicians' perceptions of quality improvement practices and infrastructure. Respondents had a greater awareness of stroke performance measures but were less aware of the neurocritical care-relevant Trauma in Quality Improvement (TQIP) and American Academy of Neurology (AAN) measures. Most respondents reported centralized quality improvement infrastructure within their institution but a lack of dedicated quality improvement programs within neurocritical care. Frequently identified barriers to quality improvement included insufficient institutional resources and lack of support to garner and sustain clinician engagement.[14]

DEFINITIONS
Approach to Quality Measurement Frameworks in Neurocritical Care

According to the quality improvement framework developed by Donabedian, quality measures encompass three distinct domains: structure, process, and outcome.[15] Structure measures reflect the infrastructure and resources necessary for care delivery to occur, including policies and protocols, equipment, and personnel. At a basic level, structure measures can be conceptualized as structural elements that are either present or not. Examples of structure measures include the presence of a designated neurocritical care unit or service, the existence of disease-specific order sets, or the incorporation of an interprofessional neurocritical care team staffing model that includes subspecialty-trained physicians, advanced practice providers, nurses, pharmacists, respiratory therapists, and rehabilitation therapists.

Process measures capture more dynamic aspects of care compared to structure measures. Process measures evaluate adherence to established processes based on guidelines and standards of care that are considered evidence-based best practice. Examples of process measures in neurocritical care include the administration of nimodipine for improved outcomes in aneurysmal subarachnoid hemorrhage, utilization of a standardized patient handoff process for neurocritical care unit patient transfers, and adherence to status epilepticus protocols to ensure rapid and appropriate treatment of seizures.

Structure and process measures drive outcome measures, without come measures that evaluate patient health and functional status considered most meaningful. Core examples of neurocritical care-relevant health outcome measures include survival, hospital-acquired complications, and readmissions. Cost, resource utilization (such as length of stay), and patient-reported outcomes (such as satisfaction and experience) also represent key outcome measures.

Despite its many strengths as a conceptual quality measures framework, the foundational Donabedian model has its limitations. First, the assumed direct causal relationship between structure and process measures driving outcomes is not necessarily the case in clinical practice, as known and unknown factors may interact in complex ways to influence outcome. Institutional culture, for example, influences how structure and care delivery processes are implemented and is a major determinant of whether a high reliability organizational state can be achieved. Another criticism of the Donabedian model is that structure, process, and outcome measures are subject to health care professional and organizational biases and may inadequately account for social determinants of health and other factors impacting health equity and quality. In addition, owing to the risk of implicit bias in measure development and application, quality measures are vulnerable to being inappropriately weighted toward practitioner and/or health care organization values and less weighted toward those of patients and families.[16]

Although it is important to be vigilant of implicit biases, there is a balance to be struck, and there are many cases in which it is appropriate and useful for practitioner-centric and health care organization-centric metrics to be emphasized. For example, the thrombolysis in cerebral infarction score, used to standardize categorization of radiographic recanalization after mechanical thrombectomy for large vessel occlusions, could be viewed as a relatively more practitioner and organization-centric outcome measure that enables institutions and credentialing agencies to track procedural success rates. It is arguably less meaningful to stroke survivors themselves, who are more likely to be concerned with ultimate functional outcome, ability to work, financial security, and psychosocial well-being. Thus, it is important to approach measurement frameworks from the perspective of multiple stakeholders to achieve a multidimensional assessment that is comprehensive and meaningful.

In neurocritical care, there is a need for the development of quality measures that are patient and family-centered. There is a relative paucity of evidence for recommended best practices pertaining to patient and family-centered care in this population. This gap is exacerbated by the heterogenous nature of neurocritical illness and challenges in neuroprognostication for patients with severe acute brain injury. Improved knowledge and understanding of the measures that matter most to patients and families will enable a transformative shift to a value-based quality measures framework (**Fig. 1**), in which care delivery assessment occurs across multiple domains inclusive of clinical outcomes, experience of care, cost, functional

- Survival
- Hospital acquired complications
- Readmission

Clinical Outcome

Cost, Efficiency, Resource Use

- Direct
  - ICU length of stay
  - Utilization of labs and studies
  - Care coordination and transitions
  - Cost variation by provider or management strategy
- Indirect
  - Patient-family financial well being
  - Caregiver missed days of work

Functional Outcome

- Physical
- Cognitive
- Psychosocial
- Ability to work
- Perceived Wellness

Patient-Family Experience

- Health care delivery
- Access to care
- Perceived benefit
- Ease of care navigation
- Education and information sharing
- Caregiver support

Fig. 1. Patient-centered value-based care framework.

status, and quality of life.[17] Emerging areas of research include shared decision-making and navigation of goals of care for neurocritically ill patients, which may shed light on important potential targets for quality measures that account for patient and family values and preferences.[18]

Benchmarking and Performance Measures

Benchmarking allows for continuous quality improvement by enabling organizations to measure and compare their own processes with similar organizations. Quality measures used for benchmarking are commonly referred to as performance measures. Although all performance measures are quality measures, not all quality measures meet the rigorous criteria necessary to achieve performance measure status for use in external benchmarking. Externally reported performance measures, if applied incorrectly, can have serious negative consequences on patient care outcomes, costs of care, institutional reputation, reimbursement, and the administrative workload of clinicians. Casalino and colleagues estimated that physician practices spend more than 15.4 billion dollars annually and an average of 785 hours per physician to report quality measures.[19] Maclean and colleagues evaluated 87 ambulatory care measures used in the Medicare Merit-based Incentive Payment Program and rated 35% of these as not valid and 28% of uncertain validity.[20] It is therefore critical that quality measures be adopted as performance measures for external benchmarking and pay-for-performance programs only if they meet the following stringent criteria:[21]

- Supported by the highest level of evidence and derived from clinical practice guidelines that use a standard methodology for assessing the quality of evidence (eg, GRADE criteria as opposed to expert opinion)
- Feasible, actionable, and meaningful, such that they can be captured without excessive administrative burden and are relevant to improving patient care delivery and health outcomes
- Validated via testing in real-world practice before adoption by credentialing agencies and payers
- Risk-adjustable to enable "apples-to-apples" comparison across organizations and avoid penalizing centers caring for higher risk patients

DISCUSSION
Performance Measure Development

In the United States, there are multiple sources of quality measure development, including governmental agencies and nonprofit third-party organizations. The largest of these are the government's Centers for Medicare and Medicaid Services (CMS), which is both a measure developer and the largest health care payer. Increasingly, performance measures are developed and used by both public and private sector payers to determine financial reimbursement in a growing effort to incentivize high-value care delivery.

The Agency for Healthcare Research and Quality (AHRQ) is a governmental organization that develops measures (including patient safety indicators, which are administratively coded identifiers of potentially preventable events) but is not a payer. Credentialing agencies such as The Joint Commission (TJC) also engage in measure development and the establishment of regulatory quality standards. The National Committee for Quality Assurance is a large nonprofit organization that contracts with both governmental and private organizations to develop and abstract quality measures. The National Quality Forum (NQF) reviews and endorses measures for public use (including those used by CMS).

Most neurocritical care disease-specific performance measures are developed by medical professional societies and organizations that often have global representation to inform best practices on an international scale. Some of these include the NCS, American Heart Association/American Stroke Association (AHA/ASA), AAN, Society for Critical Care Medicine, and Neurohospitalist Society, among others.

In the United States, of the many performance measures proposed by medical professional societies and others, only a small fraction are ultimately beta-tested and endorsed by NQF for public use. Hence, most are not tracked by CMS and are not subject to financial incentives or penalties.

Neurocritical Care Disease-Specific Performance Measures

In 2020, the NCS published "Standards for Neurologic Critical Care Units," which established several recommended structure measures as potential targets for improving care delivery to neurocritically ill patients.[22] As with tiering of stroke and trauma centers by TJC, a classification of neurocritical care centers by level of service provided was proposed, with recommendations for personnel, processes, and organizational infrastructure associated with each level:

- Level I: Provides comprehensive neurocritical care services, including advanced monitoring, surgical and medical interventions, physician fellowship training programs, and advanced practice provider (APP) training capabilities.
- Level II: Resourced to stabilize patients and manage high acuity neurocritical disease conditions.
- Level III: Capable to evaluate and stabilize neurologic emergencies and facilitate transfer to Level I or II units.

Recognizing that complex structure measures are context-dependent and not necessarily feasible in all care delivery settings, these were published with the intent of delineating aspirational quality improvement goals.[23] A criticism of the recommendations, however, was the need for more evidence to support the proposed structure measures as standards.

In 2021, the NCS published the first neurocritical care disease-specific performance measure set consisting of 21 performance measures based on the rigorous selection

Table 1
Neurocritical care society performance measures

NCS PM	Aligns with AHA PM	Aligns with AAN PM	Aligns with TJC PM	New PM
Immunomodulatory treatment of Guillain–Barré syndrome		X		
Immunomodulatory treatment of myasthenic crisis		X		
Acute interventions for ischemic stroke				X
Vascular imaging in ischemic stroke				X
Symptomatic ICH after ischemic stroke intervention	X		X	
Decompressive craniectomy in ischemic stroke				X
Coagulopathy reversal in ICH	X		X	
Avoidance of steroids in ICH	X		X	
Nimodipine in aneurysmal SAH	X		X	
Vasospasm screening in aneurysmal SAH				X
Dexamethasone in bacterial meningitis		X		
Acyclovir for herpes simplex virus encephalitis				X
Dexamethasone in tuberculosis meningitis				X
Benzodiazepine in status epilepticus		X		
Status epilepticus treatment with anticonvulsant medication		X		
Avoidance of steroids in traumatic brain injury				X
Targeted temperature management in cardiac arrest				X
Documentation of external ventricular drain insertion bundle				X
Venous thromboembolism prophylaxis				X

Abbreviations: AHA, American Heart Association; AAN, American Academy of Neurology; ICH, intracerebral hemorrhage; PM, performance measures; TJC, The Joint Commission.

criteria of quality measures backed by the highest level of evidence in clinical practice guidelines (**Table 1**).[24] To maintain patient-centeredness and promote practitioner and health organization accountability, these measures were developed with the intent of evaluating care of neurocritically ill patients based on patient care needs as opposed to the subspecialty of the clinician delivering care or the location of the patient during admission (ie, appropriate care delivery should occur regardless of whether a patient is admitted to a neurocritical unit or not, and whether the patient is under the care of an emergency medicine physician, medical intensivist, or neurointensivist). In addition, performance measures were designed to harmonize with similar measures already proposed by other organizations. Of the 21 measures put forth, 10 measures represent original performance measures, 5 are similar to preexisting AAN Inpatient and Emergency performance measures, and 6 are similar to preexisting AHA/ASA performance measures.[25,26]

High-Value Care, Pay-for-Performance and Publicly Reported Quality Rankings in Neurocritical Care

High-value care is defined by the National Academy of Medicine as care that is effective, safe, timely, efficient, equitable, and patient-centered. Value can be measured as quality divided by cost, where quality represents patient-centered health outcomes.[27] As health care costs in the United States have continued to rise without clearly demonstrated health benefit, payers are increasingly shifting from fee-for-service models to pay-for-performance programs. These programs aim to incentivize value-based care by aligning reimbursement with clinical outcome, adherence to evidence-based best practices, appropriate resource utilization, and patient and family experience.[28]

The Affordable Care Act of 2010 paved the way for CMS value-based incentive programs which greatly impact hospital reimbursement. Although these programs do not track neurocritical care-specific performance measures, neurocritical care practitioners should be aware of them, as conditions for which neurocritically ill patients are at high risk (including mortality, readmissions, and preventable hospital-acquired complications) are weighted heavily. In addition, ischemic stroke, which accounts for a significant proportion of neurocritical care admissions, is one of the major disease conditions tracked in several key CMS reimbursement programs.

Up to 6% of hospital reimbursement from CMS is at risk through three major pay-for-performance programs, including[29-31]

(1) CMS Hospital Readmission Reduction Program, where a maximum 3% penalty is applied to inpatient payments. This program penalizes the 50% of hospitals that have higher than median readmissions across each of seven clinical cohorts: stroke, myocardial infarction, chronic obstructive pulmonary diseases, heart failure, pneumonia, coronary artery bypass graft surgery, and elective primary total hip and/or knee arthroplasty.

(2) CMS Hospital Value-Based Purchasing Program, in which up to 2% of inpatient payments are at risk. In this program, hospitals have 2% of inpatient revenue withheld to fund the program. Quality is evaluated across four domains: clinical outcomes, safety, cost-effectiveness, and patient experience. Patient experience is assessed with the Hospital Consumer Assessment of Healthcare Providers and Systems survey. It includes measures evaluating communication with nurses and doctors, the responsiveness of hospital staff, the cleanliness and quietness of the hospital environment, communication about medicines, discharge information, overall rating of hospital, and whether patients would recommend the hospital.

Program funds are redistributed to hospitals in a revenue-neutral manner based on performance. Hospitals that reach some but not all quality targets will receive a portion of the 2% of funds previously withheld. Hospitals with excellent performance may earn back the full 2% of funds initially withheld and may stand to gain additional funds if top performers. For hospitals with poor performance, the full 2% of inpatient revenue is withheld.

(3) CMS Hospital-Acquired Condition (HAC) Reduction Program penalizes hospitals scoring in the lowest performing quartile for hospital-acquired conditions, applying a 1% payment reduction on inpatient reimbursement. Examples of commonly encountered neurocritical care-relevant HACs include catheter-associated urinary tract infections, central line-associated bloodstream infections, surgical site infections (including external ventricular drain (EVD)-associated ventriculitis),

respiratory failure requiring reintubation after elective surgery, iatrogenic pneumothorax incurred during vascular access procedures, venous thromboembolism, and mortality.

CMS publicly reports hospital quality rankings on their Care Compare Web site to provide health care consumers with access to transparent hospital performance data.[32] There are numerous other publicly reported quality ranking systems, including Leapfrog and US News and World Report (USNWR).[33,34] None provide ranking data at the level of individual neurocritical care service lines, although USNWR provides combined neurology and neurosurgery program rankings. All use different methodologies for defining measures and benchmarking models, such that ranking well in one system does not necessarily guarantee ranking well in others.

Risk adjustment is critically important to allow for true "apples-to-apples" comparison in pay-for-performance and publicly reported quality ranking programs. Inadequate risk adjustment can result in hospitals that care for sicker patients (such as academic medical centers and safety net hospitals) being unduly penalized for having worse outcomes. Coding terminology used for risk adjustment is often not intuitive to frontline clinicians (eg, in neurocritical care, terms such as "brain compression" and "functional quadriplegia" are not common vernacular for most clinicians), yet failure to document these precise terms has consequences at the institutional level.[35] Adding to the complexity and burden of coding for clinicians is the frequent turnover of coding terms. It is therefore essential for health care systems to invest in coding and documentation infrastructure not only for the traditional purposes of billing but also to avoid financial penalties in value-based care programs and loss of institutional reputation in publicly reported quality ranking programs. Unfortunately, this creates another potential driver of increased administrative costs in health care.[36]

FUTURE DEVELOPMENTS
Registries and Quality Improvement Collaboratives in Neurocritical Care

A challenge faced by many clinicians engaged in quality improvement efforts is access to data to inform performance initiatives. Internal institutional registries such as hospital-acquired infection registries (often maintained by a hospital's infection control or epidemiology departments) can be used to detect special cause variation, achieve consistency of care, and drive local improvement initiatives. To transform care delivery on a broader scale, external registries enable the sharing of data across institutions to improve patient safety, quality, and value-based care. External registries may be developed by quality improvement collaboratives focused on specific patient populations or disease conditions, where participating centers compare outcomes and processes to peer institutions. This allows for the detection of innovators and high performers as well as the adoption of practices that may elevate care delivery across centers.[37]

Several neurocritical care-relevant registries exist which enable benchmarking and allow institutions to target areas where they may be underperforming compared with peer institutions. A sampling of these are listed in **Table 2**. Although some registries are available for public access (such as CMS Care Compare), most require a fee to participate. Multiple registries have performance data relevant to general critical care. Relatively fewer exist with metrics specific to neurocritical care disease conditions. Examples include TQIP (which includes traumatic brain injury data) and the GWTG stroke registry.

Although there is a significant opportunity in neurocritical care for development of quality improvement collaboratives and disease-specific registries, considerable resources may be necessary to develop and sustain these, including fees for data

Table 2
Sampling of neurocritical care-relevant registries

Registries	Focus	Web site
Get With the Guidelines	• Reports stroke performance measures • Sponsored by AHA/ASA	https://www.heart.org/en/professional/quality-improvement/get-with-the-guidelines/get-with-the-guidelines-stroke
Trauma Quality Improvement Program	• Reports blunt and penetrating trauma (including brain trauma) performance measures • Sponsored by the American College of Surgeons	https://www.facs.org/quality-programs/trauma/tqp/center-programs/tqip
National Surgical Quality Improvement Program	• Reports surgical care outcomes • Sponsored by the American College of Surgeons	https://www.facs.org/quality-programs/acs-nsqip
Vizient	• Reports health care performance data on all patients from participating institutions • Merger of University Health Consortium, VHA Inc., and Novation	https://www.vizientinc.com
Healthcare Cost and Utilization Project	• Umbrella for multiple databases: National Inpatient Sample, Kids' Inpatient Database, Nationwide Emergency Department Sample • Sponsored by AHRQ	https://www.hcup-us.ahrq.gov/nisoverview.jsp https://www.hcup-us.ahrq.gov/kidoverview.jsp https://www.hcup-us.ahrq.gov/nedsoverview.jsp
Care Compare	• Reports performance measures across Medicare-certified hospitals • Used in CMS Five-Star Quality Rating System (publicly reported ranking system)	https://www.medicare.gov/care-compare

sharing platforms, data abstraction, entry, and quality assurance. International initiatives such as the Curing Coma Campaign sponsored by the NCS may pave the way forward for the formation of quality improvement collaboratives that are accessible to a global community, with the potential to improve outcomes of neurocritically ill patients worldwide.[38]

SUMMARY

Quality measures have the potential to significantly improve value-based care delivery and reduce unwarranted variation leading to health care disparities. In neurocritical care, this may translate to patients living longer with less functional impairment, and/or receiving higher quality of care that aligns with patient values and preferences. Although the landscape of quality measurement in neurocritical care is rapidly evolving, we have only begun to lay the foundation for quality and performance improvement. The first step in this process is performing thorough gap analyses, followed by carefully crafting measures to drive improvements in care delivery. It is incumbent on neurocritical care as a field to advance the implementation of these measures and continually readdress their impact on care delivery as they are incorporated broadly into health care organizations beyond the beta-testing phase. Effective measure development and implementation will guide quality improvement initiatives in clinical practice and ultimately inform whether measures are appropriate and relevant. Defining and locally implementing evidence-based quality standards for the care of neurocritically ill patients is an important first step in improving patient outcomes. Future directions include testing of proposed neurocritical care performance measures in real-world practice and establishment of disease-specific registries and quality improvement collaboratives to drive care forward.

CLINICS CARE POINTS

- There is a need to better understand variation in neurocritical care practice and the impact of this on patient outcomes and health disparities.
- Quality measurement frameworks in neurocritical care should include patient and family-centered outcomes.
- Neurocritical care performance measures have been recently developed and can be used to guide and prioritize improvement initiatives.
- The quality of neurocritical care delivery can impact pay-for-performance and public benchmarking programs, and providers should be aware of risk-adjustment and the neurocritical care-relevant measures weighted heavily in these models.
- Quality improvement collaboratives and disease-specific registries represent opportunities to advance neurocritical care practice and improve outcomes on a global scale.

DISCLOSURE

The authors have nothing to disclose.

REFERENCES

1. Institute of Medicine (IOM). Crossing the quality Chasm: a New health system for the 21st Century. Washington, (DC): National Academy Press (US); 2001.

2. Institute of Medicine (US). Committee on quality of health care in America. In: Kohn LT, Corrigan JM, Donaldson MS, editors. To Err is Human: Building a safer health system. Washington (DC): National Academy Press (US); 2000.
3. Bodenheimer T, Sinsky C. From triple to quadruple aim: care of the patient requires care of the provider. Ann Fam Med 2014;12(6):573–6.
4. Chassin MR, Loeb JM, Schmaltz SP, et al. Accountability measures - using measurement to promote quality improvement. NEJM 2010;363(7):683–8.
5. Busl KM. Healthcare-associated infections in the neurocritical care unit. Curr Neurol Neurosci Rep 2019;19:76.
6. Huijben JA, Volovici V, Cnossen MC, et al. Variation in general supportive and preventive intensive care management of traumatic brain injury: a survey in 66 neurotrauma centers participating in the Collaborative European NeuroTrauma Effectiveness Research in Traumatic Brain Injury (CENTER-TBI) study. Crit Care 2018;22(1):90.
7. Diringer MN, Edwards DF. Admission to a neurologic/neurosurgical intensive care unit is associated with reduced mortality rate after intracerebral hemorrhage. Crit Care Med 2001;29(3):635–40.
8. Thompson MP, Zhao X, Bekelis K, et al. Regional variation in 30-day ischemic stroke outcomes for Medicare beneficiaries treated in Get with the Guidelines-Stroke hospitals. Circ Cardiovasc Qual Outcomes 2017;10(8):e003604.
9. Miyares LC, Falcone GJ, Leasure A, et al. Race/ethnicity influences outcomes in young adults with supratentorial intracerebral hemorrhage. Neurology 2020; 94(12):e1271–80.
10. Greene NH, Kernic MA, Vavilala MS, et al. Variation in adult traumatic brain injury outcomes in the United States. J Head Trauma Rehabil 2018;33(1):E1–8.
11. Suarez J, Martin RH, Bauza C, et al. Worldwide organization of neurocritical care: results from the PRINCE Study Part 1. Neurocrit Care 2020;32(1):172–9.
12. Venkatasubba Rao CP, Suarez JI, Martin RH, et al. Global survey of outcomes of neurocritical care patients: analysis of the PRINCE Study Part 2. Neurocrit Care 2020;32(1):88–103.
13. Ormseth CH, Sheth KN, Saver JL, et al. The American Heart Association's Get with the Guidelines (GWTG)-stroke development and impact on stroke care. Stroke Vasc Neurol 2017;2(2):94–105.
14. Lele AV, Quality Committee of the Neurocritical Care Society, Moheet AM. Neurocritical care quality improvement practices: a survey of members of the Neurocritical Care Society. Neurocrit Care 2020;32(1):295–301.
15. Donabedian A. The quality of care: how can it be assessed? JAMA 1988;260(12): 1743–8.
16. Berwick D, Fox DM. Evaluating the quality of medical care: Donabedian's classic article 50 years later. Milbank Q 2016;94(2):237–41.
17. Nelson EC, Mohr JJ, Batalden PB, et al. Improving health care, part I: the clinical value compass. Jt Comm J Qual Impov 1996;22(4):243–58.
18. Khan MW, Muehlschlegel S. Shared decision making in neurocritical care. Neurosurg Clin N Am 2018;29(2):315–21.
19. Casalino LP, Gans D, Weber R, et al. US physician practices send more than $15.4 billion annually to report quality measures. Health Aff 2016;35(3):401–6.
20. Macleean CH, Kerr EA, Qaseem A. Time out-charting a path or improving performance measurement. NEJM 2018;378(19):1757–61.
21. Adair CE, Simpson E, Deer AB, et al. Performance measurement in healthcare: part II—state of the science findings by stage of the performance measurement process. Healthc Policy 2006;2(1):56–78.

22. Moheet AM, Livesay SL, Abdelhak T, et al. Standards for neurologic critical care units: a statement for healthcare professionals from the Neurocritical Care Society. Neurocrit Care 2018;29(2):145–60.
23. Kaplan L, Moheet AM, Livesay SL, et al. A perspective from the neurocritical care society and the society of critical care medicine: team-based care for neurological critical illness. Neurocrit Care 2020;32(2):369–72.
24. Livesay S, Fried H, Gagnon D, et al. Clinical performance measures for neurocritical care: a statement for healthcare professionals from the Neurocritical Care Society. Neurocrit Care 2020;32(1):5–79.
25. Josephson SA, Ferro J, Cohen A, et al. Quality improvement in neurology: inpatient and emergency care quality measure set: executive summary. Neurology 2017;89(7):730–5.
26. Smith EE, Saver JL, Alexander DN, et al. Clinical performance measures for adults hospitalized with acute ischemic stroke. Stroke 2014;45:3472–98.
27. Porter ME. What is value in health care? N Engl J Med 2010;363(26):2477–81.
28. Blumenthal D, Abrams M. The affordable care act at 10 years—payment and delivery system reforms. N Engl J Med 2020;382(11):1057–63.
29. Centers for Medicare & Medicaid Services. Hospital-acquired conditions [Internet] [cited 2022 Feb 11]; Available at: https://www.cms.gov/Medicare/Medicare-Fee-for-Service-Payment/HospitalAcqCond/Hospital-Acquired_Conditions.html. Accessed Feb 11 2022.
30. Centers for Medicare & Medicaid Services. The hospital value-based based Purchasing (VBP) program [Internet] [cited 2022 Feb 11]; Available at: https://www.cms.gov/Medicare/Quality-Initiatives-Patient-Assessment-Instruments/Value-Based-Programs/HVBP/Hospital-Value-Based-Purchasing.html.
31. Centers for Medicare & Medicaid Services. The hospital readmissions reduction program [Internet] [cited 2022 Feb 11]; available at: https://www.cms.gov/Medicare/Medicare-Fee-for-Service-Payment/AcuteInpatientPPS/Readmissions-Reduction-Program.
32. Centers for Medicare & Medicaid Services. Hospital compare [Internet] [cited 2022 Feb 11]; Available at: https://www.medicare.gov/care-compare/?providerType=Hospital&redirect=true.
33. Leapfrog hospital safety Grade [Internet] [cited 2022 Feb 11]; Available at: https://www.hospitalsafetygrade.org/.
34. U.S. News & World Report. U.S. News best hospitals [Internet] [cited 2022 Feb 11]; Available at: https://health.usnews.com/best-hospitals. Accessed Feb 11 2022.
35. Kessler BA, Catalino MP, Jordan JD. Reducing the reported mortality index within a neurocritical care unit through documentation and coding accuracy. World Neurosurg 2020;133:e819–27.
36. Wilensky G. The need to simplify measuring quality in health care. JAMA 2018; 319(23):2369–70.
37. Wells S, Orly T, Gray J, et al. Are quality improvement collaboratives effective? A systematic review. BMJ Qual Saf 2018;27(3):226–40.
38. Provencio JJ, Hemphill JC, Claassen J, et al. The curing coma campaign: framing initial scientific challenges-proceedings of the first curing coma campaign scientific advisory council meeting. Neurocrit Care 2020;33(1):1–12.

Neurocritical Care Education in the United States

Angela Hays Shapshak, MD, FNCS[a],*, Lori Shutter, MD, FNCS, FCCM[b]

KEYWORDS

- Graduate medical education • Neurocritical care • Critical care • Fellowship

KEY POINTS

- Neurocritical care (NCC) has evolved as a multidisciplinary specialty, which requires the development of broad critical care expertise as well as an in-depth understanding of the neurosciences.
- Several pathways for training and certification of neurointensivists are now available in the US.
- Despite a few key differences, broad similarities exist among NCC training pathways, and between NCC education and other intensive care disciplines.
- Recent advances in NCC training and certification have the potential to pave the way for improved integration of the neurointensivist workforce into mainstream critical care.

INTRODUCTION

In many respects, the evolution of neurocritical care (NCC) training as a distinct subspecialty has mirrored the development of critical care medicine as a whole. The emergence of critical care as a medical subspecialty is often attributed to the poliomyelitis (polio) epidemic that struck Europe and parts of the US in the 1950s. Anesthesiologists initially recognized that techniques used in the operating room could potentially be redeployed to save the lives of polio victims with pulmonary insufficiency and/or bulbar weakness. At the time, negative pressure ventilation techniques predominated; cuirass ventilators and "iron-lungs" were typical. Unfortunately, demand for these devices rapidly outstripped supply during the epidemic. Dr Bjorn Ibsen, an anesthesiologist in Copenhagen, was among the first to use positive pressure ventilation in the care of these patients. He pioneered the practice of early tracheostomy in this patient population, which facilitated the use of manual bag-mask ventilation, often provided by medical students as part of their clinical training. This technique proved quite

[a] Departments of Neurology and Anesthesiology, University of Alabama at Birmingham, RUWH M22, 619 19TH Street South, Birmingham, AL 35249-3280, USA; [b] Departments of Critical Care Medicine, Neurology, & Neurosurgery, UPMC Healtcare System / University of Pittsburgh School of Medicine, 3550 Terrace Street, Scaife Hall Suite 600, Pittsburgh, PA, 15261, USA
* Corresponding author.
E-mail address: ashapshak@uabmc.edu

Crit Care Clin 39 (2023) 29–46
https://doi.org/10.1016/j.ccc.2022.07.004
criticalcare.theclinics.com

successful, reducing the mortality of polio in Copenhagen by approximately 50%. However, caring for this population was labor-intensive, requiring large numbers of specialized personnel.[1]

Although early respiratory care units were devoted to the care of patients with a neurologic disease, it would be many years before NCC developed into a distinct discipline. For the most part, neurologists' involvement in the care of critically ill patients was limited to diagnostic evaluation and assessment of bulbar dysfunction. However, there were some notable exceptions, including Dr W. Ritchie Russel who, along with colleagues, pioneered the development of one of the first positive pressure ventilation systems.[2] In the United States (US), Dr A. B. Baker, chief of neurology at the University of Minnesota, reported extensively on the multisystem care of patients with polio.[3] Similarly, Dr Fred Plum took an interest in the care of critically ill patients after his sister succumbed to polio, and went on to publish one of the first comprehensive descriptions of the evaluation of patients with alterations of consciousness, which is still frequently referenced today.[4]

Neurosurgeons began to recognize the value of dedicated units providing postoperative neurosurgical care, leading to the development of ICUs to care for complex neurosurgical patients, spinal cord injury, and traumatic brain injury.[5] These efforts led to the development of protocols and procedures for the management of patients with nervous system trauma as well as other neurosurgical conditions including aneurysmal subarachnoid hemorrhage. Ultimately these early neurosurgical ICUs laid the groundwork for concepts central to the practice of modern NCC, including principles of intracranial hypertension, vascular autoregulation, and cerebral hemodynamics.[6]

By the 1980s, NCC was developing as a distinct subspecialty. Early on Dr Alan Ropper described the scope of the emerging field, which included management of intracranial hypertension; evaluation and treatment of patients with coma; cerebrovascular diseases including ischemic stroke, intracerebral hemorrhage, and aneurysmal subarachnoid hemorrhage; neuromuscular respiratory failure; status epilepticus; and central nervous system trauma.[2] Dedicated neurologic and neurosurgical intensive care units (Neuro ICUs) were beginning to develop at several academic centers, often as a collaboration between internists, neurologists, and neurosurgeons (**Fig. 1**).

HISTORY OF EDUCATION IN NEUROCRITICAL CARE

As interest in NCC grew, the need for formal education and training became apparent. Drs Peter Safar and Ake Grenvik developed the first formal multidisciplinary critical care medicine training program at the University of Pittsburgh in 1961. They initially brought together physicians from anesthesiology, internal medicine and surgery to train together to advance critical care medicine, with a focus on resuscitation and acute care. Pediatrics and emergency medicine soon followed. The introduction of neurology to critical care training programs was still delayed for a few more years.

Dr David Jackson at Case Western Reserve University was one of the few neurologists engaged in the practice of general critical care. In the 1970s, he developed one of the first general adult critical care programs in the US and went on to create an annual course on NCC administered by the American Academy of Neurology (AAN). In response to growing interest in the field, the American Academy of Neurology (AAN) approved the creation of the Critical Care and Emergency Neurology section within the organization. In 1989, Dr Daniel Hanley, a dual-trained neurologist and internist was confirmed as the inaugural chair. Simultaneously, formal training programs in NCC were being created. These training programs were collaborative efforts involving multiple medical specialties. In fact, neurologists with an interest in critical care

1970s	Dr. David Jackson, a neurologist, becomes director of one of the earliest training programs in general adult intensive care.
1980s	Dedicated neurology and neurosurgery ICUs at academic centers including Johns Hopkins University, Massachusetts General Hospital, Columbia University and the University of Virginia begin training fellows.
1980s	Critical Care Medicine is recognized as a subspecialty by ABMS & ACGME.
1983	The first textbook of neurocritical care, edited by Drs. Ropper, Kennedy and Zervas, is published.
1988	The Critical Care and Emergency Neurology Section of the AAN is established.
2002	The UCNS is founded.
2003	The Neurocritical Care Society is founded, and the certification committee established.
2005	Neurocritical care is recognized as a subspecialty by UCNS.
2007	Administration of the first UCNS neurocritical care certification exam.
2013	The CAST Committee of the Society for Neurological Surgeons begins accrediting neurosurgical fellowships.

2018 2021	Neurocritical care receives formal recognition from ABMS.
	• September:
	   o Neurocritical care program requirements receive approval from the ACGME Board of Directors, paving the way for fellowship programs to apply for accreditation.
	• October:
	   o The first ABMS Neurocritical Care certification exam is offered, administered by the ABPN.
	• December:
	   o Inaugural Recognition of Focused Practice in Neurocritical Care examination is administered by the ABNS.

2026	ABMS grandfathering window expected to close.

Fig. 1. Timeline of significant events in neurocritical care training and certification.

medicine were often required to complete 2 residencies, as there was no mechanism at the time for neurology residents to obtain sufficient intensive care exposure. The first NCC training program was established at Massachusetts General Hospital in 1978 by Drs. Allan Roper, a neurologist and internist, and Sean Kennedy, an anesthesiologist. Shortly thereafter, programs were established at the Johns Hopkins University Hospital under Drs Hanley and Cecil Borel, a neuroanesthesiologist; at Columbia University under Dr Matt Fink, a neurologist and internist; and University of Virginia with Drs E. Clark Haley and Thomas Bleck, both neurologists and internists.[5] Trainees from these first programs went on to establish additional early training programs, with Dr Darryl Gress, (MGH NCC alumnus) starting the University of California San Francisco program, and Dr Michael Diringer (Johns Hopkins NCC alumnus) starting the Washington University in St Louis program. In 1993, Dr Borel moved to Duke University to establish an NCC program and through collaboration with nursing pioneer

Joanne Hickey, PhD, RN the subspecialty training of nurse practitioners in NCC was started.

Although training programs at these and other institutions were beginning to flourish, no formal mechanism for program accreditation or physician certification would be available for approximately 20 years. In the US before the 1970s, postgraduate medical education was governed at a local level. The Accreditation Council for Graduate Medical Education (ACGME) was founded in 1981 as an independent, not-for-profit organization intended to set standards for postgraduate medical education in the US. As of 2020, the ACGME recognized more than 12,000 residency and fellowship programs across 182 disciplines and had begun to provide accreditation to some international institutions as well. Accreditation requires programs and sponsoring institutions to document that they have adequate resources to support a program including, patient volume, appropriately credentialed faculty; capacity to provide high-quality educational opportunities for residents and fellows, and establish and adhere to policies and procedures to prioritize patient safety and safeguard trainees. The ACGME works in concert with the American Board of Medical Specialties (ABMS), which provides physician credentialing for recognized specialties and subspecialties by way of various member boards.

Critical care medicine was recognized as a subspecialty by ABMS and ACGME in the 1980s, with distinct training and certification pathways recognized through the American Board of Anesthesiology (ABA), American Board of Internal Medicine (ABIM), American Board of Surgery (ABS), and the American Board of Pediatrics (ABP). Several physician specialties were eligible for ACGME-accredited critical care training and ABMS member board certification. However, neurologists and neurosurgeons were not among them. The Neurocritical Care Society (NCS), founded in 2003, was instrumental in developing criteria for the formal recognition of NCC expertise. Dr Thomas Bleck served as the inaugural president of the society, and one of the first tasks undertaken by the organization involved the establishment of a certification committee. Cochaired by Drs Jose Suarez and Cherylee Chang, this committee helped create the core curriculum and requirements for NCC training programs.[7,8] At the time, NCC did not qualify for recognition by ABMS, in part due to a lack of a sufficient number of programs and providers. Fortunately, the United Council for Neurologic Subspecialties (UCNS) offered an alternative. The UCNS was founded in 2002 by members of 5 stakeholder organizations—the AAN, Association of University Professors of Neurology, American Neurologic Association, Child Neurology Society, and Professors of Child Neurology—for the express purpose of supporting new subspecialties within the neurosciences.[8] The UCNS offered a mechanism for program accreditation, as well as the certification of qualified physicians. The AAN CCEN section, Society for Neuroscience in Anesthesiology and Critical Care (SNACC), and NCS jointly sponsored the proposal to UCNS. In October 2005, NCC was formally recognized, creating the opportunity for individuals to become certified and training programs to gain accreditation. The first certification examination was administered in 2007. Dr Chang, serving as Chair of the UCNS NCC Examination Writing Committee, took pains to emphasize the need for neurointensivists to establish a solid foundation in general critical care.[8,9] This is reflected both in the core curriculum for fellowship programs and in the certification examination. The core curriculum includes a thorough and detailed listing of general critical care principles, procedures, and disease states which are considered integral to training in NCC, in addition to an extensive list of neurologic and neurosurgical conditions.[8] The UCNS examination content is evenly split between general critical care and subspecialty topics; a passing grade in each is a requirement for certification.[9]

Table 1
Required critical care experience in residencies whose graduates are eligible for neurocritical care training

Primary Specialty	ACGME Requirements
Neurology[25]	"…must include at least 6 months of inpatient experience in adult neurology. (Core) Residents must have…exposure to and understanding of evaluation and management of patients with neurologic disorders in various settings, including an intensive care unit and an emergency department, and for patients requiring acute neurosurgical management. (Core)"
Neurosurgery[26]	"During the first 18 mo of education residents must have at least 3 months of basic clinical neuroscience education and at least 3 months of critical care education applicable to the neurosurgical patient. (Core)"
Emergency Medicine[27]	"4 months of dedicated critical care experiences, including critical care of infants and children; At least 2 months of these experiences must be at the PGY-2 level or above. (Core)"
Internal Medicine[28]	"Experiences must include required critical care rotations (medical or respiratory intensive care units, cardiac care units). (Core) These experiences cannot be fewer than 3 months and more than 6 months over the 36 mo of training. (Detail)"
Anesthesiology[29]	"Resident education must include a minimum of four 1-month rotations in critical care medicine. (Core) No more than 2 months of this experience should occur prior to the CA-1 y (Core)"
Surgery[30]	"At least 54 mo of the 60-mo program must be spent on clinical assignments in surgery, with documented experience in emergency care and surgical critical care in order to enable residents to manage patients with severe and complex illnesses and with major injuries. (Core)"
Pediatric Critical Care Medicine[31]	"Fellows must have a minimum of 12 mo of clinical experience in an ICU in which they have primary responsibility for providing patient care. (Core) a) Fellows must have a minimum of 8 months of critical care experience in the PICU. (Core) b) Fellows' clinical experience in critical care settings other than the PICU…must be no more than 4 months. (Core)"
Child Neurology[32]	at least 12 FTE months of adult neurology under the supervision of faculty members certified by the ABPN or AOBPN in neurology, that do not need to be contiguous, including: (Core) (1) "6 months on inpatient rotations…" as well as "at least 12 FTE months of clinical child neurology;" with "management responsibility for hospitalized patients with neurologic disorders, including pediatric patients with acute neurologic disorders, in an intensive care unit and in an emergency department"

In recognition of the many pathways to NCC expertise, the UCNS recognizes 8 specialties as eligible for accredited fellowships: neurology, neurosurgery, child neurology, internal medicine, pediatric critical care, general surgery, anesthesiology, and emergency medicine. Due to variable critical care exposure in each of these specialties (**Table 1**), 3 different fellowship tracks were established. For most eligible applicants, including those with prior training in pediatric critical care, the training program consists of a minimum of 24 months. This must include a minimum of

12 months spent in the direct care of critically ill patients, most of which involves caring for neurocritically ill patients. Rotations in other critical care settings are also encouraged to ensure that fellows gain expertise in general critical care principles as well. The remaining 12 months of training allow some flexibility for trainees to gain additional experience in general critical care, other neurologic subspecialties, and related fields. This enables the training program to be tailored to the needs of physicians from a variety of backgrounds to ensure that graduates can function independently both as general intensivists and as neurointensivists on graduation. In contrast, residents in neurosurgery and graduates of neurosurgery residencies are eligible for a 12-month training program that emphasizes building a general critical care skill set. Ten of the 12 months must be spent in the care of critically ill patients, and a minimum of half of this time must be spent in critical care disciplines other than NCC. In 2015 the UCNS NCC program requirements were updated to permit neurosurgical residents to complete their training as part of an "enfolded" fellowship, incorporated into their 84 months of required residency training. Rotations qualifying for credit toward fellowship training must occur after the completion of the 4th year of training and must be completed over 12 consecutive months. Finally, a different 12-month pathway is available for graduates of critical care fellowships. This track consists of a minimum of 8 months of NCC exposure, as well as relevant rotations in the neurosciences.[10]

In the 17 years since achieving recognition, the number of UCNS accredited training programs and certified physicians has grown tremendously (**Fig. 2**). As of January 2022, 1543 physicians hold UCNS certification in NCC.[11] Of these, 51% identified neurology as their primary subspecialty. Internal medicine physicians comprise the next largest group, constituting 35% of the total. Since 2012, most NCC fellowships have participated in the SF Match matching program. Data obtained from SF Match indicate that applicant interest in the field has also been rising steeply (**Fig. 3**). At present, there are more positions offered through SF Match than there are applicants; however, this data may under-represent the number of applicants seeking positions, since Match participation is voluntary.

In parallel with the UCNS accreditation mechanism, the Society of Neurologic Surgeons (SNS) has maintained a pathway for recognizing neurosurgeons with expertise in NCC. The Committee for Accreditation of Subspecialty Training was established by SNS in 1999 to oversee accreditation for various subspecialties within neurosurgery. In 2013, this group was renamed the Committee on Advanced Subspecialty Training (CAST).[12] As part of this restructuring effort, and in response to the growth in UCSN-

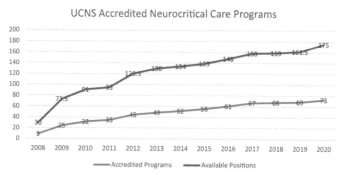

Fig. 2. Growth in UCNS-accredited neurocritical care programs over time. (Data courtesy of Ms. Brenda Riggott, United Council of Neurologic Subspecialties (UCNS), Minneapolis, MN.)

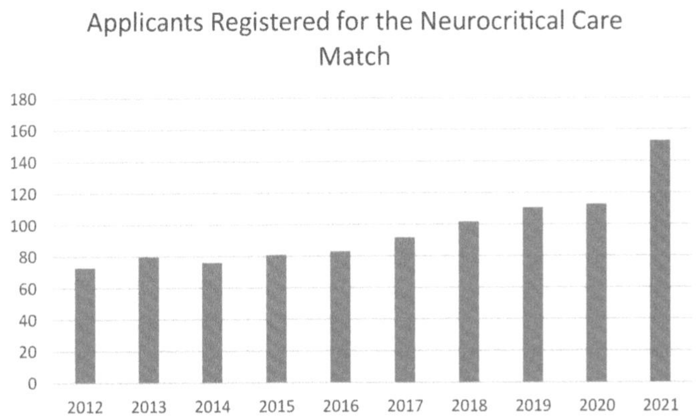

Applicants Registered for the Neurocritical Care
Match

Fig. 3. Trends in the number of applicants registered for the neurocritical care match. Reflected are the numbers of residents who registered for the neurocritical care match administered by SF Match, regardless of whether they ultimately secured positions. (Data courtesy of Mr. Dennis S. Thomatos, SF Matching Program, San Francisco, CA.)

accredited NCC fellowships, CAST developed a formal fellowship review process and began offering accreditation of NCC programs open to neurosurgeons. The CAST pathway requires 12 months of dedicated NCC training. CAST NCC program requirements, like the UCNS version, emphasize the multidisciplinary nature of the field, and reinforce the need for graduates to be prepared to address "all aspects of care, including pulmonary, cardiac, renal, gastrointestinal, hematological, infectious and other systemic problems."[13] Fellowship training may occur following the completion of residency or enfolded into residency training. In the latter case, fellowship-level experiences must occur after the 3rd year of residency training, for example, postgraduate year 4 and above, and can be divided into blocks of no less than 4 months duration. In 2019, CAST transitioned away from offering certification to individuals, in favor of the Recognition of Focused Practice (RFP), which is conferred by the American Board of Neurologic Surgeons (ABNS). Physicians who have been certified via CAST may apply to have their certification transitioned to RFP. Obtaining certification through the ABNS RFP process requires that the applicant hold ABNS certification in neurosurgery and pass a written exam. Currently, physicians may qualify to take the examination either by completing an accredited fellowship or via the practice track. Practice track eligibility requires documentation that a sufficient percentage of the applicant's time has been dedicated to the practice of NCC over the preceding 3 to 6 years.[14]

By the late 2010s, there had been sufficient growth within the NCC community that recognition by the ABMS and ACGME became feasible. Although alternate credentialing pathways have been successfully implemented, there were several arguments in favor of seeking ABMS/ACGME recognition. First, the ABMS and ACGME are the primary method of certification and accreditation among physicians in the US. Therefore, they are more widely recognized among physicians, hospital administrators, and members of the public than either UCNS or CAST. For this reason, it was argued that ABMS recognition would lend additional legitimacy to NCC and promote the continued growth of the subspecialty. Second, heterogeneity among NCC programs could potentially be exacerbated by the presence of multiple credentialing alternatives. ACGME is a robust organization with considerable resources at its disposal.

Transitioning to ACGME oversight of fellowship programs could promote improved consistency. Finally, some within the wider critical care community had expressed concern that trainees in NCC programs were not achieving the same level of competency in general critical care as intensivists from other backgrounds, and that oversight by ACGME may better ensure program quality.[9] In 2017, the Neuroscience Section of the Society of Critical Care Medicine (SCCM) published an analysis of NCC training requirements as compared with standards established for various critical care specialties accredited by ACGME.[15] This review identified considerable overlap among recognized routes to critical care certification, including a broad consensus regarding general competencies and the core knowledge base. However, there were several areas of variability, including prerequisites for fellowship, breadth of critical care exposure, procedural requirements, and administrative oversight. The authors concluded that the breadth of critical care training and substantial concordance of the core skillsets across critical care programs supported the contention that neurointensivists should be well prepared to provide high-quality critical care, as well as subspecialty expertise. At around the same time, the NCS convened the Program Accreditation, Physician Certification, and Fellowship Training (PACT) Committee, which surveyed fellowship program directors to evaluate the state of fellowship training and better understand attitudes about the potential development of an ACGME accreditation pathway.[16] The Committee surveyed program directors of existing programs and achieved a 61% response rate. Of the 33 survey respondents, 32 indicated that their institutions offered UCNS-accredited fellowships, and 12 indicated that their institutions offered both CAST and UCNS-accredited options. In institutions offering both options, 92% reported significant overlap among the faculty, though only 17% shared a common program director. Data obtained from this survey indicated that most respondents viewed ABMS/ACGME recognition as a means to better integrate NCC within the broader critical care community and support the continued growth of the subspecialty. However, the survey did reveal some variability among programs, particularly with respect to ICU coverage models and procedural requirements. Additionally, the level of institutional support for programs fell below the minimum ACGME requirements in many cases; for example, only 30% of surveyed fellowship directors reported having protected time for program administration, and only 48% reported having a designated administrative coordinator. Funding of fellow salaries represented another potential area of concern, with roughly $1/3$rd of programs indicating that fellows were funded out of clinical revenues, and $1/4$ of programs permitting fellows to bill for services and procedures. Nevertheless, most survey respondents felt that the additional requirements and administrative burden imposed by ACGME accreditation would be surmountable and had the potential to benefit the field.

CURRENT STATE OF NEUROCRITICAL CARE EDUCATION

Due largely to advocacy on the part of professional organizations such as the NCS, SCCM, and the CCEN section of the AAN, NCC was recognized as a subspecialty by ABMS in June of 2018. The first ABPN board certification examination in NCC was administered in October of 2021 to a total of 1103 candidates who qualified through practice track criteria outlined by relevant ABMS member organizations. For the initial examination administration, 450 applicants applied via the American Board of Internal Medicine (ABIM), 369 via ABPN, 237 through ABA (including anesthesiologists and surgeons), and 47 by the American Board of Emergency Medicine (ABEM) (personal communication from Patti Vondrak, MBA; Vice President of

Table 2
Comparison of UCNS, CAST and ACGME program requirements for neurocritical care fellowships

Domain	UCNS[33]	CAST/ABNS[34]	ACGME[35]
Fellow Eligibility: Accreditation of prior training: Eligible Specialties: Other Requirements:	• ACGME, RCPSC, or CanERA • 24-mo track: Graduates of neurology, general internal medicine, general surgery, emergency medicine, pediatric critical care, or child neurology programs. • 12-mo track (intensivists): Graduates of critical care medicine fellowships (anesthesia, surgery, internal medicine, and/or emergency medicine). • 12-mo track (neurosurgeons): Neurosurgery residents or graduates (see later in discussion). • All fellows must be certified ACLS providers or instructors.	• ACGME	• ACGME, ACGME-I, AOA, RCPSC, or CFPC • NCC-1 (24-mo track): Graduates of neurology, internal medicine, anesthesiology, child neurology, emergency medicine, or general surgery programs. • NCC-2 (intensivists): Must have completed a fellowship in anesthesiology critical care medicine, internal medicine critical care medicine, or pediatric critical care medicine, or a surgical critical care residency. • NCC-2 (neurosurgeons): Must have completed or be currently enrolled in a neurosurgery residency. • Programs must verify the level of competence in the relevant specialty-specific milestones before matriculation. • An exception is available for exceptionally qualified international graduates in neurosurgery who's prior training does not meet the criteria specified above.
Sponsoring Institution:	Institution must be accredited by ACGME or CanERA.	Institution must be accredited by ACGME, must have a dedicated neuro-ICU, and must offer an ACGME-accredited neurosurgery residency.	Institution must be accredited by ACGME. The institution must have a dedicated neuro-ICU or dedicated beds in a general critical care unit for the care of neurologic and neurosurgical patients. The average census of neurocritical care patients must be at least 5 patients per fellow.

(continued on next page)

Table 2
(continued)

Domain	UCNS[33]	CAST/ABNS[34]	ACGME[35]
Recognized Pathways:	• 24-mo track: Includes 12 mo of critical care, more than half of which are devoted to the care of neuro-critically ill patients. • 12-mo track for neurosurgeons: 10 mo of critical care, no less than half of which focus on general critical care. The remaining 2 mo must be spent in noncritical patient care or research. All clinical activities, including call, must take place within the UCNS neurocritical care fellowship. *Enfolded fellowships* must occur after the completion of the 4th post-graduate year, and must consist of 12 consecutive months. • 12-mo track for intensivists: 8 mo of critical care focused on neuro-critically ill patients, with the remainder of the time spent in noncritical neuroscience experiences.	• Postgraduate 12-mo track: occurs after the completion of an ACGME-accredited neurosurgery residency. • Enfolded fellowship: Consists of no <12 mo of training during the course of a neurosurgery residency which must take place in the PGY-4 y or later. The training may occur in blocks of no <4 mo in duration. • No specific requirements for time spent in general critical care rotations are stated. A continuous presence in the ICU should be maintained, "except for night and weekend on-call experiences in surgery."	• NCC-1 Level (24-mo track): Includes a minimum of 12 mo of critical care, at least 8 mo of which focuses on the care of neurologic and neurosurgical patients. • NCC-2 Level (12-mo track) for neurosurgeons: Includes a minimum of 8 mo of critical care focused on neurologic and neurosurgical patients. The remaining time, no more than 4 mo, may be spent on noncritical care medicine or on research. Enfolded training must occur in the PGY-4 y or later. • NCC-2 Level (12-mo track) for intensivists: Consists of a minimum of 8 mo of critical care focused on neurologic and neurosurgical patients. A maximum of 4 mo may be spent in rotations dedicated to the noncritical neurosciences.
Didactic Conferences:	There must be structured, fellow-specific educational experiences, and fellows must regularly attend seminars and conferences in neurology, neurosurgery, neuroradiology and critical care.	A didactic curriculum sufficient to allow trainees to acquire advanced knowledge of neurologic/neurosurgical care, including complex coexisting medical problems.	Fellows must participate in weekly didactic conferences, including conferences on neurology, neurosurgery, neuroradiology, and neurocritical care. Regularly scheduled research seminars, journal clubs, and basic science conferences are also required.

Program Director Qualifications:	• Must be certified by the ABMS, RCPSC, AOA, or CFPC in an eligible primary specialty. • Must hold UCNS certification in neurocritical care. • Must devote a minimum of 50% of his/her clinical effort to the care of neurocritical care patients.	The PD must hold certification in NCC by an appropriate certifying body, which may include ABNS/SNS-CAST for neurosurgeons, and UCNS or ABPN/ABMS for other disciplines.	• Must be board certified in NCC by the appropriate ABMS board, or ABNS certification in neurosurgery with RFP in NCC. • Must spend no <25% of his/her responsibilities in NCC clinical care and administration. • Must have a minimum of 0.1 FTE protected time. The required amount increases according to fellow complement. • Must have a minimum of 3 y' experience as an attending neurointensivist.
Core Faculty:	• Must be certified by ABMS, RCPSC, AOA, or CFPC in an eligible specialty (see above). • Must also possess either: UCNS NCC certification, ABMS certification in critical care, or ABMS certification in neurosurgery. • Must include at least one neurologist.	Must be board certified in their primary discipline. A minimum of 2 NCC-certified faculty in addition to the PD is required.	• Core faculty must be board certified in NCC by the appropriate ABMS board, or ABNS certification in neurosurgery with the recognition of focused practice (RFP) in NCC. • There must be at least one neurologist and at least one neurosurgeon. • Core faculty must complete the ACGME faculty survey.
Faculty to Fellow Ratio:	At least 1 NCC-certified faculty member for every 2 fellows.	None specified. A minimum of 3 NCC-certified faculty, including the PD, is required regardless of fellow complement.	At least 1 NCC-certified core faculty member for every 2 fellows.
Administrative Support:	There must be a single program director responsible for overseeing the program, and adequate technical, professional, and administrative support.	There must be a designated program coordinator, who may also serve as the coordinator for the neurosurgical residency. The program must also have sufficient clerical support.	There must be a designated program coordinator. The minimum FTE requirement ranges from 0.25 to 0.5 FTE depending on the number of fellows.
Patient case mix:	Not specified	Training must include both adult and pediatric experience, though most of the training is expected to involve adults.	Not specified

(continued on next page)

Table 2
(continued)

Domain	UCNS[33]	CAST/ABNS[34]	ACGME[35]
Fellow Evaluation:	Must occur at least semiannually. A final evaluation must incorporate faculty input to assess the fellow according to NCC milestones and must include a statement about the fellow's ability to practice independently on the completion of the program.	Faculty must evaluate fellows according to core competencies in a timely manner, and include at least semiannual written evaluations. The final evaluation must include a statement addressing the fellow's ability to practice independently.	Evaluation must occur at least semiannually and must address the fellow's progress according to the ACGME Core Competencies and the subspecialty milestones. The final evaluation must be prepared with the input of the faculty and include a statement regarding the fellow's ability to practice independently on graduation.
Faculty Evaluation:	PDs must evaluate faculty at least annually, incorporating input from confidential fellow evaluations of the faculty.	Faculty must be evaluated by the program regularly. To preserve confidentiality in small programs, this should occur no less frequently than the midpoint of the accreditation cycle.	Faculty must be evaluated by the PD at least annually, and the evaluation must incorporate confidential evaluations from fellows.
Program Evaluation:	The program must be evaluated in a systematic manner, incorporating confidential evaluations from fellows. The process should address the degree to which program goals and objectives have been met, and should use outcome measures including performance on the UCNS board examination.	The effectiveness of the program and rotations should be evaluated in a systemic manner in such a way as to maintain fellow confidentiality. The effectiveness of the PD must be evaluated by the fellows and faculty no less than semiannually.	The PD must appoint a formal program evaluation committee (PEC), including at least 1 fellow and a minimum of 2 faculty. The PEC should conduct an annual review of the program effectiveness including data from fellow and faculty evaluations, prior PEC reviews, ACGME surveys, fellow well-being, program diversity, and so forth. An action plan must be generated and distributed to faculty, fellows and DIO. The PEC must also conduct a self-study prior to the 10-y accreditation site visit.

Abbreviations: ABMS, American Board of Medical Specialties; ABNS, American Board of Neurologic Surgeons; ACGME, Accreditation Council on Graduate Medical Education; ACGME-I, ACGME International; ACLS, Advanced Cardiac Life Support; AOA, American Osteopathic Association; CanERA, Canadian Excellence in Residency Accreditation; CAST, Committee on Advanced Subspecialty Training; CFPC, College of Family Physicians of Canada; FTE, full-time equivalent; NCC, neurocritical care; PD, program director; PGY, postgraduate year; RCPSC, Royal College of Physicians and Surgeons of Canada; RFP, recognition of focused practice (conferred by ABNS); SNS, Society of Neurologic Surgeons; UCNS, unitized council of neurologic subspecialties.

Operations at ABPN, October 13, 2021). ABMS recognition paved the way for ACGME accreditation of NCC fellowships. In 2019, the ACGME Board of Directors approved the petition from the ABPN regarding the training guidelines and competency-based milestones. The ACGME convened a working group consisting of medical educators from all relevant specialty boards to draft program requirements, which were submitted for public comment in December 2020 and ultimately approved by the ACGME Board of Directors in September 2021.[17]

Therefore, currently, there are 3 mechanisms for NCC program accreditation and physician certification that coexist. Considerable overlap exists between the various organizations, with some important differences, summarized in **Table 2**. Many are attributable to the incorporation of elements from the ACGME Common Program Requirements, which are standard expectations pertaining to all accredited programs, regardless of specialty. These include stipulations about institutional resources, administrative support, faculty qualifications, trainee wellness, and policies surrounding supervision and grievances. Fortunately, the UCNS and CAST organizations have taken pains to adhere to ACGME policies and procedures when developing their program requirements. For example, both have implemented duty hours restrictions that mirror ACGME, and have similar requirements for fellow evaluation and program improvement.[10,13] In fact, UCNS requires that programs be affiliated with an ACGME-accredited sponsoring institution under the supervision of the Designated Institutional Official (DIO), and CAST programs are only permitted within the auspices of an ACGME-accredited neurosurgery program. UCNS has also established NCC-specific milestones, which were based on the ACGME milestones established for other critical care disciplines; and developed faculty and fellow surveys modeled after the ACGME. Areas of divergence worth noting include that the ACGME imposes a greater administrative burden on programs, including maintenance of duty hours logs, semiannual competency committee meetings, verification of specific competencies for incoming fellows, and periodic self-study visits as well as external audits. To ensure that programs have sufficient support to comply with these requirements, program directors are required to have a minimum amount of protected time as well as dedicated coordinator support, which some existing programs may not currently meet. The ACGME also outlines specific requirements for the clinical learning environment, including stipulations regarding transitions of care, fatigue mitigation, and mechanisms to ensure patient safety. Although these stipulations are not explicitly included in CAST and UCNS requirements, it is likely that most existing programs are substantially in compliance with these requirements, because CAST and UCNS programs occur in the context of ACGME-accredited institutions. Perhaps more significantly, there are discrepancies pertaining to fellow eligibility for the various clinical pathways, as well as the required curricular components. For example, pediatric intensivists are eligible for appointment at an NCC-2 level, requiring only 12 months of additional training, under ACGME requirements, whereas they qualify for the 24-month pathway under UCNS guidelines. Although there is considerable overlap among resident specialties eligible for 24-month fellowships accredited by UCNS and ACGME, board eligibility is governed by the relevant ABMS member board, which is dependent on the applicants' primary field. Both ABIM and ABS have indicated that, after the closure of the practice track in 2026, applicants will only be considered eligible for the NCC board examination after obtaining ABIM or ABS certification in critical care.[18,19] Therefore, the ACGME 24-month training program will only confer board eligibility to graduates of neurology, child neurology, anesthesiology, and emergency medicine programs after 2026. There are also significant differences with respect to the enfolded fellowships available for neurosurgery residents. The UCNS requires that all 12 months of fellowship training be completed continuously and that fellows be excused from clinical obligations associated with their residency training for the duration of the enfolded fellowship. The CAST and ACGME requirements permit enfolded fellowship training to begin in the fourth postgraduate year, whereas UCNS stipulates that neurosurgery residents are eligible to begin fellowship only after the completion of 4 years of accredited training. It is also important to note that, unlike UCNS, ACGME and CAST do not require neurosurgical fellows to rotate in "off-service" ICUs, such as medical, surgical, or cardiac intensive care units, though general critical care topics are listed among the core medical knowledge competencies. CAST programs are unique in the requirement for pediatric NCC exposure, which is optional under the other 2 accrediting bodies. Finally, the ACGME program requirements include a description of various medical knowledge and patient care skills that fellows are expected to acquire, which is substantially consistent with the UCNS and CAST curricula. However, the requirements are fairly general for specific procedural skills and do little to ameliorate the concern for training variability expressed by Marcolini et al. and Dhar et al.[15,16] Some of these questions may be addressed by the ACGME Neurocritical Care Milestones and the accompanying supplemental guide, which are currently in development.

FUTURE DIRECTIONS

ABMS recognition, and development of an ACGME process for accrediting training programs, no doubt represent a significant milestone for the NCC community. However, it remains to be seen how many current NCC training programs will choose to apply for ACGME accreditation. UCNS has indicated that it will continue to offer both accreditation and certification for NCC in the foreseeable future, and the ABNS continues to offer the RFP credential to qualifying neurologic surgeons. It is, therefore, likely that the 3 certification mechanisms will continue to coexist and may promote increased heterogeneity among programs in the short term rather than decreasing it.

Efforts on the part of professional societies to ensure the quality of training in NCC dovetail with efforts in the mainstream critical care community to develop a core critical care curriculum conserved across subspecialties. A version of this has been realized in Europe through the work of the Competency-Based Training in Intensive Care in Europe (CoBaTrICE) Collaboration, an international collaboration of critical care stakeholders convened by the European Society of Intensive Care Medicine (ESICM) in 2003 to establish a common set of critical care competencies.[20] The ESICM initiative was motivated by the need to ensure a consistent minimum level of competency among critical care providers in Europe, and to permit the free movement of professionals throughout the European Union, as required by law. During the initial stages of the project, the collaborators surveyed intensive care educators internationally to characterize various training pathways. Of the 54 programs identified, only 3 at that time were competency based. The investigators characterized critical care training into 4 broad categories:

1. A supra-specialty model, which entails advanced critical care that is accessible from a variety of primary specialties
2. A single subspecialty model, in which critical care training is restricted to physicians from a single primary specialty
3. A multi-specialty model, in which multiple primary specialties offer disparate mechanisms for critical care training

4. A primary specialty model, in which stand-alone critical care programs are available to graduates immediately on the completion of undergraduate medical training.[21]

The multi-specialty model most closely reflects the state of critical care training in the US,[22] though in some respects NCC more closely aligns with the supraspecialty model. The CoBaTrICE Collaboration undertook the development of a consensus set of core competencies essential for intensivists, which would apply to these various training models internationally.[23] In the US, professional societies have been contemplating a similar endeavor. In 2015, the SCCM convened the Critical Care as a Specialty Task Force, with the goal of drafting recommendations for critical care training programs in the future. Unlike the ESCIM project, the SCCM initiative was motivated by an interest in streamlining critical care training, to ensure a competent critical care workforce sufficient to keep pace with the needs of an aging population.[24] The Task Force concluded that the silo-ing of intensivists in the US system was exacerbating the workforce shortage, by limiting intensivists to practice within ICUs dedicated to caring for patients within a particular base specialty, and that the duration of training under the current model may deter interested residents from seeking critical care certification. Proposed solutions included the development of a common certification examination; the creation of a unified pathway for the training of critical care fellows; and/or promoting the growth of intensive care medicine as a primary specialty. The task force recommended incremental changes in the current training paradigm, beginning with the development of multidisciplinary training curricula, and the consideration of a common certification examination. Efforts are currently underway to develop a proposed set of core competencies applicable to all intensivists, regardless of their primary specialty.

SUMMARY

The recent recognition of the NCC subspecialty by ABMS and ACGME represents an opportunity to further integrate NCC training into the broader critical care community. As noted by Marcolini et al.,[15] considerable overlap exists between the curricula in NCC programs and those in place within other intensive care disciplines. Uniting all US critical care specialties under the auspices of ABMS/ACGME offers the opportunity to promote harmonization between the various intensivist programs while affording the flexibility to enable the development of subspecialty expertise. The NCC community should work to harmonize training and certification requirements between the CAST/ABNS, UCNS, and ACGME/ABMS credentialing mechanisms, to ensure a high standard for training and certification within NCC. The continued evolution of NCC training and certification should take place in the context of broader trends toward common curricular elements in intensive care medicine as a whole.

CLINICS CARE POINTS

- Neurocritical care is an evolving, multidisciplinary subspecialty with multiple potential training pathways and routes to certification.
- Although significant overlap exists between the different neurocritical care training pathways, some significant differences persist.
- Continued collaboration between neurointesivists, relevant professional societies, and accrediting agencies will be necessary to ensure consistent program quality.

DISCLOSURE

Drs A.H. Shapshak and L. Shutter have no financial conflicts of interest to disclose.

REFERENCES

1. Kelly FE, Fong K, Hirsch N, et al. Intensive care medicine is 60 years old: the history and future of the intensive care unit. clin Med (Lond) 2014;14(4):376–9.
2. Wijdicks EF. The history of neurocritical care. Handbook Clin Neurol 2017; 140:3–14.
3. Posner JB. Fred Plum, MD (1924-2010). Arch Neurol 2010;67(11):1409–10.
4. Plum F, Posner JB. The diagnosis of stupor and coma. Contemp Neurol Ser 1972; 10:1–286.
5. Bleck TP. Historical aspects of critical care and the nervous system. Crit Care Clin 2009;25(1):153–64, ix.
6. Rabelo NN, da Silva Brito J, da Silva JS, et al. The historic evolution of intracranial pressure and cerebrospinal fluid pulse pressure concepts: two centuries of challenges. Surg Neurol Int 2021;12:274.
7. Mayer SA, Coplin WM, Chang C, et al. Program requirements for fellowship training in neurological intensive care: United Council for Neurologic Subspecialties guidelines. Neurocrit Care 2006;5(2):166–71.
8. Mayer SA, Coplin WM, Chang C, et al. Core curriculum and competencies for advanced training in neurological intensive care: United Council for Neurologic Subspecialties guidelines. Neurocrit Care 2006;5(2):159–65.
9. Chang CWJ. Focused subspecialty critical care training is Superior for trainees and patients. Crit Care Med 2019;47(11):1645–7.
10. The united Council of neurologic subspecialties subspecialty program requirements for neurocritical care. United Council of neurologic subspecialties. 2022. Available at: https://www.ucns.org/common/Uploaded%20files/Accreditation/Program%20Requirements/NCC%20Program%20Requirements%20APPROVED%2020210721.pdf. Accessed January 14, 2022.
11. United Council for neurologic subspecialties Diplomate directory. The united Council of neurologic subspecialties. 2022. Available at: https://www.ucns.org/Online/Diplomate_Directory/Online/Diplomate_Directory.aspx?hkey=f8f00552-f924-4ef6-a9bb-6023b1cd341b. Accessed January 14, 2022.
12. Committee on Advanced Subspecialty Training: History. Society of Neurological Surgeons, 2022. Accessed January 14, 2022. https://sns-cast.org/cast-history/.
13. CAST program requirements for fellowship education in neurocritical care. Society of neurological surgeons. 2022. Available at: https://sns-cast.org/wp-content/uploads/2021/02/CASTrequirementsNCC2021.pdf. Accessed January 14, 2022.
14. ABNS RFP in neurocritical care. American board of neurological surgeons. Available at: https://abns.org/rfp-neurocritical-care/. Accessed January 18, 2022.
15. Marcolini EG, Seder DB, Bonomo JB, et al. The present state of neurointensivist training in the United States: a Comparison to other critical care training programs. Crit Care Med 2018;46(2):307–15.
16. Dhar R, Rajajee V, Finley Caulfield A, et al. The state of neurocritical care fellowship training and attitudes toward accreditation and certification: a survey of neurocritical care fellowship program directors. Front Neurol 2017;8:548. https://doi.org/10.3389/fneur.2017.00548.
17. ACGME program requirements for graduate medical education in neurocritical care. 2021. https://www.acgme.org/globalassets/pfassets/programrequirements/550_neurocriticalcare_2021-09-26.pdf. Accessed January 20, 2022.

18. Neurocritical care policies. American board of internal medicine. Available at: https://www.abim.org/certification/policies/internal-medicine-subspecialty-policies/neurocritical-care/. Accessed January 21, 2022.

19. Subspecialty certification in neurocritical care. American board of surgery. Available at: https://www.absurgery.org/default.jsp?certscc_ncc. Accessed January 22, 2022.

20. CoBaTrICE: competency based training in intensive care medicine in Europe. European society for intensive care medicine. Available at: http://www.cobatrice.org/data/ModuleGestionDeContenu/PagesGenerees/en/07-divers/52.asp. Accessed January 22, 2022.

21. Barrett H, Bion JF. An international survey of training in adult intensive care medicine. Intensive Care Med 2005;31(4):553–61.

22. Napolitano LM, Rajajee V, Gunnerson KJ, et al. Physician training in critical care in the United States: Update 2018. J Trauma Acute Care Surg 2018;84(6):963–71.

23. CoBaTr ICEC, Bion JF, Barrett H. Development of core competencies for an international training programme in intensive care medicine. Intensive Care Med 2006;32(9):1371–83.

24. Tisherman SA, Spevetz A, Blosser SA, et al. A case for change in adult critical care training for physicians in the United States: a white Paper developed by the critical care as a specialty task force of the society of critical care medicine. Crit Care Med 2018;46(10):1577–84.

25. ACGME Program Requirements for Graduate Medical Education in Neurology. ACGME Specialties: Neurology 2021. Available at: https://www.acgme.org/globalassets/pfassets/programrequirements/180_neurology_2021.pdf. Accessed January 18, 2022.

26. ACGME Program Requirements for Graduate Medical Education in Neurological Surgery. In: ACGME Subspecialties: Neurosurgery. ACGME Specialties: Neurological Surgery 2020. Available at: https://www.acgme.org/globalassets/pfassets/programrequirements/160_neurologicalsurgery_2021.pdf. Accessed January 18, 2022.

27. ACGME Program Requirements for Graduate Medical Education in Emergency Medicine. In: ACGME Specialties: Emergency Medicine. 2021. Available at: https://www.acgme.org/globalassets/pfassets/programrequirements/110_emergencymedicine_2021.pdf. Accessed January 18, 2022.

28. ACGME Program Requirements for Graduate Medical Education in Internal Medicine. In: ACGME Specialties: Internal Medicine. 2021. Available at: https://www.acgme.org/globalassets/pfassets/programrequirements/140_internalmedicine_2021.pdf. Accessed January 18, 2022.

29. ACGME Program Requirements for Graduate Medical Education in Anesthesiology. In: ACGME Specialties: Anesthesiology. 2021. Available at: https://www.acgme.org/globalassets/pfassets/programrequirements/040_anesthesiology_2021.pdf. Accessed January 18, 2022.

30. ACGME Program Requirements for Graduate Medical Education in General Surgery. In: ACGME Specialties: Surgery. 2021. Available at: https://www.acgme.org/globalassets/pfassets/programrequirements/440_generalsurgery_2021.pdf. Accessed January 18, 2022.

31. ACGME Program Requirements for Graduate Medical Education in Pediatric Critical Care Medicine. In: ACGME Specialties: Pediatrics. 2021. Available at: https://www.acgme.org/globalassets/pfassets/programrequirements/323_pediatriccriticalcaremedicine_2021v2.pdf. Accessed January 18, 2022.

32. ACGME Program Requirements for Graduate Medical Education in Child Neurology. In: ACGME Specialties: Neurology. 2021. Available at: https://www.acgme.org/globalassets/pfassets/programrequirements/185_childneurology_2021.pdf. Accessed January 18, 2022.

33. The United Council of Neurologic Subspecialties Subspecialty Program Requirements for Neurocritical Care. In: United Council of Neurologic Subspecialties: Accreditation. 2021. Available at: https://www.ucns.org/common/Uploaded%20files/Accreditation/Program%20Requirements/NCC%20Program%20Requirements%20APPROVED%2020210721.pdf. Accessed January 14, 2022.

34. CAST Program Requirements for Fellowship Education in Neurocritical Care. In: Society of Neurological Surgeons: Committee on Advanced Subspecialty Training. 2021. Available at: https://sns-cast.org/wp-content/uploads/2021/02/CASTrequirementsNCC2021.pdf. Accessed January 14, 2022.

35. ACGME Program Requirements for Graduate Medical Education in Neurocritical Care. In: ACGME Specialties: Neurology. 2021. Available at: https://www.acgme.org/globalassets/pfassets/programrequirements/550_neurocriticalcare_2021-09-26.pdf. Accessed January 19, 2022.

Neurocritical Care Research
Collaborations for Curing Coma

Jose Javier Provencio, MD

KEYWORDS

• Research gaps • Curing coma • Disorders of consciousness • Collaborations

KEY POINTS

- Research in the field of Neurocritical Care is contributing to advances in the medical care of critically ill patients with neurological conditions.
- Neurocritical care research must be collaborative and multidisciplinary to address the spectrum of clinical needs.
- The Curing Coma Campaign is an international effort to identify and address research gaps in Neurocritical Care.

Family members of brain-injured patients in the intensive care unit (ICU) share a more complicated analysis than other families in the ICU. In *non-neurological injuries and illnesses*, families contend with the possibility of their loved ones not surviving the illness/injury. Families of brain-injured patients have similar worries but also must contend with the question "will my loved one wake up?". Much of our self-identity as humans depends on the ability to interact with the outside world and coordinate information we take in from the outside world. As such, the question of whether consciousness will be restored after an injury is important in the assessment of the acceptability of "quality of life." Despite the centrality of this issue in decisions families and medical care teams make, we struggle to identify patients who may have a better outcome or to impact patients with impaired consciousness through treatment.

This review will attempt to understand the current state of science in the field of coma and disorders of consciousness. Research in consciousness and consciousness recovery is not new, there has been extensive work conducted by consciousness researchers from the brain mapping world as well as coma recovery research conducted in the setting of rehabilitation. The novel aspect of the current research is that this effort focuses on addressing issues of coma and consciousness in the setting of the intensive care unit and acute critical illness. Until now, much of the work in the ICU setting has focused on the prognosis of recovery in the setting of hypoxic brain injury. In the conclusion,

Department of Neurology, University of Virginia, PO Box 800394, Charlottesville, VA 22908, USA
E-mail address: Jp3b@virginia.edu

Crit Care Clin 39 (2023) 47–54
https://doi.org/10.1016/j.ccc.2022.08.001
0749-0704/23/

this work will also summarize the development of the Curing Coma Campaign that outlines gaps in the research.

WHAT ARE COMA AND DISORDERS OF CONSCIOUSNESS?

Part of the challenge of studying disorders of consciousness (DoC), of which coma is the most severe form, is the challenge of determining if a patient who does not respond is conscious or not. This presents both a definitional problem and a measurement issue. Posner and colleagues[1] proposed that "consciousness is the state of full awareness of the self and one's relationship to the environment." Young (1998) proposed that there are 4 conceptual levels of consciousness: (1) "Crude consciousness (or alertness)"; (2) "Phenomenal consciousness where the brain registers internal or external phenomena"; (3) "Access consciousness" (directed attention and decision making); and (4) "Philosophic" consciousness which he termed as "nondimensional awareness of the harmony of the universe.[2]" Defining consciousness is less important clinically than describing DoC. Sanders and colleagues[3] proposed that DoC can be characterized within the framework of "consciousness, environmental connectedness, and responsiveness (C-EC-R)." This framework has been helpful in characterizing differences between patients in different states of injury.

Traditionally, clinical working definitions of DoC such as coma, persistent vegetative state, and minimally conscious state have been defined by the patient's ability to respond or interact with their environment. Although, as a practical matter, this conforms to the limits of physical examination at the bedside, there is no requirement to outwardly interact with the environment to be conscious. In fact, in so far as interaction with the outside world is partly voluntary, a completely conscious person could in fact choose not to interact with their environment (albeit with a great deal of practice). In patients with impaired output function (motor, speech, autonomic such as crying), consciousness can be extremely challenging to detect. This is magnified in the intensive care setting where recovery of some neurological functions returns slowly and nonlinearly after acute injury.[4]

Outside of clinical evaluation, efforts have focused on neuromonitoring techniques that can detect the processing of information without the need for patient participation. Among the new techniques, 2 broad strategies are evolving.[5] *Confrontational testing* relies on administering a stimulus or prompt while concurrently employing visualization techniques, while *resting-state techniques* employ prolonged monitoring to compare periods of relative increased and decreased activity.[6] Several technologies show promise: magnetic resonance imaging, both functional (fMRI) and diffusion tensor (DTI MRI), continuous electroencephalography (cEEG), specialized positron emission spectroscopy (PET) and transcranial magnetic stimulation (TMS). These techniques require a great deal of postprocessing that limits real-time assessment.

In addition to neuromonitoring, there have been efforts to correlate protein biomarkers and recovery from DoC.[4,7] This has been best studied in the setting of DoC from hypoxic-ischemic injury after cardiac arrest. Although there are several biomarkers that predict the return of consciousness, these markers are less helpful in understanding the mechanism of abnormal consciousness and therefore are limited. Elevated levels of neuron-specific enolase have been shown to predict prolonged coma and DoC after cardiac arrest.[8,9]

THE CURRENT CONCEPTIONS OF DISORDERS OF CONSCIOUSNESS

The most elusive aspect of DoC has been to define what parts of the brain hold consciousness and, more importantly, what parts of the brain in a patient with brain injury and DoC are required to improve to regain consciousness. Several theories (not all mutually exclusively) are painting a picture of how consciousness is held and how it can be recovered. This review will focus on the ICU implications with an understanding that this work has grown from the robust work in subacute and chronic injury.

The best-known brain injury that leads to loss of consciousness is damage to the ascending reticular activating system of the brainstem (ARAS). The structures of the ARAS were first identified in the 19th century but their function in wakefulness was elucidated in the 1940s and 1950s when the interruption of the brainstem was found to lead to coma that could be experimentally overridden by electrical stimulation of the rostral midline brainstem structures. Anatomical studies have shown that the ARAS is diffusely distributed through the medulla, pons, and midbrain and sends projections through the intralaminar nucleus of the thalamus to cortical structures of all the cerebral lobes. It is easiest to conceptualize the ARAS as a battery that leads to the alertness of all parts of the brain. In fact, the ARAS sends rhythmic pulses to the cortex that can be discerned using cEEG. How this system interacts with its cortical outputs is still poorly understood.

After the brainstem, current theories of consciousness and by default DoC have to do with how subcortical and cortical portions of the brain work. This concept of connectivity between specific brain regions has led to several theories about how the cerebrum, following ARAS activation, integrates information to lead to a conscious person. Work is ongoing but several prominent theories merit discussion.

Focal lesioning experiments in animals help describe a system called the *mesocircuit* that implicates information flow from the basal ganglia to the thalamus and then to the cortex in consciousness.[10] There have been several refinements to this theory that have included direct pathways from the basal ganglia to the cortex. Although this theory has benefits, particularly well-defined structures that serve as treatable targets in DoC, the mesocircuit does not predict all of consciousness. This is likely due to the limitations of individual lesioning experiments to describe an extremely complex system.

Newer theories are based on imaging and mathematical modeling. A widely used approach is to combine structural connectivity, which looks for areas of disrupted brain tracts by diffusion tensor imaging, with functional connectivity, which uses cEEG and fMRI. This has led to interesting findings in patients with DoC. This technique has led to the discovery of interconnected "nodes" of cortex that affect consciousness. This concept of the "connectome" of consciousness has become central to our understanding of how structure affects function. Importantly, impairment of an already-described resting connectivity network in the brain known as the default mode network (DMN) has been found by fMRI to correlate with consciousness in patients with comatose [11] More importantly, in a small study of acutely ill patients with comatose, the DMN was preserved in all patients who later regained any level of consciousness.[12]

Other consciousness theories have also been implicated in DoC but with less rigorous study.[13] For example, integrated information theory (ITT) presumes that spatial and time domains play a role in how information is integrated.[14] Conversely, the global neuronal workspace model of consciousness suggests that different processes in the brain compete for access to a global workspace analogous to articles on your desk competing for space in the line of sight.[15] Tests of these theories in patients with comatose have not been published.

Excitingly, how these competing theories of consciousness control interact with each other is now being tested. A recent report on the interaction between the mesocircuit and DMN suggests that damage to the mesocircuit inhibits the DMN further suggesting that there is a hierarchical control of consciousness among the deep brain structures that influence cortical networks.[16,17] It is not hard to the image that the ARAS is a top-level control of consciousness leading to a hierarchy of control from the ARAS to the mesocircuit to the DMN. As a more cohesive picture of the functional organization of consciousness circuits is understood, implications for DoC may lead to interventions.

The Curing Coma Campaign

The Curing Coma Campaign (CCC) is an initiative started by the Neurocritical Care Society (NCS) to "(1) focus the science of acute DoC on identifying and testing therapeutic interventions and (2) form an enduring community of medical providers, scientists, and advocates to test and implement these advances.[18]" Although there was already a significant body of research around consciousness and DoC, this initiative is focused on the acute phase of illness, whereas much of the current work in the field is focused on consciousness absent injury, chronic injury, or anesthetized patients as a model of unconsciousness. Although the initiative was started under the auspices of NCS, it quickly grew to include scientists in the fields of consciousness, rehabilitation, and traumatic brain injury.

The 3 main accomplishments of the CCC so far have been to: (1) develop a community of researchers to investigate gaps in our knowledge of coma and DoC (particularly in the early injury stage), (2) develop an infrastructure upon which research studies can be conducted in a streamlined fashion, and (3) develop the awareness of coma as a global entity. A fourth goal is to help researchers develop studies to both understand and treat patients with DoC.

The gap analysis has been derived from several white articles investigating the gaps from different perspectives.[4,13,18,19] In addition, there have been 2 National Institutes of Health (NIH) symposia jointly sponsored by the National Institute of Neurological Disorders and Stroke (NINDS) and the CCC where gaps in knowledge that are amenable to funding priorities for the NIH were discussed.[20,21] Finally, the CCC did an evaluation of the ethical parameters that should guide investigation of gaps and testing of treatments.[22]

As part of developing infrastructure, the CCC worked with investigators to develop baseline data about medical practice around patients in the ICU with DoC[23] and patient and family perspectives of coma (article in preparation). In addition, the CCC has developed a community of investigators from the fields of neurocritical care, neurology, neurosurgery, rehabilitation medicine, translational and basic science that scientists can call on to be site leaders in multicenter trials. There is an active plan to develop a database that can be used by all investigators associated with the CCC which can be interrogated for patterns based on common data elements.

GAPS IN OUR KNOWLEDGE THAT ARE AMENABLE TO FURTHER RESEARCH

The most important function the CCC has conducted so far is to thoughtfully outline gaps in our current knowledge that can be studied. Importantly, the group has published several publications identifying challenges around which investigators from all fields can start to generate testable hypotheses (**Table 1**).[4,13,20,21,24] It is useful to outline the types of gaps in our knowledge of acute injury DoC.

The gaps can be grouped into 4 different categories: (1) infrastructure and technical challenges that must be advanced to address coma issues, (2) a better understanding of the similarities and differences between patients with DoC, (3) mechanistic understanding of consciousness and how it is affected by brain injury, and (4) understanding

Table 1	
Examples of knowledge gaps in critical illness DoC research	
Category	**Knowledge Gap**
Infrastructure and technical challenges	1. Combining both hypothesis-driven and data-driven approaches to understanding of DoC. 2. Develop a shared database with common elements that all studies can populate.
A better understanding of the similarities and differences between patients with DoC.	1. A framework for differentiating clinical subtypes of DoC 2. Develop prognostic indicators for patients with various mechanisms of DoC 3. Establish global incidence, prevalence, and etiology of coma, the natural history of disease progression, and impact of current practices on acute post/acute outcomes and resource allocation 4. Develop proxy biomarkers that allow for trials with small patient numbers to inform larger trials on the timing of treatment and promising strategies 5. Correctly characterize patients in terms of the 3 dimensions described in the C-EC-R framework.
Mechanistic understanding of consciousness and how it is affected by the brain	1. A comprehensive understanding of the structural–functional relationship of the brain on a macroscale and microenvironment 2. Identify the most relevant anatomic and biochemical pathways should be identified that indicate the ability to emerge from coma and improve cognition. 3. Precisely map the consciousness centers as they pertain to acute brain injuries. This can be achieved by overlaying the structural correlates of DOC with the healthy human connectome (both structural and functional) to derive likely locations for a diaschisis effect (defining changes that affect consciousness in brain injury).
Understanding the variability of care of patients with DoC and how this affects patient outcome.	1. To standardize coma assessment battery throughout the continuum of care to provide a consistent approach to clinical examination, indicators for advanced imaging, and better accuracy 2. Establish new best practices, reinforce existing practices, and eliminate ineffective practices and timing for assessment, monitoring, treatment, and care transitions. 3. Assess current variabilities in care and trial resources across collaborating sites.

Data from Refs.[4,13,21]

the variability of care of patients with DoC and how this affects patient outcome. Each group will be addressed in turn.

Infrastructure and technical challenges: Both Provencio, and colleagues and Mainali and colleagues suggested the need to establish a comprehensive database that can house both common data elements and more complicated data such as processed functional imaging and EEG.[4,21] Mainali and colleagues[21] also suggested a "tier-based network" that would allow large, complicated studies and smaller limited studies to be accomplished in parallel with institutions participating at the appropriate level considering access to technology and expertise. Luppi and colleagues[13] suggested developing a whole-brain computational model of consciousness incorporating both structural and functional imaging for initial hypothesis testing that could later be tested in human subjects with DoC. All the authors suggested developing a community of researchers, families, and medical providers to work toward understanding the breadth of impact of DoC.[4,13,20,21]

A better understanding of the similarities and differences between patients with DoC. All authors agreed that a better understanding of the different "endotypes" of DoC is critical to better understand the disease. Impaired consciousness is a consequence of several types of injuries, it is critical to understand how much of the mechanism, prognosis, and recovery is specific to the disease and how much is common among all patients with DoC. Luppi and colleagues suggested conceptualizing coma, DoC, and recovery in a construct proposed by Sanders, and colleagues.[3,13] This construct groups patients along different stages of disease progression based on the characteristics of consciousness, environmental connectedness, and responsiveness (C-EC-R). They proposed that the common language of this construct can bridge the divide between different investigator definitions, and allow for easy quantification of recovery.

Mechanistic understanding of consciousness and how it is affected by the brain. It is clear that to understand DoC, it is imperative to understand how consciousness is regulated in the brain. Much work in this area is already underway by a community of researchers who study the brain mechanisms behind consciousness. Much of our understanding has been informed by studying patients with impaired consciousness but much has also been learned by studying consciousness in animal and human models of anesthesia. Mainali and colleagues[21] suggest that "A comprehensive understanding of the structural–functional relationship requires understanding the brain on a macroscale and a deep dive into the microenvironment consisting of genetic, cellular, molecular, microcircuits, and neurotransmitter substrates."

Understanding the variability of care of patients with DoC and how this affects patient outcome. It is clear that there exists a great deal of variability in the care of patients with DoC. A recent survey of practitioners of critical care medicine throughout the world (the COME TOGETHER) survey showed that "There is wide heterogeneity among health care professionals regarding the clinical definition of coma and limited routine use of advanced coma assessment techniques in the acute care setting.[23]" This baseline variability has the potential to hide meaningful differences in outcome between interventions simply by muddying the statistical analysis. A better understanding of the types of variability and how to standardize care will make the investigation more meaningful.

These "gap analyses" should generate testable questions that researchers can use to develop studies. The goal of the Curing Coma Campaign is to invigorate research at all levels. It is unlikely that a single interventional study is going to "solve" the DoC problem in critical care units around the world. Instead, it is most likely that complex trials to better differences in cerebral metabolism in patients with DoC will need to occur alongside smaller studies of bedside interventions to decrease delirium in the ICU and animal experiments to understand the critical networks of neurons that allow consciousness. It is the hope of the group that this research effort will be diffuse and fast-moving but integrated so that each study serves as a small section of the DoC tapestry and will together form the whole picture.

In conclusion, our understanding of coma and DoC in the intensive care unit patient builds on research traditions from both the brain mapping and rehabilitation recovery communities. Our understanding of both consciousness and DoC has improved due to improved technology. The Curing Coma Campaign aims to harness the energy of the previous work and expand the scope to address DoC in the intensive care unit early after the injury. The group has identified important gaps in our knowledge highlighting great opportunities for research in the field.

REFERENCES

1. Posner JB, Saper CB, Schiff ND, et al. Plum and Posner's diagnosis and treatment of stupor and coma. Fifth edition. Oxford ; New York: Oxford University Press; 2019.
2. Young GB, Ropper AH, Bolton CF. Coma and impaired consciousness : a clinical perspective. New York: McGraw-Hill, Health Professions Division; 1998.
3. Sanders RD, Tononi G, Laureys S, et al. Unresponsiveness not equal unconsciousness. Anesthesiology 2012;116(4):946–59.
4. Provencio JJ, Hemphill JC, Claassen J, et al. The curing coma campaign: framing initial scientific challenges-proceedings of the first curing coma campaign scientific advisory council meeting. Neurocrit Care 2020;33(1):1–12.
5. Giacino JT, Fins JJ, Laureys S, et al. Disorders of consciousness after acquired brain injury: the state of the science. Nat Rev Neurol 2014;10(2):99–114.
6. Kondziella D, Bender A, Diserens K, et al. European Academy of Neurology guideline on the diagnosis of coma and other disorders of consciousness. Eur J Neurol 2020;27(5):741–56.
7. Giacino JT. The vegetative and minimally conscious states: consensus-based criteria for establishing diagnosis and prognosis. NeuroRehabilitation 2004; 19(4):293–8.
8. Dauberschmidt R, Zinsmeyer J, Mrochen H, et al. Changes of neuron-specific enolase concentration in plasma after cardiac arrest and resuscitation. Mol Chem Neuropathol 1991;14(3):237–45.
9. Bangshoj J, Liebetrau B, Wiberg S, et al. The value of the biomarkers neuron-specific enolase and S100 calcium-binding protein for prediction of mortality in children resuscitated after cardiac arrest, Pediatr Cardiol, 2022: 1-7 (epub ahead of print).
10. Schiff ND. Recovery of consciousness after brain injury: a mesocircuit hypothesis. Trends Neurosci 2010;33(1):1–9.
11. Norton L, Hutchison RM, Young GB, et al. Disruptions of functional connectivity in the default mode network of comatose patients. Neurology 2012;78(3):175–81.
12. Kondziella D, Fisher PM, Larsen VA, et al. Functional MRI for assessment of the default mode network in acute brain injury. Neurocrit Care 2017;27(3):401–6.
13. Luppi AI, Cain J, Spindler LRB, et al. Mechanisms underlying disorders of consciousness: bridging gaps to move toward an integrated translational science. Neurocrit Care 2021;35(Suppl 1):37–54.
14. Oizumi M, Albantakis L, Tononi G. From the phenomenology to the mechanisms of consciousness: integrated information theory 3.0. PLoS Comput Biol 2014; 10(5):e1003588.

15. Mashour GA, Roelfsema P, Changeux JP, et al. Conscious processing and the global neuronal workspace hypothesis. Neuron 2020;105(5):776–98.
16. Lant ND, Gonzalez-Lara LE, Owen AM, et al. Relationship between the anterior forebrain mesocircuit and the default mode network in the structural bases of disorders of consciousness. Neuroimage Clin 2016;10:27–35.
17. Coulborn S, Taylor C, Naci L, et al. Disruptions in effective connectivity within and between default mode network and anterior forebrain mesocircuit in prolonged disorders of consciousness. Brain Sci 2021; 11(6): 749.
18. Olson DM, Hemphill JC 3rd, Curing Coma C, et al. The curing coma campaign: challenging the paradigm for disorders of consciousness. Neurocrit Care 2021; 35(Suppl 1):1–3.
19. Kondziella D, Menon DK, Helbok R, et al. A Precision medicine framework for classifying patients with disorders of consciousness: advanced classification of consciousness endotypes (ACCESS). Neurocrit Care 2021;35(Suppl 1):27–36.
20. Claassen J, Akbari Y, Alexander S, et al. Proceedings of the first curing coma campaign NIH symposium: challenging the future of research for coma and disorders of consciousness. Neurocrit Care 2021;35(Suppl 1):4–23.
21. Mainali S, Aiyagari V, Alexander S, et al. Proceedings of the second curing coma campaign nih symposium: challenging the future of research for coma and disorders of consciousness. Neurocrit Care 2022;37(1):326-350.
22. Lewis A, Claassen J, Illes J, et al. Ethics priorities of the curing coma campaign: an empirical survey. Neurocrit Care 2022;37(1):12-2123.
23. Helbok R, Rass V, Beghi E, et al. The curing coma campaign international survey on coma epidemiology, evaluation, and therapy (COME TOGETHER). Neurocrit Care 2022;37, pages 47-59. (2022)
24. Hammond FM, Katta-Charles S, Russell MB, et al. Research needs for prognostic modeling and trajectory analysis in patients with disorders of consciousness. Neurocrit Care 2021;35(Suppl 1):55–67.

Neurocritical Care Aspects of Ischemic Stroke Management

Dania Qaryouti, MD, Diana Greene-Chandos, MD, FNCS*

KEYWORDS

- Stroke • Fibrinolysis • Neurointensive care • Cerebral thrombectomy
- Cerebral edema • Decompressive hemicraniectomy • Poststroke hemorrhage
- Carotid endarterectomy

KEY POINTS

- Care of ischemic stroke in the intensive care unit (ICU) begins with postfibrinolytic and/or thrombectomy care, through the management of cerebral edema and hemorrhagic conversion, and finally to prolonged ICU issues such as common infections and immobility complications.
- Acute management of blood pressure (BP) is critical with goals individualized for each type of stroke treatment and revascularization score.
- Familiarity with postcraniotomy complications is important in caring for patients following surgical treatment of malignant cerebral edema in both the anterior and posterior fossa.
- Key differences in the management of embolic strokes caused by infective endocarditis include urgent initiation of antibiotics, avoiding anticoagulation, and evaluation of possible associated mycotic aneurysms.
- Following carotid endarterectomy (CEA) intensivists must anticipate and monitor for the life-threatening complications of expanding wound hematoma, hemodynamic instability, and hyperperfusion injury with hemorrhage and seizures.

INTRODUCTION

Numerous factors contribute to outcomes after acute ischemic stroke (AIS). Neurointensive care (Neuro ICU) management of patients with AIS calls for an individualized approach considering factors such as the size and location of infarct, presenting blood pressure (BP), and National Institute of Health Stroke Scale (NIHSS). The main goals of admission to specialized intensive care units (ICU) for patients with stroke are divided into supportive care and management and prevention of specific complications.

Department of Neurology, University of New Mexico, MSC10 5620, 1 University of New Mexico, Albuquerque, NM 87131, USA
* Corresponding author.
E-mail address: DGreenechandos@salud.unm.edu
Twitter: @DianaGCMD (D.G.-C.)

Crit Care Clin 39 (2023) 55–70
https://doi.org/10.1016/j.ccc.2022.07.005
0749-0704/23/© 2022 Elsevier Inc. All rights reserved.
criticalcare.theclinics.com

Supportive care includes airway watch, ventilatory support, and close BP monitoring. Management of specific complications addresses cerebral edema and hemorrhagic transformation, timely recognition of indications for, and postoperative management of decompressive hemicraniectomy (DHC) and carotid endarterectomy (CEA), and prevention of postthrombectomy reocclusion, stroke expansion, and recurrence.[1,2] Additional circumstances such as the management of endocarditis-related strokes, common infectious, and cardiac complications of critically ill stroke patient are presented. All aspects discussed require intensive bedside neuromonitoring in a Neuro ICU to optimize stroke outcomes. NIHSS-trained staff is key for proper clinical monitoring and is thus a Joint Commission Association of Hospital Organization (JCAHO) requirement for primary and comprehensive stroke center certifications.

GENERAL SUPPORTIVE CARE
Respiratory Support

Intubation
Stroke volume and location play a critical role in determining the need for respiratory support. Large hemispheric infarctions (LHI) can cause impairments in the level of consciousness (LOC), respiratory drive, and protective and swallowing reflexes, thus leading to respiratory failure. Per The Neurocritical Care Society guidelines for Large Hemispheric Stroke, intubation is strongly recommended.[3]

With respect to location, brainstem and thalamic strokes affect both LOC and respiratory centers. Erratic respiratory patterns causing ventilatory issues lead to acid/base imbalance. Furthermore, strokes that impair swallowing functions, have a high risk of aspiration and associated complications. Large cerebellar strokes with cytotoxic edema can cause direct brainstem compression resulting in secondary microischemia and dysfunction, or effacement of the fourth ventricle, resulting in obstructive hydrocephalus. Cortical strokes, particularly those with hemorrhagic conversion, can cause status epilepticus with resultant loss of airway protection.[4]

One prospective study in AIS identified GCS less than 10 or respiratory failure, history of hypertension (HTN), and infarct size more than 2/3rd of the MCA territory or LHI as independent risk factors for intubation and mechanical ventilation.[4] Other risk factors frequently considered include[3]:

- Loss of airway protective reflexes
- Signs and symptoms of increased intracranial pressure (ICP)
- Midline shift
- Pulmonary edema or pneumonia
- Imminent need for surgical management

This subset of patients with stroke is at high risk of aspiration and subsequent acute hypoxic or hypercarbic respiratory failure, thus warranting monitoring in a Neuro ICU.

Extubation
Delays in extubation after successful ventilator weaning are associated with higher rates of pneumonia, increased need for tracheostomy, longer ICU length of stay, and increased mortality.[5] However, extubation failure (EF) and subsequent need for emergent reintubation are associated with similar sequelae.

The following general extubation criteria should be considered before the extubation of patients with stroke with adequate airway protection[6]:

- Glasgow Coma Scale greater than 8
- No signs/symptoms of elevated ICP

- Body temperature 36°C to 38.5°C
- Heart rate 60 to 120 bpm
- Systolic blood pressure (SBP) 90 to 185 mm Hg

Additionally, the following respiratory parameters should be considered for the same subpopulation[6]:

- Spontaneous respiratory minute volume ($\leq$12 L)
- Positive end-expiratory pressure ($\leq$5 mm Hg)
- Pao_2/Fio_2 (>200)
- Rapid shallow breathing index (<105).

Specific criteria for extubation in LHI have been identified[3]:

- Successful spontaneous breathing trials
- Absence of oropharyngeal saliva collections
- Suctioning required less than every 4 hours
- Presence of cough reflex and tube intolerance (ie, if the patient is comfortably tolerating the endotracheal tube off sedation and analgesia, this should give pause for extubation).
- Free of analgesia and sedation

Ultimately, tracheostomy should be considered if there has been one failure of extubation that was not due to an immediately reversible cause (ie, fluid overload, inadequate time off sedation) and if extubation has not been possible in 7 days after intubation. Placing a tracheostomy should be completed by the fourteenth day of intubation, given the increased risk of injury to the posterior oropharynx, vocal cords, and trachea.[6]

Blood Pressure Goals and Monitoring

Stroke etiology and modality of treatment are key factors in setting BP goals. Commonly encountered scenarios are detailed later in discussion and summarized in **Table 1** with antihypertensive options summarized in **Table 2**.

Table 1 Blood pressure targets versus type of stroke treatment used	
Stroke Treatment	**Blood Pressure Target**
Acute Ischemic Stroke, not eligible for tpA	Permissive hypertension (SBP up to 220, DBP up to 120) for first 24–48 h
Acute Ischemic Stroke, tpA eligible before tpA administration	SBP <180 mm Hg and DBP< 105 mm Hg
Acute Ischemic Stroke, tpA eligible post tpA administration	SBP < 185 mm Hg and DBP <110 mm Hg for 24 h
Acute Ischemic Stroke, Postthrombectomy TICI 2a or <	SBP 120–180
Acute Ischemic Stroke, Postthombectomy TICI 2b-3	SBP 120–160

Please note TICI stands for thrombolysis in cerebral infarction score.
Data from Powers WJ, Rabinstein AA, Ackerson T, Adeoye OM, Bambakidis NC, Becker K, et al. 2018 Guidelines for the early management of patients with acute ischemic stroke: a guideline for healthcare professionals from the American Heart Association/ American Stroke Association. Stroke 2018;49:e46-110; and Matusevicius M, Cooray C, Bottai M, Maza M, Tsivgoulis G, Nunes AP, Moreira T, Ollikainen J, Tassi R, Strbian D, Toni D, Holmin S, Ahmed, N. Blood Pressure After Endovascular Thrombectomy.Stroke 2020; 51(2): 519-525.

Table 2	
Antihypertensives used in acute ischemic stroke to achieve blood pressure goals	
Labetalol	10 mg IV over 1–2 min. Can repeat Q 5–10 min
Nicardipine	5 mg/h IV, titrate up by 2.5 mg/h every 5–15 min, maximum 15 mg/h; when desired BP reached, adjust to maintain proper BP limits
Clevidipine	1–2 mg/h IV, titrate by doubling the dose every 90 s until desired BP reached; recommended maximum 21 mg/h
Enalapril	Starting dose 1.25 mg IV give over 5 min. Repeat every 20 min. Maximum 5 mg
Hydralazine	Starting dose 10 mg to 20 mg IV. May repeat every 15 min for a total of 3 doses

Data from Refs.[10,24,27]

Tissue plasminogen activator/tenecteplase eligible strokes

Blood pressure goals before tissue plasminogen activator (tPA) per the 2013 American Heart Association guidelines are SBP less than 185 mm Hg and diastolic BP (DBP) less than 110 mm Hg. Post-tPA BP should be SBP less than 180 and DBP less than 105. Guidelines for antihypertensive medication use in this acute phase are provided in **Table 2**. [7–12]

Frequent measurement of BP every 10 to 15 minutes for the first 60 minutes following the administration of tPA can establish a trajectory and guide management of BP before transferring to another unit.[7]

Current guideline recommendations for post-tPA monitoring are close monitoring in an ICU or stroke unit for at least 24 hours after the infusion. Parameters to be monitored include BP and neurologic examination every 15 minutes for the first 2 hours, then every 30 minutes for the next 6 hours, and then every hour for the next 16 hours.[13] The importance of BP control should prompt the initiation of a continuous antihypertensive infusion once 2 to 3 intravenous push doses have been administered.[7]

Mechanical thrombectomy eligible strokes

Current AHA/ASA guidelines recommend maintaining BP < 180/105 mm Hg during and for 24 hours after mechanical thrombectomy (MT) (class IIa, *level of evidence B*). If successful reperfusion is achieved, guidelines recommend that BP be maintained at less than 180/105 mm Hg (class IIb, *level of evidence B*).[14,15]

The protocol from the endovascular treatment of small core and anterior circulation proximal occlusion with emphasis on minimizing CT to recanalization times (ESCAPE) trial stated that if reperfusion failed, an SBP ≥ 150 mm Hg may be useful in maintaining adequate collateral flow, and if successful reperfusion was achieved, normal BP was then targeted.[16]

Permissive hypertension in large vessel occlusions not eligible for tissue plasminogen activator or mechanical thrombectomy

Patients may be ineligible for MT (outside of a clinical trial) despite large vessel occlusion for the following reasons: presentation beyond the 24-h time window, Alberta Stroke Program Early Computed Tomography (ASPECT) score </ = 6, and Computed Tomography Perfusion (CTP) ratio of less than 1.7. For these patients, permissive hypertension up to 220/120 for the initial 24 to 48 hours is targeted as tolerated.[7]

However, controversy exists regarding the possible contribution of such hypertension to cerebral edema and risk of hemorrhagic conversion. Several studies have looked at lowering BP goals poststroke. The recommended goals for lowering BP vary but are consistent in limiting reduction by < 10–15% from baseline.[7]

Per AHA guidelines it is reasonable to lower BP by 15% during the first 24 hours after stroke onset. Lower BP targets are often initiated if there is evidence of end-organ damage or exacerbating of comorbid conditions.[7]

Blood pressure augmentation/induced hypertension in acute ischemic strokes
Although BP augmentation is sometimes used in AIS, no large, randomized control studies have assessed the safety and efficacy of this treatment.[7] Koenig *and colleagues* showed the relative safety of induced hypertension therapy when moderate elevation was targeted, but data on clinical outcomes were insufficient.[17]

Hypotension was associated with worse neurologic outcomes in 3 separate studies.[7] The Safety and Efficacy of Therapeutic INduced HYPERTENSION in noncardioembolic AIS (SETIN-HYPERTENSION) trial is a multicenter, randomized, open-label, prospective, phase-III trial that aims to determine safety and efficacy of induced hypertension (IH) using phenylephrine in patients with noncardioembolic AIS. There is potential for this study to further inform the practice of IH for AIS, and subjects are currently being enrolled.[7]

Hemorrhagic transformation of ischemic stroke
The frequency of hemorrhagic transformation (HT) is associated with epidemiologic factors (eg, age, prestroke treatment, and conditions), characteristics of the infarct (core volume and timing of follow-up), reperfusion techniques (intravenous thrombolysis with or without mechanical thrombectomy), radiological diagnosis (CT or MRI techniques), and subsequent use of antithrombotics.[18]

The recent Enhanced Control of Hypertension and Thrombolysis Stroke Study (ENCHANTED) trial has shown that intensive BP control potentially reduces the risk of major intracranial hemorrhage in patients with AIS receiving intravenous thrombolytic therapy.[18]

Health care providers should determine BP targets by weighing the risk of worsening ischemia versus the risk of expansion based on the severity of hemorrhage. Patients with incomplete recanalization may need higher BP targets to maintain sufficient blood flow to the ischemic bed to reduce infarct growth. Conversely, these same patients may need tighter BP control to avoid impending HT.[18]

MANAGEMENT OF SPECIFIC COMPLICATIONS
Management of Cerebral Edema

The development of cerebral edema after an AIS is secondary to cytotoxic cell injury resulting in intracellular water influx. The timeline of cytotoxic cerebral edema development begins a few hours postictus and peaks 2 to 5 days. This "watch period" necessitates close monitoring for a decline in neurologic examination due to secondary brain and brainstem compression.[5,6] Malignant cerebral edema is identified with large hemispheric strokes. The mortality rate of malignant cerebral edema is high (40%–80%) if not thoughtfully managed.[5,6] Recent studies have shown that imaging can be helpful in predicting outcomes. A midline shift of more than 3 mm can be a predictor of poor outcome.[19]

The following are risk factors for malignant edema[3]:

- Younger age
- Presenting NIHSS greater than 20 and greater than 15 for dominant and nondominant hemisphere strokes, respectively
- Early development of encephalopathy

- Systolic BP (SBP) > 180 within 12 hours of stroke onset
- CT scan showing hypodensity in 50% or more of the MCA territory
- Involvement of multiple major vascular territories
- MRI with Diffusion Weighted Imaging (DWI) volume of 82 cm or more if conducted within 6 hours of initial stroke onset

Current therapies include both medical and surgical options.[3]

Hyperosmolar Therapy

Hyperosmolar therapy, that is, mannitol or hypertonic saline (HTS), can lower elevated ICP and reverse herniation by extracting water from intracellular and interstitial spaces. This secondarily increases cerebral perfusion to peri-infarct areas at risk for secondary ischemia from compression.[1,20]

HTS and mannitol carry conditional recommendations with low-quality evidence for the initial management of cerebral edema with or without elevated ICP in AIS. Overall, there is insufficient evidence to recommend either, though both are used when neurologic worsening occurs while awaiting surgical rescue, when surgery is not offered, and in cases of impending herniation.[1,20]

Surprisingly, few clinical studies have assessed mannitol use in AIS, and no randomized clinical trial has evaluated the effect of mannitol on clinical outcomes after LHI with edema. Thus, mannitol is used based on experimental studies, or observations in small nonrandomized case series in humans.[20,21]

Historically, HTS was administered as continuous infusion titrated to serum sodium concentration; however, recent data suggest better outcomes with intermittent boluses. Desired target sodium is determined on individual bases typically ranging between 140 and 155 mEq/L. There is no therapeutic value of serum sodium levels greater than 160 mEq/L and mental status can be further negatively affected beyond this threshold.[20,22]

Temperature Management

Fever with AIS is known to worsen outcomes. Therefore, normothermia is an important goal in ICU stroke care. When cerebral edema is refractory to all measures including advanced cooling devices, hypothermia is sometimes tried. We are still lacking evidence from randomized trials regarding the effect of hypothermia on malignant MCA strokes. Five observational case series showed decreased mortality with hypothermia compared with other methods of ICP management in preliminary analysis. This data remains experimental, and no evidence-based recommendations can be provided.[1,23]

SURGICAL METHODS
Decompressive Craniectomy

Anterior fossa strokes

DHC is an option in LHI for most patients under the age of 60 and some patients under the age of 75.[3] The key to maximizing surgical outcomes is timing the decompression to avoid secondary brain injury. Secondary injury can occur from significant and prolonged mass effect, and before clinical signs of brainstem compression. Trials have shown that patients up to 60 years of age with a large stroke burden greater than 2/3 of brain volume that also presents with a decreased level of consciousness experience better outcomes if decompressed in the first 24 to 48 hours after presentation. Careful identification of those patients is essential.[1] Most recent studies have shown that DHC improves survival and functional outcome, but most survivors live with at least a moderately severe disability. The proportion of survivors with moderately severe to severe disability increases in the elderly.[23] **Fig. 1** demonstrates a case of successful DHC.

Optimization of neurocritical care may reduce the need for surgery. It should also be noted that advancement in other therapies for AIS such as thrombolytics and thrombectomy may further mitigate the need. Another aspect of medical care that requires further evaluation is the optimal provider setting in which these patients should receive care. While most of the RCTs admitted enrolled patients to ICUs, there was a higher proportion of surgical patients in ICU, compared with medical patients. The differences in the level of care alone could have confounded outcomes.[19]

DESTINY II was a randomized controlled trial in patients 61 years and older with LHI.[1,18] The results showed a decrease in mortality rate from 70% to 33% in the DHC group, but 32% and 28% of patients who survived remained in a very poor neurologic status quantified as Modified Rankin Scale (mRS) of 4 and 5, respectively. Only 7% of patients showed a mRS of 3 as the best outcome that could be achieved. Although the authors concluded that DHC significantly increased the probability of survival without the most severe disability, data clearly show that an increased survival rate was achieved by a significant increase of patients with poor and very poor outcomes (mRS5).[23]

In summary, DHC as a potential therapy to improve survival after large hemispheric strokes is recommended with the following special considerations[3]:

- In patients older than 60 years, it is recommended to consider patient and family wishes, since in this age group, DHC can reduce mortality rate but with a higher likelihood of being severely disabled

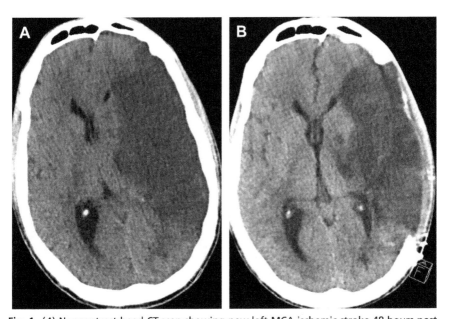

Fig. 1. (*A*) Noncontrast head CT scan showing new left MCA ischemic stroke 48 hours post-onset of symptoms, with cerebral edema and midline shift. (*B*) Noncontrast head CT of same patient 24 hours post-DHC with near resolution of shift. (*Courtesy of* The University of New Mexico, Albuquerque, NM.)

- There are insufficient data to recommend against DHC based on hemispheric dominance
- To achieve the best neurologic outcome, it is recommended to perform DHC within 24 to 48 h hours of symptom onset and before any herniation symptoms
- The minimal size for DHC should be 12 cm, with larger sizes of 14 to 16 cm being associated with better outcomes

Postoperative care for patients with DHC involves monitoring the flap site for sudden expansion which can occur with a post-DHC subdural hematoma or hemorrhagic conversion. The head should be positioned to take the weight off the DHC side. The patient should not be out of bed without an othortically fitted protective helmet. The wound should be examined daily for leakage or erythema suggesting infection.

Cerebellar Strokes

Up to 20% of patients with cerebellar infarcts are at risk of developing malignant edema. Initial infarct size on imaging helps identify those at risk. The kinetics of edema in the posterior fossa is not well characterized. The infarct–edema growth rate over the first 48 h independently predicted the need for surgical intervention in patients with cerebellar infarction.[24,25] The AHA recommends that Neuro ICU monitoring is indicated when $1/3^{rd}$ of one cerebellar hemisphere is affected by a stroke. The most concerning issues related to cerebellar infarcts are brainstem and fourth ventricle compression. When either is present, it is recommended that medical therapy serves as a bridge to early suboccipital craniectomy (SOC). Care must be taken when obstructive hydrocephalus is present, that ventriculostomy placement is timed with surgical decompression to avoid inducing upward herniation.[24,26]

Fig. 2A demonstrates brainstem and fourth ventricular compression in the setting of bilateral cerebellar strokes and **Fig.** 2B shows resolution after SOC.

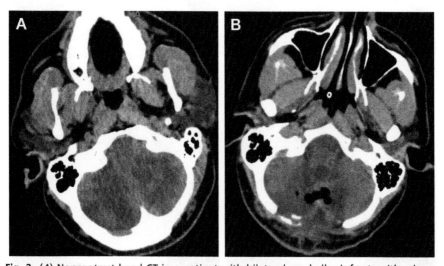

Fig. 2. (*A*) Noncontrast head CT in a patient with bilateral cerebellar infarcts with edema, fourth ventricular compression, and brainstem compression. (*B*) Noncontrast head CT in the same patient post-suboccipital decompression with a resolution of brainstem compression and ventricular compression. (*Courtesy of* The University of New Mexico, Albuquerque, NM.)

Management of Hemorrhagic Transformation

HT can be classified clinically and radiographically.

Clinical classification distinguishes symptomatic intracranial hemorrhage (sICH) from asymptomatic intracranial hemorrhage (aICH). sICH is defined as a worsening of the NIHSS by ≥ 4 points attributable to HT, within 36 hours of ictus. Clinical classification may be unreliable in cases of severe stroke whereby significant decline may be difficult to discern.[13]

Radiographic classification of HT distinguishes small petechial hemorrhagic infarction (HI1), confluent petechial hemorrhagic infarction (HI2), small parenchymal hemorrhage (PH1) (<30% of infarct, mild mass effect), and large parenchymal hemorrhage (PH2, >30% of infarct, marked mass effect). The Heidelberg Bleeding Classification scale has been proposed to address some of the challenges and limitations of the ECASS classification, outlined in **Table 3**.[13,27] **Fig. 3** illustrates PH1 hemorrhagic transformation of a left MCA stroke post tPA treatment.

The use and reversal of antiplatelets and anticoagulants in AIS are discussed in other chapters of this text. This article is additive by specifically addressing the reversal of fibrinolytic agents used in AIS.

Post tPA/TNK reversal: Prompt diagnosis and early correction of coagulopathy after fibrinolytic therapy has remained the mainstay of treatment.[13,28] The options for reversal of an HT after fibrinolytics are included in **Table 4** later in discussion:

Table 3 A and B: Radiologic classification of hemorrhagic conversion	
ECASS Classification for Hemorrhagic Conversion	
Petechial hemorrhage	
HI1	Small petechial hemorrhages that are scattered
HI2	Petechial hemorrhages that are confluent
Parenchymal Hemorrhage	
PH1	Parenchymal hemorrhage <30% of infarct, only mild mass effect
PH2	Parenchymal hemorrhage more than 30% of infarct, marked mass effect
3B Heidelberg Bleeding Classification	
1a HI1	Scattered small petechia, no mass effect
1b HI2	Confluent petechia, no mass effect
1c PH1	Hematoma with infarcted tissue occupying <30% without mass effect
2 PH2	Hematoma occupying 30% or more of infarcted tissue with mass effect
3	ICH, outside infarcted tissue or intracranial-extracerebral hemorrhage
3a	Parenchymal hematoma away from infarction tissue
3b	Parenchymal hematoma away from infarction tissue with: IVH
3c	Parenchymal hematoma away from infarction tissue with: Subarachnoid Hemorrhage
3d	Parenchymal hematoma away from infarction tissue with: Subdural Hemorrhage

Data from Spronk E, Sykes G, Falcione S, Munsterman D, Twinkle J, Kamtchum-Tatuene J, Jickling GC. Hemorrhagic Transformation in Ischemic Stroke and the Role of Inflammation. Frontiers in Neurology vol. 12, 2021; and Yaghi S, Willey JZ, Cucchiara B, Goldstein JN, Gonzales NR, Khatri P, Kim LJ, Mayer SA, Sheth KN, Schwamm LH; Treatment and Outcome of Hemorrhagic Transformation After Intravenous Alteplase in Acute Ischemic Stroke: A Scientific Statement for Healthcare Professionals From the AHA/ASA. Stroke. 2017 Dec;48(12):e343-e361.

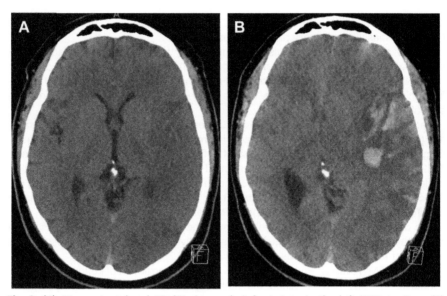

Fig. 3. (*A*): Noncontrast head CT showing early infarct signs in the left MCA territory (*B*) Noncontrast head CT showing hemorrhagic conversion within 24 hours of first head CT. Note that the ECASS score here would be PH1 using definitions in **Table 3**A and the Heidelberg Bleeding Classification would be 1cPH1 using definitions in **Table 3**B. (*Courtesy of* The University of New Mexico, Albuquerque, NM.)

Table 4		
Options for reversal of an HT after fibrinolytics		
Agent	**Amount**	**Comments**
Cryoprecipitate	Initial dose: 10 U cryoprecipitate. Additional given as needed	Derived from FFP and contains fibrinogen. A fibrinogen level should be sent immediately. Goal fibrinogen level >150 mg/dL. Each 10 U cryoprecipitate increases fibrinogen by nearly 50 mg/dL
Platelets	6–8 units	Unclear benefit except in thrombocytopenia <100 that was not known on admission
Fresh Frozen Plasma	12 mL/kg	INR = 1.6
Prothrombin Complex Concentrate	25–50 U/Kg	Dose depends on the INR level
Vitamin K:	10 mg IV	
Recombinant Factor VIIa	20–160 μg/kg	
Antifibrinolytic agents:		
Aminocaproic acid	4 g IV during the first hour followed by 1 g/h for 8 h	
Tranexamic acid:	1000 mg IV x once[13,14]	

Strokes Secondary to Infective Endocarditis

Cerebrovascular complications (ie, AIS, transient ischemic attack, silent cerebral embolism) frequently occur in patients with infective endocarditis (IE) and result from cerebral septic embolization of an endocardial vegetation.[29]

Treatment recommendations include[30–32]:

- Starting antibiotics as soon as possible (reduces the risk of neurologic complications by more than 50%).
- Avoid anticoagulation, if possible, due to the risk of hemorrhagic transformation
- Obtain CT angiogram to look for mycotic aneurysms warranting endovascular coiling
- If cardiac valvular surgery is indicated, timing will depend on the presence and severity of AIS.

Optimal surgical timing is unknown and is recommended to be individualized based on embolic risk factors including[30–33]:

- Age
- Diabetes
- Presence of atrial fibrillation
- Size, mobility, and location of vegetations
- Changing the size of the embolism *on* antibiotics
- Prior embolism
- Organisms such as Staphylococcus aureus

In general, it is recommended to wait 2 weeks before surgical intervention.[32]

Management of Patients Postcarotid Revascularization

Revascularization via open CEA or endovascular carotid artery stenting (CAS) is indicated for symptomatic internal carotid stenosis of greater than 70%.[34,35] Ideally, depending on the size of stroke (if one has occurred) revascularization is completed within 2 weeks following the heralding event. For the initial 2 to 48 hours postprocedure, these patients benefit from monitoring in the Neuro ICU.[14,35]

Postoperative Care for Carotid Endarterectomy Procedures

Significant postoperative complications to anticipate include wound hematoma, uncontrolled hypertension, hemodynamic depression with hypotension and bradycardia, hyperperfusion syndrome with postoperative ICH, and seizures. Due to the seriousness of these complications, perioperative care in a Neuro ICU is recommended. For those who remain stable for 24 hours after surgery, direct discharge from the ICU is often possible. However, if instability is demonstrated, continued close observation is recommended.[14]

- Wound hematoma

Wound hematomas are relatively common following CEA. In the NASCET study, 5.5% of patients had documented wound hematomas. The majority are small but large hematomas may require emergency treatment. If the trachea is not compromised, emergency evacuation of hematoma in the operating room is warranted. Once the hematoma begins obstructing the trachea, emergent bedside revision is best.[14]

- Hypertension

BP control post-CEA is vital. Neck hematoma, hyperperfusion syndrome, and intra-cerebral hemorrhage are associated with poor control. Preoperative hypertension is the single most important predictive factor for postoperative hypertension. Baroreflex failure syndrome with either unilateral or bilateral CEA can occur. Yet, even of those who were normotensive preprocedure, 21% had postsurgically induced abnormalities of baroreceptor sensitivity during the dissection of the common carotid artery and vagus nerve. Careful BP management in the initial post-CEA period is essential in avoiding further complications.[14]

- Hemodynamic depression: hypotension and bradycardia

Hemodynamic depression with hypotension and bradycardia occurs predominately after CAS with a frequency between 13% and 76%. Critical care management of hypotension includes fluid infusion and low dose phenylephrine or norepinephrine, dependent on heart rate. Bradycardia is frequently benign but can become symptomatic or severe (heart rate < 40) requiring treatment with atropine or glycopyrrolate. In very severe cases transient external pacing may need to be considered. Typically, the course is self-limited to 24 to 48 hours[14,36]

- Hyperperfusion syndrome

Post-CEA, hyperperfusion syndrome is a critical entity resulting from impaired cerebral autoregulation in the ipsilateral carotid territory. Chronic hypoperfusion distal to the stenotic segment causes tonic compensatory maximal collateral vasodilation. Postoperatively these beds remain unable to vasoconstrict. The ensuing luxury perfusion leads to edema followed by hemorrhage. A progression is similar to hemorrhagic PRES (Posterior Reversible Encephalopathy Syndrome) but isolated to the affected carotid territory. Tight BP control is the mainstay of treatment along with hourly observation of the neurologic exam.[14]

- Intracerebral hemorrhage

Risk factors for post-CEA and CAS hemorrhage include advanced age, presence of pre-existing hypertension, presence of poor collaterals, and evidence of slow MCA territory flow on angiography. Angiographic hypoperfusion is the strongest risk factor. The ICH that develops postrevascularization is typically large and often fatal.[14]

- Seizures

Post-CEA and CAS seizures are managed with BP control in addition to antiseizure medications and may be attributed to one or more of the following 3 mechanisms.[14]

- Postoperative cortical ischemic strokes
- Postoperative intracranial hemorrhage
- Cerebral hyperperfusion syndrome

Common Medical/Intensive Care Unit-Related Complications After Stroke

Strokes and cardiac issues

Cardiac ischemia and arrhythmias are known risk factors for complications after AIS. Involvement of the insular cortex, particularly on the right, is associated with cardiac events due to its role in autonomic control. The most common of these is subendocardial myonecrosis, or non-ST elevation myocardial infarction clinically.[21]

Screening for cardiac ischemia in AIS includes obtaining a 12-lead ECG and at least 2 sets of troponin levels 8 hours apart. If the troponin is elevated, it needs to be followed until the level peaks. All patients with AIS in the ICU should be on continuous cardiac monitoring. Common abnormal ECG changes after AIS include prolonged QT, ST segment changes, prominent U waves, atrial fibrillation, and supraventricular tachycardia.

Other Aspects of Care for Patients with Stroke in Critical Care Unit

Deep venous thrombosis prevention

The incidence of deep venous thrombosis (DVTs) in AIS is high and typically manifests clinically between 2 and 7 days. Pulmonary Embolism is the most common cause of death (25%) in AIS.

Venous thromboembolism (VTE) prophylaxis recommendations are as follows[33]:

- Initiate VTE prophylaxis as soon as feasible in all patients with AIS.
- Prophylaxis with low molecular weight heparin (LMWH) is recommended over unfractionated heparin (UFH) in AIS with restricted mobility.
- Those undergoing hemicraniectomy or endovascular procedure are suggested to use UFH, LMWH, and/or intermittent pneumatic compression devices for VTE prophylaxis in the immediate postsurgical or endovascular epoch. Administration of thrombolytics is the exception when prophylaxis can be delayed for 24 hours.[33,37,38]

Strokes and aspiration pneumonia

Coughing and swallowing reflexes are crucial protective mechanisms to prevent aspiration pneumonia and are frequently impaired in patients with poststroke. Pneumonia impacts stroke outcomes even without respiratory failure. Although pneumonia is a common complication, antibiotic prophylaxis is not recommended. Conversely, beta-blockers and statins are linked to a lower risk of pneumonia. Other drugs, such as benzodiazepines and antiacid medications, are associated with an increased risk of pneumonia and should be used judiciously.[37]

Strokes and urinary tract infection

Patients with AIS have a high risk of infection in general. Several factors have been identified as predictors for the development of UTI, including age, elevated procalcitonin, interleukin-6, CRP levels, higher presenting NIHSS, comorbid diabetes, and presenting hemoglobin level.[39] Early removal of indwelling Foley catheters is the mainstay of prevention, as well as protocolized postvoid bladder scanning for early identification of acute retention.

Glycemic control

Among patients with AIS and hyperglycemia, treatment with intensive (blood glucose <120) versus standard glucose control (blood glucose <180) for up to 72 hours did not result in a significant difference in favorable functional outcomes at 90 days. These findings do not support using intensive glucose control in this setting.[40]

SUMMARY PARAGRAPH

AIS management in the Neuro ICU addresses several cornerstones of patient care. Management of airway compromise and BP are critical first steps. Monitoring for iatrogenic complications preoccupies the early phase of care. Management of stroke-related sequelae such as cerebral edema and secondary ischemia are critically important. Early surgical intervention for malignant poststroke edema, in appropriate cases, is also important for survival and functional outcome for some. Patients with poststroke are at risk for cardiopulmonary, thromboembolic, and infectious complications. Detailed ICU checklists to address these issues assist in the prevention of these common complications that can significantly impact stroke recovery.

CLINICS CARE POINTS

- Loss of airway control requiring intubation poststroke depends mainly on the size and/or location of stroke, GCS assessment (<10 at risk), loss of cough or gag reflex, and degree of cerebral edema with midline shift in anterior fossa or brainstem compression in posterior fossa strokes.

- Targeted BP control in patients with ischemic stroke reduces the risk of hemorrhagic conversion postfibrinolytics and interventional thrombectomy reduces the risk of hemorrhagic conversion

- Management of poststroke cerebral edema includes early surgical management, appropriate use of hypertonic saline or mannitol, temperature control, blood glucose, and BP control to improve mortality and outcome.

- Patients with post-CEA have the greatest risk of complications in the first 24 hours after the procedure. BP control will reduce the risk of neck hematoma and exacerbation of reperfusion injury complications.

- The most common ICU-related complications include aspiration pneumonia, deep venous thromboses, cardiac arrhythmias, and urinary tract infections. Implementation of mechanisms to prevent these complications is an important part of stroke ICU care.

DISCLOSURE

The authors have nothing to disclose.

REFERENCES

1. Bevers MB, Kimberly WT. Critical care management of acute ischemic stroke. Curr Treat Options Cardiovasc Med 2017;19(6):41.
2. Herpic F, Rincon F. Management of acute ischemic stroke. Crit Care Med 2020; 48(11):1654–63.
3. Torbey MT, Bösel J, Rhoney DH, et al. Evidence-based guidelines for the management of large hemispheric infarction: a statement for health care professionals from the NCS and the German Society for Neuro-intensive Care and Emergency Medicine. Neurocrit Care 2015;22(1):146–64.
4. Milhaud D, Popp J, Thouvenot E, et al. Mechanical ventilation in ischemic stroke. J Stroke Cerebrovasc Dis 2004;13(4):183–8.
5. Coplin WM, Pierson DJ, Cooley KD, et al. Implications of extubation delay in brain-injured patients meeting standard weaning criteria. Am J Respir Crit Care Med 2000;161:1530–6.
6. Krueger S, Schmidt S, Warnecke T, et al. Extubation Readiness in critically ill stroke patients. Stroke 2019;50(8):1981–8.
7. McManus M, Liebeskind DS. Blood pressure in acute ischemic stroke. J Clin Neurol 2016;12(2):137–46. https://doi.org/10.3988/jcn.2016.12.2.137.
8. Jauch EC, Saver JL, Adams HP Jr, et al. Guided early Management for patients with acute ischemic stroke: a guideline for Healthcare professionals AHA/ASA Stroke 2013;44(3):870–947.
9. Saldana S, Breslin J 2nd, Hanify J, et al. Comparison of Clevidipine and nicardipine for acute blood pressure reduction in hemorrhagic stroke. Neurocrit Care 2021;36(3):983–92.
10. Rosenbaum DM, Grotta JC, Yatsu FM, et al. Pilot study of nicardipine for acute ischemic stroke. Angiology 1990;41(11 Pt 2):1017–22.

11. Li J, Zhang P, Wu S, et al. Factors associated with favourable outcome in large hemispheric infarctions. BMC Neurol 2018;18:152.

12. Yaghi S, Willey JZ, Cucchiara B, et al. Treatment and outcome of hemorrhagic transformation after intravenous Alteplase in acute ischemic stroke: a Scientific statement for healthcare professionals from the AHA/ASA. Stroke 2017;48(12): e343–61.

13. Yee J, Kaide CG. Emergency reversal of anticoagulation. West J Emerg Med 2019;20(5):770–83. https://doi.org/10.5811/westjem.2018.5.38235.

14. Powers WJ, Rabinstein AA, Ackerson T, et al. 2018 Guidelines for the early management of patients with acute ischemic stroke: a guideline for healthcare professionals from the AHA/ASA. Stroke 2018;49:e46–110.

15. Matusevicius M, Cooray C, Bottai M, et al. Blood pressure after endovascular thrombectomy. Stroke 2020;51(2):519–25.

16. Goyal M, Demchuk AM, Menon BK, et al. ESCAPE Trial Investigators. Randomized assessment of rapid endovascular treatment of ischemic stroke. N Engl J Med 2015;372(11):1019–30.

17. Koenig MA, Geocadin RG, de Grouchy M, et al. Safety of induced hypertension therapy in patients with acute ischemic stroke. Neurocrit Care 2006;4:3–7.

18. Hong JM, Kim DS, Kim M. Hemorrhagic transformation after ischemic stroke: mechanisms and management. Front Neurol 2021;12:703258.

19. Lin J, Frontera J. Decompressive hemicraniectomy for large hemispheric strokes. Stroke 2021;52(4):1500–10.

20. Kamel H, Navi BB, Nakagawa K, et al. Hypertonic saline versus mannitol for the treatment of elevated intracranial pressure - a meta-analysis of randomized clinical trials. Crit Care Med 2011;39:554–9.

21. Zazulia AR. Critical care management of acute ischemic stroke. Continuum Lifelong Learn Neurol 2009;15(3):68–82.

22. Aiyagari V, Diringer MN. Management of large hemispheric strokes in the neurological intensive care unit. Neurologist 2002;8:152–62.

23. Cook AM, Morgan Jones G, Hawryluk GWJ, et al. Guidelines for the acute treatment of cerebral edema in neurocritical care patients. Neurocrit Care 2020;32(3): 647–66.

24. Wang Y, Binkley MM, Qiao M, et al. Rate of infarct–edema growth on CT Predicts need for surgical intervention and clinical outcome in patients with cerebellar infarction. Neurocrit Care 2021. https://doi.org/10.1007/s12028-021-01414-x.

25. McKeown ME, Prasad A, Kobsa J, et al. Midline shift greater than 3 mm independently Predicts outcome after ischemic stroke. Neurocrit Care 2022;36(1):46–51.

26. Kim MJ, Park SK, Song J, et al. Preventive suboccipital decompressive craniectomy for cerebellar infarction: a retrospective-Matched case-control study. Stroke 2016;47(10):2565–73.

27. Spronk E, Sykes G, Falcione S, et al. Hemorrhagic transformation in ischemic stroke and the role of Inflammation. Front Neurol 2021;12.

28. Frontera JA, Lewin JJ 3rd, Rabinstein AA, et al. Guideline for reversal of antithrombotics in intracranial hemorrhage: a statement for healthcare professionals from the neurocritical care Society and Society of critical care medicine. Neurocrit Care 2016;24(1):6–46.

29. Juttler E, Bosel J, Amiri H, et al. Destiny II: decompressive surgery for the treatment of malignant infarction of the middle cerebral artery II. Int J Stroke 2011; 6(1):79–86.

30. Lee SJ, Oh SS, Lim DS, et al. Clinical significance of cerebrovascular complications in patients with acute infective endocarditis: a retrospective analysis of a 12-year single-center experience. BMC Neurol 2014;14:30.
31. Rodriguez Tori. LPC infective endocarditis: best practices for treating neurologic complications. https://www.neurologyadvisor.com/topics/general-neurology/infective-endocarditis-best-practices-for-treating-neurologic-complications.
32. Oh THT, Wang TKM, Pemberton JA, et al. Early or late surgery for endocarditis with neurological complications. Asian Cardiovasc Thorac Ann 2016;24(5): 435–40.
33. Nyquist P, Jichici D, Bautista C, et al. Prophylaxis of venous thrombosis in neurocritical care patients: an Executive summary of evidence-based guidelines: a statement for healthcare professionals from the neurocritical care Society and Society of critical care medicine. Crit Care Med 2017;45(10). 1097/CCM.0000000000002247.
34. Tan K, Cleveland T, Berczi V, et al. Timing frequency Complications after carotid Artery stenting: what is optimal period observation J Vasc Surg 2003;38(2): 236–43.
35. Biller J, Feinberg WM, Castaldo JE, et al. Guidelines for carotid endarterectomy. Stroke 1998;29(2):554–62.
36. Cao Q, Zhang J, Xu G. Hemodynamic changes and baroreflex sensitivity associated with carotid endarterectomy and carotid artery stenting. Interv Neurol 2015; 3(1):13–21.
37. Grossmann I, Rodriguez K, Soni M, et al. Stroke and pneumonia: mechanisms, risk factors, management, and prevention. Cureus 2021;13(11):e19912.
38. Li YM, Xu JH, Zhao YX, Predictors of urinary tract infection in acute stroke patients: A cohort study. Medicine (Baltimore) 2020;99(27):e20952.
39. Yan T, Liu C, Li Y, et al. Prevalence and predictive factors of urinary tract infection among patients with stroke: a meta-analysis. Am J Infect Control 2018;46:402–9.
40. Johnston KC, Bruno A, Pauls Q, et al. Intensive vs standard treatment of hyperglycemia and functional outcome in patients with AIS: The SHINE Randomized Clinical Trial. JAMA 2019;322(4):326–35.

Advances in Intracranial Hemorrhage

Subarachnoid Hemorrhage and Intracerebral Hemorrhage

Salvatore A. D'Amato, MD[a], Tiffany R. Chang, MD[b,c],*

KEYWORDS

- Intracranial hemorrhage • Subarachnoid hemorrhage • Intracerebral hemorrhage
- Delayed cerebral ischemia

KEY POINTS

- Aneurysmal subarachnoid hemorrhage requires clinicians to address potential neurologic sequalae as well as cardiopulmonary complications.
- Delayed cerebral ischemia is a major determinant of functional outcome following aneurysmal subarachnoid hemorrhage and occurs more frequently in higher grade hemorrhages.
- Blood pressure control and coagulopathy reversal are paramount in efforts to minimize hematoma expansion during the acute management of intracerebral hemorrhage.
- Surgical management of supratentorial intracerebral hemorrhage is considered on a case-by-case basis, with minimally invasive procedures potentially on the horizon.

ANEURYSMAL SUBARACHNOID HEMORRHAGE
Background

In North America, aneurysmal subarachnoid hemorrhage (aSAH) incidence is estimated at approximately 6.9 per 1,000,000 people.[1] Cerebral aneurysms generally form at arterial bifurcations. Over time, vessel wall remodeling leads to thinning of the tunica media layer.[2] Risk factors for aneurysm formation and rupture are the same. Key modifiable risk factors include hypertension, active tobacco, and heavy

[a] Department of Neurosurgery, Neurocritical Care Fellowship Program, University of Texas Health Science Center at Houston, 6431 Fannin Street, MSB 7.154, Houston, TX 77030, USA; [b] Department of Neurosurgery, University of Texas Health Science Center at Houston, 6431 Fannin Street, MSB 7.154, Houston, TX 77030, USA; [c] Department of Neurology, University of Texas Health Science Center at Houston, 6431 Fannin Street, MSB 7.154, Houston, TX 77030, USA
* Corresponding author. Department of Neurosurgery, University of Texas Health Science Center at Houston, 6431 Fannin Street, MSB 7.154, Houston, TX 77030.
E-mail address: tiffany.r.chang@uth.tmc.edu

Crit Care Clin 39 (2023) 71–85
https://doi.org/10.1016/j.ccc.2022.06.003
0749-0704/23/© 2022 Elsevier Inc. All rights reserved.

criticalcare.theclinics.com

alcohol use. Female sex and family history of aSAH are non-modifiable risk factors.[3–5] Furthermore, certain genetic conditions, including autosomal dominant polycystic kidney disease,[6] glucocorticoid remediable aldosteronism,[7] Marfan syndrome, Ehlers–Danlos, and neurofibromatosis type I increase risk of cerebral aneurysm formation and aSAH as well.[8]

Diagnosis and Imaging

Classically, aSAH presents as the "worst headache of life" or a "thunderclap headache." Associated signs include nuchal rigidity, cranial nerve palsies, and/or focal neurologic deficits. Hemiparesis or hemiplegia is more common with an intraparenchymal component. Signs of increased intracranial pressure (ICP) may be present and include nausea, emesis, and decreased level of arousal. Of note, one international population study estimated that 12.4% of patients with aSAH present with sudden cardiac death before medical attention.[9]

Diagnosis of aSAH via imaging is time-dependent on symptom onset. Non-contrast computed tomography (CT) has a sensitivity near 100% within 6 hours of rupture but decreases to 93% within 24 hours and less than 60% after 1 week.[10] MRI, particularly the combination of fluid attenuated-inversion recovery, gradient echo, and/or susceptibility-weighted imaging sequences, has been suggested to be superior to CT for this indication.[10,11] However, the availability and rapidity with which MRI can be obtained limits its utility. Negative imaging with continued suspicion for aSAH prompts lumbar puncture to assess for xanthochromia.[12] Combinations of clinical and radiographic features yield grading scales with important management and prognostic implications (**Table 1**).[13–15] Once aSAH is confirmed, vessel imaging via CT angiography (CTA) is preferred for identification of the aneurysm and surgical planning. Digital subtraction angiography (DSA) remains the gold standard for diagnosis when CTA is negative and may be an initial imaging option for simultaneous aneurysm identification and treatment with endovascular interventions.

Initial Management

Neurologic

Early neurologic stabilization focuses on addressing elevated ICP and minimizing risk of re-rupture. External ventricular drain (EVD) is recommended for reduced levels of consciousness and/or evidence of acute obstructive hydrocephalus. Immediate cerebrospinal fluid (CSF) diversion can be associated with improvement in clinical status.[12] This also allows for ICP measurement and management. Several weaning strategies exist for EVDs, and weaning failure warrants chronic CSF diversion via a ventriculoperitoneal shunt.

Society guidelines recommend targeting systolic blood pressure (SBP) less than 160 mm Hg[12] and mean arterial pressure (MAP) less than 110 mm Hg[16] to lower hydrostatic forces within the aneurysm dome. Prompt reversal of coagulopathy and/or antithrombotic medication should be undertaken. Seizure prophylaxis is optional and, if used, is generally administered for only 3 to 7 days.[12,16] If the patient experiences seizures at any point, ongoing anti-seizure therapy is often warranted.

Cardiovascular

Although aSAH is a neurologic emergency, medical stabilization must take priority because of the concurrent life-threatening nature of its systemic complications. Cardiovascular injury due to aSAH exists on a spectrum ranging from leakage of troponin-I with preserved cardiac function to myocardial infarction and cardiac arrest.[17] Neurogenic stunned myocardium occurs in up to 30% of cases and is more common in

Table 1
Summary of common clinical and radiographic grading scales for aneurysmal subarachnoid hemorrhage

Hunt and Hess		Fisher		Modified Fisher	
Grade	Features	Grade	Features	Grade	Features
1	Asymptomatic, mild headache	1	No SAH detected	0	No blood or IVH detected
2	Severe headache; nuchal rigidity; cranial nerve palsy	2	Thin layer of SAH	1	Thin SAH, (−) IVH
3	Lethargic; mild neurologic deficit (eg, extremity drift)	3	Thick layer of SAH, +/− IPH, no IVH	2	Thin SAH, (+) IVH
4	Stupor; moderate to severe deficit (eg, hemiplegia)	4	IVH and/or IPH with thin or no SAH detected	3	Thick SAH, (−) IVH
5	Comatose; posturing			4	Thick SAH, (+) IVH

Abbreviations: IPH, intraparenchymal hemorrhage; IVH, intraventricular hemorrhage; Thick, >1 mm; Thin, <1 mm.

Data from Hunt WE, Hess RM. Surgical risk as related to time of intervention in the repair of intracranial aneurysms. J Neurosurg. Jan 1968;28(1):14-20. https://doi.org/10.3171/jns.1968.28.1. 0014 Fisher CM, Kistler JP, Davis JM. Relation of cerebral vasospasm to subarachnoid hemorrhage visualized by computerized tomographic scanning. Neurosurgery. Jan 1980;6(1):1-9. https://doi. org/10.1227/00006123-198001000-00001 and Claassen J, Bernardini GL, Kreiter K, et al. Effect of cisternal and ventricular blood on risk of delayed cerebral ischemia after subarachnoid hemorrhage: the Fisher scale revisited. Stroke. Sep 2001;32(9):2012-20. https://doi.org/10.1161/hs0901. 095677.

higher grade aSAH.[18] Resulting acute left heart failure requires ionotropic and vasopressor support. The phenomenon is theorized to result from massive catecholamine release by injured brain leading to cardiac myocyte calcium overload, contraction band necrosis, and possible epicardial coronary vasospasm.[18] Although cardiac recovery often occurs, association with increased morbidity and mortality exists.[19] Additional cardiac manifestations include electrocardiogram (ECG) abnormalities, such as section between the end of the S wave and the beginning of the T wave (ST) segment changes, T-wave inversions, time from the start of the Q wave to the end of the T wave, corrected for heart rate (QTc) prolongation, and U waves as well as various arrythmias, such as atrial fibrillation or flutter, ventricular tachycardia, and torsades de pointe.[17]

Pulmonary
Endotracheal intubation may be required in patients with aSAH because of the reduced level of consciousness, hypoxemia from aspiration, and/or pulmonary edema secondary to acute heart failure or primary neurogenic mechanisms. Similar to its effect on cardiac function, the catecholamine surge following aSAH may result in vasoconstriction of the pulmonary circulation, causing increased pulmonary venous and capillary pressures. This consequently leads to increased hydrostatic forces, alveolar endothelial cell damage, and subsequent increased capillary permeability. In addition, damage of the blood–brain barrier results in release of inflammatory cytokines, including interleukin (IL)-1, IL-6, IL-8, and tumor necrosis factor alpha, further increasing pulmonary capillary permeability.[20] The mainstay of therapy is ventilatory support in severe cases, with diuretics and cardiac support if concurrent cardiac dysfunction exists.

Aneurysm Treatment

Once medically stabilized, aneurysm treatment occurs as soon as possible, but usually not later than 72 hours. The risk of re-rupture is estimated as high as 13% and is greatest within the first 2 to 12 hours, peaking at 6 hours from symptom onset.[12] Associated risk factors for re-rupture include Hunt/Hess grade 3 or higher, larger aneurysm size, presence of intraparenchymal or intraventricular hemorrhage (IVH), and higher SBP (>160 mm Hg).[21] Historically, aneurysm treatment was accomplished via craniotomy and surgical clipping across the neck of the aneurysm obliterating flow within the dome. In recent decades, endovascular procedures have emerged as the treatment modality of choice for many ruptured aneurysms. The International Subarachnoid Aneurysm Trial (ISAT) trial demonstrated decreased death and disability, but higher rebleeding risk, within the endovascular compared with surgical clipping group.[22] During a 10-year follow-up, a composite outcome of survival and Modified Rankin Scale (mRS) 0 to 2 again favored the endovascular group.[23] Given the immense variety and location of cerebral aneurysms, the decision to undergo coiling or clipping is often determined via multidisciplinary discussion.

Delayed Cerebral Ischemia

Neuronal injury results from initial aneurysm rupture. Secondary injury may also develop several days later by a phenomenon known as delayed cerebral ischemia (DCI), which represents a major source of morbidity and mortality. DCI is defined as a new focal neurologic deficit or a decrease in a patient's Glasgow Coma Scale (GCS) by two points for at least 1 hour in the absence of another attributable cause. The DCI window is generally considered to be between day 4 and 14, but ultra-early and delayed DCI has been described. Historically, cerebral vasospasm was thought to be the sole cause of DCI, but further understanding of the pathophysiological mechanisms of DCI have implicated both macro-vasospasm and micro-vasospasm, microthrombosis, thromboinflammation, autoregulation failure, and cortical spreading depolarizations as likely contributors.[24] Consistent risk factors for DCI include a higher grade aSAH, especially Hunt/Hess grade 4 to 5, and modified Fisher grade 3 to 4, with these patients having increased morbidity and mortality.[25,26]

Delayed cerebral ischemia monitoring

Various noninvasive monitoring options have emerged for early detection of DCI, particularly in patients without a reliable neurologic examination. Among these, continuous electroencephalogram (cEEG) has been used to assess electrical changes within the brain due to ischemia. Electrical rhythms slow as the ischemic threshold is approached, moving from the alpha to delta frequency, with corresponding ischemic changes at the cellular level.[27] A ratio to assess for these changes, termed the alpha–delta ratio, in addition to the relative alpha variability, has shown correlation with DCI and angiography-confirmed vasospasm.[28] Furthermore, various cEEG patterns, such as nonconvulsive status epilepticus, generalized periodic epileptiform discharges, and periodic lateralized epileptiform discharges, have been suggested to indicate a poor prognosis, especially in high-grade aSAH.[29] Consequently, cEEG has been used in many centers as an adjunct in monitoring for DCI.

Transcranial Doppler (TCD) is a form of ultrasonography focusing on measurement of blood velocity through the anterior and posterior cerebral circulation. As arterial diameter narrows, blood velocity increases, making TCD a useful screening tool for detection of vasospasm, before development of irreversible ischemia. Detection of vasospasm with TCDs has been most studied within the middle cerebral artery (MCA), with mild vasospasm beginning at a mean flow velocity (MFV) of greater than 120 cm/s and severe being greater than 200 cm/s.[30] Parameters such as blood pressure, hematocrit, and partial pressure of carbon dioxide within the arterial system can influence cerebral velocity measurements independent of vasospasm. Furthermore, other causes of hyperemia may give the appearance of vasospasm from the flow velocities alone. The Lindegaard ratio (LR), a ratio of MFV of the MCA to the ipsilateral internal carotid artery, is calculated to correct for this. An LR greater than 6.0 indicates severe vasospasm.[30]

CT perfusion (CTP) is another imaging modality used in the diagnosis of DCI and vasospasm following aSAH. It may be particularly helpful when sonographic windows are poor, limiting the utility of TCDs. In addition, it guides medical decision-making when clinical examination is limited. There is no clear consensus of diagnostic criteria for vasospasm via CTP, but using an increased mean transient time (>6.0 second) and decreased cerebral blood flow (<30%) has shown correlation with vasospasm.[31] Taken together, clinical examination, when available, is paramount in detecting DCI, but clinicians must use a combination of resources to detect DCI.

Delayed cerebral ischemia treatment

Nimodipine, a calcium channel blocker, is the only medication demonstrated to improve functional outcomes following aSAH in clinical trials.[32] The mechanism of such neuroprotection is unclear but occurs independent of improving vasospasm.[33] It is administered beginning on admission for a period of up to 21 days, with transient hypotension being the only usual adverse effect. For treatment of DCI, society guidelines recommend increasing MAP with vasopressors if needed, until clinical improvement is observed. However, there have not been large-scale clinical trials investigating this.[12,16] It is theorized that augmentation of MAP assists in maximizing cerebral blood flow and possibly results in arterial dilation at the macroscale and microscale levels. Maintenance of euvolemia, normothermia, normoglycemia, and normal electrolyte levels, especially normonatremia, are also important in the prevention and treatment of DCI. Patients with DCI often undergo repeat DSA for angioplasty or infusion of vasodilators, such as nicardipine, verapamil, and milrinone, directly into the cerebral vasculature (**Fig. 1**). Also, repeat DSA is performed in poor grade aSAH, when clinical change suggestive of DCI is difficult to detect. Systemic options are emerging as well, with milrinone potentially leading to reduced DCI and functional disability, though randomized trials are required for confirmation.[34,35] Furthermore, intrathecal options exist, such as nicardipine, which has shown efficacy in non-randomized trials,[36] and others are under investigation.

INTRACEREBRAL HEMORRHAGE
Background

Worldwide, intracerebral hemorrhage (ICH) accounts for nearly 18 million cases of stroke annually, leading to 39.4 million disability-adjusted life years lost.[37] In the United States, review of a nationwide database for hospital admissions estimates inpatient mortality from ICH at 24% as of 2015.[38] Hypertension is considered the greatest risk factor.[39] Chronic hypertension induces lipohyalinosis in small blood vessels, loss of autoregulation, decreased vessel compliance, and formation of microaneurysms, which all contribute to vessel rupture.[40] Classically, hypertensive ICH occurs within deep structures, namely the basal ganglia, thalamus, pons, and cerebellum, where perforator vessels penetrate. Lobar ICH is considered another type of hypertensive hemorrhage, though cerebral amyloid angiopathy is a major contributor to ICH in this location, particularly in the elderly. Other risk factors for ICH include age, with significant increase beyond 45 year old,[41] obesity through its secondary effect on

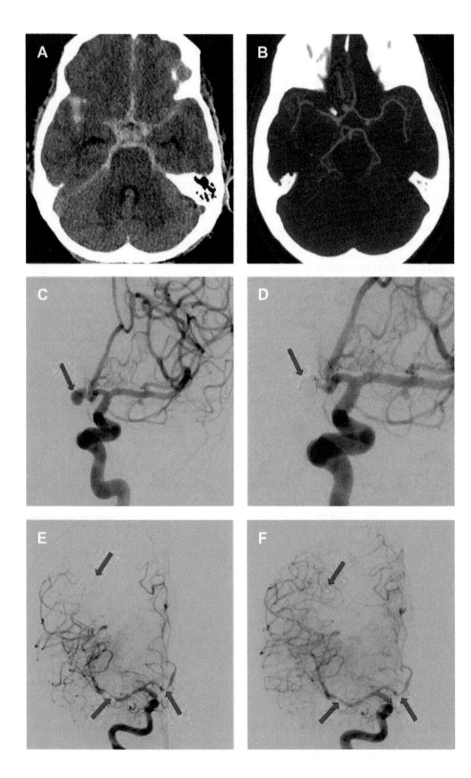

hypertension,[42] heavy alcohol intake,[43] and stimulant use. Other conditions that may underlie ICH include cerebral venous sinus thrombosis, reversible cerebral vasoconstriction syndrome, malignancies, arteriovenous malformations or fistulas, and cavernous malformations.

Diagnosis and Imaging

Patients with ICH present with a variety of symptoms but often have focal neurologic deficits localizing to the affected territory. They may also present with new onset seizures or signs of increased ICP similar to aSAH, particularly if accompanied by IVH resulting in obstructive hydrocephalus. CT of the brain should be performed emergently. If ICH is confirmed, CTA of the head and neck can further evaluate for vascular malformations, particularly in younger patients. Non-contrast CT is repeated 4 to 6 hours from the initial scan to assess hematoma stability. A "spot sign," or a focus of enhancement within the hematoma on CTA representing active contrast extravasation, has been associated with early hematoma expansion and worse functional outcomes (**Fig. 2**).[44] Numerous imaging features on non-contrast CT have similar association, including irregular shape of the hematoma, "island sign" (multiple smaller, satellite hematomas), "black hole" sign (focus of hypodensity within hematoma), and the "swirl sign" (larger areas of isodense or hypodense within hematoma).[45] The presence of these imaging features should increase clinician concern for possible neurologic deterioration due to early hematoma expansion and may prompt earlier stability imaging.

Initial Management

ICH is a neurologic emergency, and medical stabilization must be prioritized over neuroimaging. This includes assessing the need for airway protection, ensuring hemodynamic stability and obtaining an ECG to assess for cardiac pathology. Particular attention should be paid to platelet count, prothrombin time, international normalized ratio (INR), and activated partial thromboplastin time, as these will assist in guiding management of concomitant coagulopathy. Seizure prophylaxis in the setting of ICH is not currently recommended by the AHA, but anti-seizure medication is indicated if seizures occur.[46] Once neuroimaging confirms ICH, it is crucial to assess for the presence of IVH and obstructive hydrocephalus and possible need for an EVD. Overall incidence of ICH with IVH varies, but post hoc analyses of larger clinical trials involving management of ICH yield an estimate of 28%.[47]

Blood Pressure Management

Blood pressure control in ICH has been subject to numerous clinical trials, as early observational studies suggested elevated SBP may lead to hematoma expansion and neurologic deterioration.[48] The two largest clinical trials examining the influence of blood pressure reduction in ICH and patient outcomes are INTERACT-2 and ATACH-2. In INTERACT-2, patients with ICH were randomized to intensive SBP control of less than 140 mm Hg versus less than 180 mm Hg, with a goal of achieving this within

---

Fig. 1. (*A*) Diffuse subarachnoid hemorrhage involving the basal cisterns. (*B*) CTA demonstrating an inferiolateral projecting anterior communicating artery (AComA) aneurysm. (*C*) Digital subtraction angiography of the same AComA aneurysm. (*D*) Status post coil embolization of the aneurysm. (*E*) Moderate vasospasm of the distal M1 and A1 arterial segments. (*F*) Improvement in vasospasm following infusion of vasodilators, including increased filling within the distal MCA branches.

1 hour of randomization.[49] There was no significant difference in the primary outcome of death or major disability (defined as mRS 3–6 at 90 days) between groups. However, in a secondary analysis, there was a significant difference in overall improved functional outcome and quality of life based on the health utility scale, favoring the intensive SBP group. In ATACH-2, an SBP goal of 110 to 139 mm Hg versus 140 to 179 mm Hg was compared, with the primary outcome being death or major disability, defined as mRS 4 to 6 at 90 days.[50] There again was no significant difference between groups. However, there was a significantly higher proportion of patients in the intensive blood pressure group who experienced adverse renal events within 7 days of randomization. ATACH-2 stopped enrollment early due to futility. Compared with INTERACT-2, patients in ATACH-2 had higher enrollment SBP, used only intravenous antihypertensive medication, had a lower mean SBP within the first few hours after randomization and were maintained at goal SBP for 24 hours compared with 7 days.[50]

In a pooled analysis of individual patient data from INTERACT-2 and ATACH-2, there was a 10% increase in odds of good functional recovery (defined as mRS 0–3) for every 10 mm Hg smooth reduction of SBP until an approximate threshold of 130 mm Hg.[51] In a systematic review and meta-analysis involving five studies investigating intensive SBP control in ICH, there was a nonsignificant trend toward lower death and dependency at 3 months, in addition to less hematoma expansion, in the intensive blood pressure groups, but overall mortality was the same.[52] Furthermore, a post hoc analysis of ATACH-2 found that patients in the intensive SBP group who presented with an SBP ≥220 mm Hg had higher rates of neurologic deterioration within 24 hours and adverse kidney events.[53]

Variation in blood pressure following ICH also may influence prognosis, as increased variability has been associated with worse functional outcomes.[54] Given these variable relationships between blood pressure control and outcomes, future trials will need to delineate not only SBP targets, but safe times-to-goal SBP and a tiered approach to gradual decrement of SBP target based on presenting blood pressure.

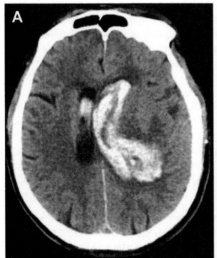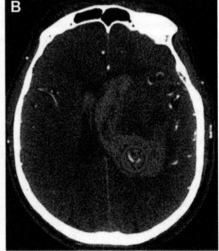

Fig. 2. (A) Left thalamic intracerebral hemorrhage with intraventricular extension causing obstructive hydrocephalus. (B) Computed tomography angiogram demonstrating a focus of enhancement within the hematoma indicating active extravasation.

Based on current evidence, the most recent AHA recommendations for blood pressure management in ICH include lowering the SBP to 140 mm Hg for any patient with an initial SBP between 150 to 220 mm Hg, provided there are no contraindications,[46] though the time period to achieve this is unclear.

Correction of Coagulopathy

Patients presenting with ICH and concurrent use of anticoagulant medications require immediate reversal. Common anticoagulation medications, the recommended reversal agent, and their mechanism of action are shown in **Table 2**.[55] Of note, in addition to intravenous vitamin K, prothrombin complex concentrate (PCC), when available, should be used over fresh frozen plasma (FFP) in reversal of warfarin-associated ICH. Four-factor PCC has been demonstrated to result in more rapid normalization of INR, greater restoration of coagulation factor levels,[56] and less hematoma expansion at the 3- and 24-h mark compared with FFP.[57]

Platelet transfusions are not routinely recommended for patients with ICH and concurrent use of antiplatelet agents. In the PATCH trial, platelet transfusion seemed to increase the risk of dependence (mRS 4–5) and death compared with standard care.[58] Of note, important patient groups excluded in this study were those undergoing an intracranial surgical procedure and patients with thrombocytopenia. In addition, patients with larger hematomas (>30 mL) and low GCS (3–4) were underrepresented. Thus, platelet transfusion in these contexts should be considered on a case-by-case basis. The overall level of evidence for administration of desmopressin in the setting of antiplatelet agent use and ICH is considered to be low, but may be considered in certain situations, such as patients undergoing a surgical procedure or those suspected of having uremic platelet dysfunction.[55]

Surgical Intervention

In addition to mass effect, increases in ICP and direct neuronal injury from acute blood extravasation, hematoma formation leads to an inflammatory response that has been implicated in secondary brain injury and possibly incomplete recovery.[59] As such, significant attention has been given to surgical evacuation of the hematoma. The surgical treatment of intracerebral hemorrhage (STICH) II trial was one of the first phase III trials to investigate supratentorial hematoma evacuation and found there was no difference in favorable outcome at 6 months among patients who underwent evacuation versus nonsurgical management.[60] Important limitations of this study included inclusion of larger volume hematomas than trended toward deriving benefit from early surgery based on early studies, a mean time to surgery of 26.7 hours from ICH symptom onset, and 21% of patients in the initial conservative group crossing over to undergo delayed surgery.

In the minimally invasive surgery plus alteplase for intracerebral hemorrhage evacuation (MISTIE) III trial, patients were randomized to undergo minimally invasive catheter-based hematoma evacuation followed by local thrombolysis with tissue plasminogen activator. There was no difference in a favorable outcome at 1 year; however, there was a decrease in mortality at 7 and 365 days in favor of the interventional group.[61] However, only about 60% of patients in the surgical group achieved the end of treatment goal volume of less than 15 mL. When comparing this group with the control group, there was a 10.5% increase in good functional outcome (mRS 0–3) at 1 year. Since MISTIE, there have been a number of clinical trials, some ongoing, investigating different minimally invasive surgical techniques, and subgroups of patients with supratentorial ICH who may benefit from such intervention.[62] Although awaiting results of trials, current AHA recommendations include considering evacuation of a supratentorial hematoma as a lifesaving measure in a deteriorating patient.[46]

Table 2
Available reversal agents and their mechanism of action for coagulopathy correction

Reversal Agent	Mechanism of Action	Agent Reversed
Andexanet alfa	Recombinant factor Xa, acting as decoy to cause sequestration of anticoagulant agent	Apixaban, rivaroxaban, edoxaban, enoxaparin
Cryoprecipitate	Replenishes factor VIII, XIII, vWF, and fibrinogen	Tissue plasminogen activator
Desmopressin	Increases plasma concentration of vWF and factor VIII via endothelial cell release	Antiplatelets (eg, aspirin, clopidogrel)
Fresh frozen plasma	Contains all coagulation factors, separated from cellular components	Warfarin
Idarucizumab	Humanized antibody fragment	Dabigatran
Protamine	Cation which binds and sequesters anionic anticoagulant agent	Heparin, enoxaparin
Prothrombin complex concentrate	A 3-factor concentrate: replenishes factor II, IX, and X A 4-factor concentrate: replenishes factor II, VII, IX, and X	Apixaban, dabigatran, fondaparinux, rivaroxaban, warfarin
Vitamin K	Promotes synthesis of factor II, VII, IX, and X	Warfarin

Abbreviations: vWF, von Willebrand Factor.

Adapted from Frontera JA, Lewin JJ, 3rd, Rabinstein AA, et al. Guideline for Reversal of Antithrombotics in Intracranial Hemorrhage: A Statement for Healthcare Professionals from the Neurocritical Care Society and Society of Critical Care Medicine. Neurocrit Care. Feb 2016;24(1):6-46. doi:10.1007/s12028-015-0222-x

For cerebellar hemorrhages, surgical evacuation has been found to be associated with improved mortality, but not with improved functional outcome compared with those who survived with medical management alone.[63] However, for any deteriorating patient, those with brainstem compression and/or signs of hydrocephalus, immediate evacuation of the cerebellar hematoma is currently recommended by the AHA.[46] Of note, placement of an EVD for hydrocephalus without concurrent suboccipital craniectomy may be harmful and lead to upward herniation. Further considerations for infratentorial hematoma evacuation include hematomas greater than 3 cm or 30 mL and effacement of the fourth ventricle.

Mobile Stroke Units for Early Treatment and Triage

Aside from possible surgical interventions on the horizon, an emerging area of interest in management of ICH has been on preventing early hematoma expansion, which can be responsible for acute decompensation among patients within the first 24 to

48 hours. Over the past several years, mobile stroke units (MSUs) have received attention in treatment and triage of ischemic stroke patients, demonstrating increased administration of thrombolytics to eligible patients compared with the standard group as well as improved functional outcomes.[64] Small studies have demonstrated the feasibility of using MSUs in triage and treatment of ICH patients as well.[65] In particular, the ultra-early diagnosis of ICH may assist with earlier reversal of coagulopathy when indicated, initiation of blood pressure control and triage to specialized centers equipped for the multidisciplinary care required by these patients, with the ultimate goal of improving long-term functional outcomes.

SUMMARY

Both aSAH and ICH remain devastating neurologic events, however, advances in imaging, medical management, and surgical techniques have improved survival after either event. Common to both processes, clinicians must work toward ensuring cardiopulmonary stability, coagulopathy correction, and addressing issues of increased ICP and/or acute hydrocephalus on presentation to reduce mortality and secondary injury. Treatment-specific strategies for aneurysm securement or hematoma management by medical and/or surgical techniques involve a multidisciplinary team. For the foreseeable future, research will continue toward elucidating mechanisms of neuronal injury in aSAH and ICH, culminating in new strategies to improve functional outcomes among survivors.

CLINICS CARE POINTS

- Aneurysmal rupture exerts widespread effects on the body that require immediate management, ranging from acute hydrocephalus to neurogenic stunned myocardium, myocardial infarction, cardiac arrest, and/or neurogenic pulmonary edema.
- Delayed cerebral ischemia is a major cause of morbidity and mortality following aneurysmal subarachnoid hemorrhage, occurring most commonly between days 4 and 14 following aneurysm rupture.
- In addition to nimodipine initiation on admission, treatment of delayed cerebral ischemia consists of induced hypertension and consideration of repeat angiography for intra-arterial infusion of vasodilators or angioplasty.
- Immediate management of intracerebral hemorrhage (ICH) entails ensuring adequate blood pressure control, with a goal systolic blood pressure of $\leq$140 mm Hg in most circumstances and correction of any coagulopathy.
- Decompressive craniectomy is recommended for cerebellar ICH with signs of brainstem compression and/or hydrocephalus, whereas surgical management of supratentorial ICH is considered on a case-by-case basis.

DISCLOSURE

Neither author has financial or commercial conflicts of interest to disclose.

REFERENCES

1. Etminan N, Chang HS, Hackenberg K, et al. Worldwide incidence of aneurysmal subarachnoid hemorrhage according to region, time period, blood pressure, and smoking prevalence in the population: a systematic review and meta-analysis. JAMA Neurol 2019;76(5):588–97.

2. Brisman JL, Song JK, Newell DW. Cerebral aneurysms. N Engl J Med 2006; 355(9):928–39.

3. Muller TB, Vik A, Romundstad PR, et al. Risk factors for unruptured intracranial aneurysms and subarachnoid hemorrhage in a prospective population-based study. Stroke 2019;50(10):2952–5.

4. Yao X, Zhang K, Bian J, et al. Alcohol consumption and risk of subarachnoid hemorrhage: a meta-analysis of 14 observational studies. Biomed Rep 2016;5(4): 428–36.

5. Vlak MH, Rinkel GJ, Greebe P, et al. Lifetime risks for aneurysmal subarachnoid haemorrhage: multivariable risk stratification. J Neurol Neurosurg Psychiatry 2013;84(6):619–23.

6. Cagnazzo F, Gambacciani C, Morganti R, et al. Intracranial aneurysms in patients with autosomal dominant polycystic kidney disease: prevalence, risk of rupture, and management. A systematic review. Acta Neurochir (Wien) 2017;159(5): 811–21.

7. Litchfield WR, Anderson BF, Weiss RJ, et al. Intracranial aneurysm and hemorrhagic stroke in glucocorticoid-remediable aldosteronism. Hypertension 1998; 31(1 Pt 2):445–50.

8. Kim ST, Brinjikji W, Kallmes DF. Prevalence of intracranial aneurysms in patients with Connective tissue diseases: a retrospective study. AJNR Am J Neuroradiol 2016;37(8):1422–6.

9. Huang J, van Gelder JM. The probability of sudden death from rupture of intracranial aneurysms: a meta-analysis. Neurosurgery 2002;51(5):1101–5 [discussion: 1105–7].

10. de Oliveira Manoel AL, Mansur A, Murphy A, et al. Aneurysmal subarachnoid haemorrhage from a neuroimaging perspective. Crit Care 2014;18(6):557.

11. da Rocha AJ, da Silva CJ, Gama HP, et al. Comparison of magnetic resonance imaging sequences with computed tomography to detect low-grade subarachnoid hemorrhage: role of fluid-attenuated inversion recovery sequence. J Comput Assist Tomogr 2006;30(2):295–303.

12. Connolly ES Jr, Rabinstein AA, Carhuapoma JR, et al. Guidelines for the management of aneurysmal subarachnoid hemorrhage: a guideline for healthcare professionals from the American Heart Association/american Stroke Association. Stroke 2012;43(6):1711–37.

13. Hunt WE, Hess RM. Surgical risk as related to time of intervention in the repair of intracranial aneurysms. J Neurosurg 1968;28(1):14–20.

14. Fisher CM, Kistler JP, Davis JM. Relation of cerebral vasospasm to subarachnoid hemorrhage visualized by computerized tomographic scanning. Neurosurgery 1980;6(1):1–9.

15. Claassen J, Bernardini GL, Kreiter K, et al. Effect of cisternal and ventricular blood on risk of delayed cerebral ischemia after subarachnoid hemorrhage: the Fisher scale revisited. Stroke 2001;32(9):2012–20.

16. Diringer MN, Bleck TP, Claude Hemphill J 3rd, et al. Critical care management of patients following aneurysmal subarachnoid hemorrhage: recommendations from the Neurocritical Care Society's Multidisciplinary Consensus Conference. Neurocrit Care 2011;15(2):211–40.

17. Behrouz R, Sullebarger JT, Malek AR. Cardiac manifestations of subarachnoid hemorrhage. Expert Rev Cardiovasc Ther 2011;9(3):303–7.

18. Kerro A, Woods T, Chang JJ. Neurogenic stunned myocardium in subarachnoid hemorrhage. J Crit Care 2017;38:27–34.

19. Kilbourn KJ, Levy S, Staff I, et al. Clinical characteristics and outcomes of neurogenic stress cadiomyopathy in aneurysmal subarachnoid hemorrhage. Clin Neurol Neurosurg 2013;115(7):909–14.

20. Zhao J, Xuan NX, Cui W, et al. Neurogenic pulmonary edema following acute stroke: the progress and perspective. Biomed Pharmacother 2020;130:110478.

21. Tang C, Zhang TS, Zhou LF. Risk factors for rebleeding of aneurysmal subarachnoid hemorrhage: a meta-analysis. PLoS One 2014;9(6):e99536.

22. Molyneux AJ, Kerr RS, Yu LM, et al. International subarachnoid aneurysm trial (ISAT) of neurosurgical clipping versus endovascular coiling in 2143 patients with ruptured intracranial aneurysms: a randomised comparison of effects on survival, dependency, seizures, rebleeding, subgroups, and aneurysm occlusion. Lancet 2005;366(9488):809–17.

23. Molyneux AJ, Birks J, Clarke A, et al. The durability of endovascular coiling versus neurosurgical clipping of ruptured cerebral aneurysms: 18 year follow-up of the UK cohort of the International Subarachnoid Aneurysm Trial (ISAT). Lancet 2015;385(9969):691–7.

24. Dodd WS, Laurent D, Dumont AS, et al. Pathophysiology of delayed cerebral ischemia after subarachnoid hemorrhage: a review. J Am Heart Assoc 2021; 10(15):e021845.

25. Duan W, Pan Y, Wang C, et al. Risk factors and clinical impact of delayed cerebral ischemia after aneurysmal subarachnoid hemorrhage: analysis from the China national stroke registry. Neuroepidemiology 2018;50(3–4):128–36.

26. Lee H, Perry JJ, English SW, et al. Clinical prediction of delayed cerebral ischemia in aneurysmal subarachnoid hemorrhage. J Neurosurg 2018;1–8. https://doi.org/10.3171/2018.1.JNS172715.

27. Foreman B, Claassen J. Quantitative EEG for the detection of brain ischemia. Crit Care 2012;16(2):216.

28. Claassen J, Mayer SA, Hirsch LJ. Continuous EEG monitoring in patients with subarachnoid hemorrhage. J Clin Neurophysiol 2005;22(2):92–8.

29. Claassen J, Hirsch LJ, Frontera JA, et al. Prognostic significance of continuous EEG monitoring in patients with poor-grade subarachnoid hemorrhage. Neurocrit Care 2006;4(2):103–12.

30. Bonow RH, Young CC, Bass DI, et al. Transcranial Doppler ultrasonography in neurological surgery and neurocritical care. Neurosurg Focus 2019;47(6):E2.

31. Greenberg ED, Gobin YP, Riina H, et al. Role of CT perfusion imaging in the diagnosis and treatment of vasospasm. Imaging Med 2011;3(3):287–97.

32. Pickard JD, Murray GD, Illingworth R, et al. Effect of oral nimodipine on cerebral infarction and outcome after subarachnoid haemorrhage: British aneurysm nimodipine trial. BMJ 1989;298(6674):636–42.

33. Petruk KC, West M, Mohr G, et al. Nimodipine treatment in poor-grade aneurysm patients. Results of a multicenter double-blind placebo-controlled trial. J Neurosurg 1988;68(4):505–17.

34. Lakhal K, Hivert A, Alexandre PL, et al. Intravenous milrinone for cerebral vasospasm in subarachnoid hemorrhage: the MILRISPASM controlled Before-after study. Neurocrit Care 2021;35(3):669–79.

35. Santos-Teles AG, Ramalho C, Ramos JGR, et al. Efficacy and safety of milrinone in the treatment of cerebral vasospasm after subarachnoid hemorrhage: a systematic review. Rev Bras Ter Intensiva 2020;32(4):592–602. Eficacia e seguranca da milrinona no tratamento do vasoespasmo cerebral apos hemorragia subaracnoidea: uma revisao sistematica.

36. Sadan O, Waddel H, Moore R, et al. Does intrathecal nicardipine for cerebral vasospasm following subarachnoid hemorrhage correlate with reduced delayed cerebral ischemia? A retrospective propensity score-based analysis. J Neurosurg 2022;136(1):115–24.

37. Virani SS, Alonso A, Benjamin EJ, et al. Heart disease and stroke statistics-2020 update: a report from the American heart association. Circulation 2020;141(9): e139–596.

38. Javalkar V, Kuybu O, Davis D, et al. Factors associated with inpatient mortality after intracerebral hemorrhage: updated information from the United States nationwide inpatient sample. J Stroke Cerebrovasc Dis 2020;29(3):104583.

39. Zia E, Hedblad B, Pessah-Rasmussen H, et al. Blood pressure in relation to the incidence of cerebral infarction and intracerebral hemorrhage. Hypertensive hemorrhage: debated nomenclature is still relevant. Stroke 2007;38(10):2681–5.

40. Vedicherla SV, Foo AS, Sharma VK, et al. The "Blush" sign on computed tomography angiography is an independent predictor of hematoma progression in primary hypertensive hemorrhage. J Stroke Cerebrovasc Dis 2018;27(7):1878–84.

41. van Asch CJ, Luitse MJ, Rinkel GJ, et al. Incidence, case fatality, and functional outcome of intracerebral haemorrhage over time, according to age, sex, and ethnic origin: a systematic review and meta-analysis. Lancet Neurol 2010;9(2): 167–76.

42. Pezzini A, Grassi M, Paciaroni M, et al. Obesity and the risk of intracerebral hemorrhage: the multicenter study on cerebral hemorrhage in Italy. Stroke 2013;44(6): 1584–9.

43. Larsson SC, Wallin A, Wolk A, et al. Differing association of alcohol consumption with different stroke types: a systematic review and meta-analysis. BMC Med 2016;14(1):178.

44. Wada R, Aviv RI, Fox AJ, et al. CT angiography "spot sign" predicts hematoma expansion in acute intracerebral hemorrhage. Stroke 2007;38(4):1257–62.

45. Morotti A, Arba F, Boulouis G, et al. Noncontrast CT markers of intracerebral hemorrhage expansion and poor outcome: a meta-analysis. Neurology 2020;95(14): 632–43.

46. Hemphill JC 3rd, Greenberg SM, Anderson CS, et al. Guidelines for the management of spontaneous intracerebral hemorrhage: a guideline for healthcare professionals from the American heart association/American stroke association. Stroke 2015;46(7):2032–60.

47. Chan E, Anderson CS, Wang X, et al. Significance of intraventricular hemorrhage in acute intracerebral hemorrhage: intensive blood pressure reduction in acute cerebral hemorrhage trial results. Stroke 2015;46(3):653–8.

48. Broderick JP, Brott TG, Tomsick T, et al. Ultra-early evaluation of intracerebral hemorrhage. J Neurosurg 1990;72(2):195–9.

49. Anderson CS, Heeley E, Huang Y, et al. Rapid blood-pressure lowering in patients with acute intracerebral hemorrhage. N Engl J Med 2013;368(25):2355–65.

50. Qureshi AI, Palesch YY, Barsan WG, et al. Intensive blood-pressure lowering in patients with acute cerebral hemorrhage. N Engl J Med 2016;375(11):1033–43.

51. Moullaali TJ, Wang X, Martin RH, et al. Blood pressure control and clinical outcomes in acute intracerebral haemorrhage: a preplanned pooled analysis of individual participant data. Lancet Neurol 2019;18(9):857–64.

52. Boulouis G, Morotti A, Goldstein JN, et al. Intensive blood pressure lowering in patients with acute intracerebral haemorrhage: clinical outcomes and haemorrhage expansion. Systematic review and meta-analysis of randomised trials. J Neurol Neurosurg Psychiatry 2017;88(4):339–45.

53. Qureshi AI, Huang W, Lobanova I, et al. Outcomes of intensive systolic blood pressure reduction in patients with intracerebral hemorrhage and Excessively high initial systolic blood pressure: post hoc analysis of a randomized clinical trial. JAMA Neurol 2020;77(11):1355–65.
54. Chung PW, Kim JT, Sanossian N, et al. Association between Hyperacute stage blood pressure variability and outcome in patients with spontaneous intracerebral hemorrhage. Stroke 2018;49(2):348–54.
55. Frontera JA, Lewin JJ 3rd, Rabinstein AA, et al. Guideline for reversal of antithrombotics in intracranial hemorrhage: a statement for healthcare professionals from the neurocritical care society and society of Critical care medicine. Neurocrit Care 2016;24(1):6–46.
56. Sarode R, Milling TJ Jr, Refaai MA, et al. Efficacy and safety of a 4-factor prothrombin complex concentrate in patients on vitamin K antagonists presenting with major bleeding: a randomized, plasma-controlled, phase IIIb study. Circulation 2013;128(11):1234–43.
57. Steiner T, Poli S, Griebe M, et al. Fresh frozen plasma versus prothrombin complex concentrate in patients with intracranial haemorrhage related to vitamin K antagonists (INCH): a randomised trial. Lancet Neurol 2016;15(6):566–73.
58. Baharoglu MI, Cordonnier C, Al-Shahi Salman R, et al. Platelet transfusion versus standard care after acute stroke due to spontaneous cerebral haemorrhage associated with antiplatelet therapy (PATCH): a randomised, open-label, phase 3 trial. Lancet 2016;387(10038):2605–13.
59. Shi K, Tian DC, Li ZG, et al. Global brain inflammation in stroke. Lancet Neurol 2019;18(11):1058–66.
60. Mendelow AD, Gregson BA, Rowan EN, et al. Early surgery versus initial conservative treatment in patients with spontaneous supratentorial lobar intracerebral haematomas (STICH II): a randomised trial. Lancet 2013;382(9890):397–408.
61. Hanley DF, Thompson RE, Rosenblum M, et al. Efficacy and safety of minimally invasive surgery with thrombolysis in intracerebral haemorrhage evacuation (MISTIE III): a randomised, controlled, open-label, blinded endpoint phase 3 trial. Lancet 2019;393(10175):1021–32.
62. Hannah TC, Kellner R, Kellner CP. Minimally invasive intracerebral hemorrhage evacuation techniques: a review. Diagnostics (Basel) 2021;11(3). https://doi.org/10.3390/diagnostics11030576.
63. Kuramatsu JB, Biffi A, Gerner ST, et al. Association of surgical hematoma evacuation vs conservative treatment with functional outcome in patients with cerebellar intracerebral hemorrhage. JAMA 2019;322(14):1392–403.
64. Grotta JC, Yamal JM, Parker SA, et al. Prospective, multicenter, controlled trial of mobile stroke units. N Engl J Med 2021;385(11):971–81.
65. Cooley SR, Zhao H, Campbell BCV, et al. Mobile stroke units Facilitate prehospital management of intracerebral hemorrhage. Stroke 2021;52(10):3163–6.

Status Epilepticus
A Neurologic Emergency

Patrick J. Coppler, PA-C[a], Jonathan Elmer, MD, MS[a,b,c,]*

KEYWORDS

- Status epilepticus • Seizure • Electroencephalography • Antiseizure drugs
- Brain injury • Neurocritical care

KEY POINTS

- Status epilepticus is a common neurologic emergency defined as abnormal, prolonged seizures lasting greater than 5 to 10 minutes, or recurrent seizure activity without recovery to the patient's baseline mental status.
- First-line treatment of status epilepticus is benzodiazepines, with multiple second-line agents available.
- Refractory and super refractory status epilepticus are defined as continued seizure activity despite administration of appropriate doses of initial and second-line therapies and medication-refractory seizure activity lasting longer than 24 hours, respectively.
- Many conditions can cause new onset status epilepticus, mandating a broad diagnostic evaluation.

INTRODUCTION

Status epilepticus (SE) is a life-threatening emergency requiring rapid treatment and diagnostic evaluation. Initial interventions include administration of medications to terminate seizures, early empiric management of presumed causes, cardiopulmonary monitoring, and potentially mechanical ventilation and other organ support. In the United States, SE develops most commonly in outpatients and is initially encountered by prehospital and emergency providers. Inpatients may also develop SE (either convulsive or nonconvulsive) as a complication of acute illness with or without a primary neurologic injury. Diagnosis requires a high index of suspicion and electroencephalography (EEG) monitoring.

[a] Department of Emergency Medicine, University of Pittsburgh, Iroquois Building, Suite 400A, 3600 Forbes Avenue, Pittsburgh, PA 15213, USA; [b] Department of Critical Care Medicine, University of Pittsburgh, Iroquois Building, Suite 400A, 3600 Forbes Avenue, Pittsburgh, PA 15213, USA; [c] Department of Neurology, University of Pittsburgh, Iroquois Building, Suite 400A, 3600 Forbes Avenue, Pittsburgh, PA 15213, USA
* Corresponding author. Iroquois Building, Suite 400A, 3600 Forbes Avenue, Pittsburgh, PA 15213.
E-mail address: elmerjp@upmc.edu

Crit Care Clin 39 (2023) 87–102
https://doi.org/10.1016/j.ccc.2022.07.006
criticalcare.theclinics.com
0749-0704/23/© 2022 Elsevier Inc. All rights reserved.

Here, we provide an overview of SE pathophysiology, diagnostic criteria, treatments, etiologies, and specific considerations based on underlying cause. We focus on several patient populations with unique clinical considerations including undifferentiated intensive care unit (ICU) patients, patients with acute brain injury, toxicity, autoimmune conditions, pediatrics, and pregnancy.

PATHOPHYSIOLOGY AND CRITERIA

Seizures are abrupt, synchronous, and pathologic depolarizations of cortical neurons that can affect a single region (focal) or the entire brain (generalized). Manifestations of focal seizures vary based on the function of affected cortex and include decreased level of consciousness, visual changes, automatisms, and tonic-clonic movements.[1] Nonconvulsive seizures (NCS) may have subtle clinical findings. NCS and nonconvulsive status epilepticus (NCSE) are more common with a history of epilepsy, persistent altered mental status, and acute brain injury.[2] Most seizures are self-terminating because of protective cellular, local, and remote network mechanisms.[3] Failure of these mechanisms marks a critical transition where neuronal inflammation, blood–brain barrier dysfunction, endocytosis of drug-sensitive gamma-aminobutyric acid (GABA) subunits, and shuttling of alpha-amino-3-hydroxy-5-methyl-4-isoxazolepropionic acid (AMPA) and N-methyl-D-aspartic acid (NMDA) receptors toward the synapse propagate further synchronization and seizure activity.[4] Thus antiseizure drug (ASD) responsiveness decreases over time.[5–7] Seizures longer than 5 minutes are less likely to terminate without ASDs.[8] Brain injury worsens with longer seizure duration, ultimately resulting in cell death.[9]

The International League Against Epilepsy defines SE as abnormally prolonged seizures greater than 5 minutes in the presence of generalized tonic-clonic activity, greater than 10 minutes of focal seizures with impaired consciousness and greater than 10 to 15 minutes of absence seizures.[10] The Neurocritical Care Society defines SE as 5 or more minutes of continuous clinical and/or electrographic seizures, or recurrent seizure without recovery to baseline.[11] The American Clinical Neurophysiology Society (ACNS) Critical Care EEG Terminology offers standardized definitions of electrographic and electroclinical SE.[12]

EPIDEMIOLOGY

The reported incidence of SE in the United States has increased from 3.5 to 41 per 100,000 during the past 35 years.[13] Increased awareness, availability of EEG monitoring, and better long-term survival of patients with chronic conditions that predispose to seizure are contributing factors. SE presents a significant financial and logistical burden to the health-care system. The average length of stay for SE is 2 weeks, whereas for refractory-(RSE) and super-refractory status epilepticus (SRSE), the average length of stay is weeks to months.[14,15] Mortality estimates vary based on underlying cause.[16] Multiorgan failure, preexisting functional dependence, advanced age, and resistance to treatment predict worse outcomes.[17] Withdrawal of life-sustaining therapies for perceived poor prognosis is a significant contributor to mortality.[18] Among long-term survivors, risk of recurrent SE maybe as high as 55%.[19]

INITIAL TREATMENT

Protocols for SE treatment should exist for hospitals or health-care systems. **Fig. 1** is a modified version of our local protocol. Benzodiazepines are the recommended initial

A

**Initial evaluation and management:
Confirmed or suspected status epilepticus**

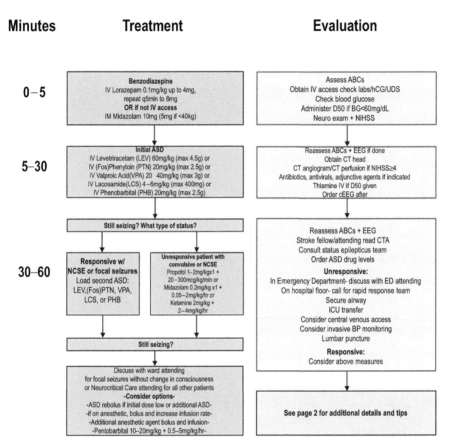

Minutes	Treatment	Evaluation

0–5

Treatment:
Benzodiazepine
IV Lorazepam 0.1mg/kg up to 4mg,
repeat q5min to 8mg
OR if not IV access
IM Midazolam 10mg (5mg if <40kg)

Evaluation:
Assess ABCs
Obtain IV access check labs/hCG/UDS
Check blood glucose
Administer D50 if BG<60mg/dL
Neuro exam + NIHSS

5–30

Treatment:
Initial ASD
IV Levetiracetam (LEV) 60mg/kg (max 4.5g) or
IV (Fos)Phenytoin (PTN) 20mg/kg (max 2.5g) or
IV Valproic Acid(VPA) 20 40mg/kg (max 3g) or
IV Lacosamide(LCS) 4–6mg/kg (max 400mg) or
IV Phenobarbital (PHB) 20mg/kg (max 2.5g)

Evaluation:
Reassess ABCs + EEG if done
Obtain CT head
CT angiogram/CT perfusion if NIHSS≥4
Antibiotics, antivirals, adjunctive agents if indicated
Thiamine IV if D50 given
Order cEEG after

Still seizing? What type of status?

30–60

**Responsive w/
NCSE or focal seizures**
Load second ASD:
LEV,(Fos)PTN, VPA,
LCS, or PHB

**Unresponsive patient with
convulsive or NCSE**
Propofol 1–2mg/kgx1 +
20–300mcg/kg/min or
Midazolam 0.2mg/kg x1 +
0.05–2mg/kg/hr or
Ketamine 2mg/kg +
2–4mg/kg/hr

Evaluation:
Reassess ABCs + EEG
Stroke fellow/attending read CTA
Consult status epilepticus team
Order ASD drug levels
Unresponsive:
In Emergency Department- discuss with ED attending
On hospital floor- call for rapid response team
Secure airway
ICU transfer
Consider central venous access
Consider invasive BP monitoring
Lumbar puncture
Responsive:
Consider above measures

Still seizing?

Discuss with ward attending
for focal seizures without change in consciousness
or Neurocritical Care attending for all other patients
-Consider options-
-ASD rebolus if initial dose low or additional ASD-
-if on anesthetic, bolus and increase infusion rate-
-Additional anesthetic agent bolus and infusion-
-Pentobarbital 10–20mg/kg + 0.5–5mg/kg/hr-

See page 2 for additional details and tips

Fig. 1. (*A*) Example status epilepticus treatment and diagnosis protocol and (*B*) additional helpful references. (Created with Biorender.com.)

abortive therapy.[11,20] In the Veterans Affairs cooperative trial, lorazepam (LZP) was equivalent to both phenobarbital (PHB) and diazepam (DZP) followed by phenytoin (PHT), and more efficacious than PHT alone, in achieving clinical and/or electrographic seizure control within 20 minutes and no recurrent activity within 60 minutes of treatment. LZP administration was faster than other treatment arms. Regardless of therapy, successful seizure termination occurred in two-thirds of subjects.[21]

When adult patients with greater than 5 minutes of continuous seizure activity in the prehospital setting received either 2 mg intravenous (IV) LZP, 5 mg IV DZP, or placebo, with the option for second dose if needed, SE terminated before emergency department arrival in 59%, 42%, and 21% of patients, respectively.[6] Moreover, administration of 10 mg of intramuscular midazolam (MDZ) is noninferior to 4 mg IV LZP.[22] Subtherapeutic dosing of benzodiazepines is common and associated with treatment

B

> **Additional considerations**
> This protocol is not intended for the management of simple partial status
>
> Some types of post-anoxic myoclonus (myoclonic status epilepticus) do not benefit from treatment with this protocol, discuss with Neurocritical Care attending or Post Cardiac Arrest Service

> **Initial ASD selection**
> Prefer home ASD if epilepsy with noncompliance
> LEV 1st choice if: stocked on floor (i.e. immediately available); liver disease; pregnancy
> VPA 1st choice if: renal disease, myoclonic status, absence status
> (Fos)PTN preferred to PTN if available (less infusion-associated hypotension)
> Prefer to avoid combination VPA + (Fos)PTN
>
> **Common acute adverse drug effects**
> (Fos)PHT: hypotension, cardiac arrhythmias, somnolence
> VPA: hyperammonemia, hepatotoxicity, thrombocytopenia, teratogenic
> LCS: AV block, bradycardia, hypotension

> **Empiric antibiotics, antivirals, and adjunctive agents**
> Vancomycin 25mg/kg x1 (max 2.5g)
> Ceftriaxone 2g x1
> Acyclovir 10mg/kg x1
> Ampicillin 2g x1 if >50y/o or immunocompromised
> Penicillin allergic patients: Bactrim 5mg/kg IV + aztreonam 2g IVx1
> Pyridoxine 25mg/kg 5g max dose. If isoniazid toxicity suspected, 1g per 1g of isoniazid ingested
> Thiamine 100–500mg IV

> **Other diagnostic pointers**
> A history, past medical history, medication list, physical examination and review of basic labs should be obtained before calling the Neurocritical Care attending
>
> If possible, discuss cases with senior resident, however, care should not delayed
>
> Review CT head neck angiogram imaging with stroke fellow/attending. If patient has a contrast allergy, dicuss imaging options with stroke fellow/attending. Defer brain imaging until convulsive activity controlled Defer lumbar puncture if CT has mass effect
>
> If continuous EEG is ordered, call the EEG techs to get monitor to bedside
>
> Be suspicious of ongoing non-convulsive status if patient dose not return to baseline after seizure
>
> Draw at least 10mL of CSF on LP. Consider sending cells, protein, glucose, bacterial culture, fungal culture, viral PCRs (HSV 1/2, VZV, EBV, CMV), and in certain cases autoimmune panel (send out testing)

Fig. 1. (*continued*)

failure and progression to RSE.[23–26] Although respiratory compromise is a concern, a trend toward fewer respiratory complications with adequate dosing is reported.[27]

SECOND-LINE INTERMITTENT ANTISEIZURE DRUGS

Second-line ASDs are administered to all SE patients regardless of benzodiazepine response to prevent seizure recurrence. Options include PHT, valproic acid (VPA), levetiracetam (LEV), PHB, or lacosamide (LCS). The Established Status Epilepticus Treatment Trial (ESETT) was the largest randomized trial of PHT, VPA, and LEV for adults and children with benzodiazepine-refractory SE.[28] The trial was stopped early for equivalence, with no difference in primary outcome of cessation of seizures and improving mental status within 60 minutes of medication administration, or safety profile. LCS has similar efficacy compared with PHT, although it has been tested in fewer patients.[29] In a recent meta-analysis, PHB was the most effective second-line ASD,

Table 1
Considerations for choosing an anesthetic infusion

Anesthetic Infusion	Considerations
Midazolam	• Favorable hemodynamic profile[115] • Tachyphylaxis with infusions >24–48 h[116] • May deposit into adipose, cause prolonged sedation[116]
Propofol	• Rapid drug clearance • May cause dose dependent hypotension, myocardial depression • Propofol infusion syndrome (PRIS) with extended use and in children
Ketamine	• N-methyl-ᴅ-aspartate (NMDA) blockade is unique mechanism compared with other anesthetic options • Favorable hemodynamic profile and intracranial hypertension concerns not observed in contemporary work[117] • Unclear half-life in high dose, prolonged infusions • Less studies compared with other agents
Pentobarbital	• Reserved for cases where other anesthetic options fail to control seizures • Prolonged half-life in adults[118] • Cardiac depression, bone marrow suppression, ileus[119,120]

Data from Refs.[115–120]

followed by VPA, LCS, LEV, and finally PHT. However, the most cost-effective was LEV, followed by VPA, then PHB. Neither LSC, nor PHT were cost-effective.[30] Our practice is to administer the medication that is most rapidly available with secondary consideration of potential adverse effect profiles, drug–drug interactions, and past medical history.

REFRACTORY STATUS EPILEPTICUS

Seizures that continue after adequate doses of first-line and second-line ASDs are deemed RSE. Based on expert opinion, guidelines suggest intubation and seizure

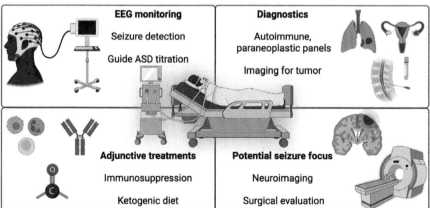

Special considerations for refractory and super refractory status epilepticus

EEG monitoring
Seizure detection
Guide ASD titration

Diagnostics
Autoimmune, paraneoplastic panels
Imaging for tumor

Adjunctive treatments
Immunosuppression
Ketogenic diet

Potential seizure focus
Neuroimaging
Surgical evaluation

Fig. 2. Failure of conventional antiseizure drugs should prompt additional workup and treatment. (Created with Biorender.com.)

suppression with anesthetics for SE continuing 20 to 60 minutes after loading a second-line ASD. Several medications are effective in this setting, with little data available to guide optimal choice (**Table 1**). EEG monitoring is needed to detect ongoing NCS and to guide titration of anesthetic infusions to effect, with options for seizure control, burst suppression, or isoelectric suppression.[31] Loading a third ASD before considering intubation may be reasonable in patients with advanced directives limiting aggressive care, when there is clinical suspicion for a rapidly reversible cause such as hypoglycemia, or ASD noncompliance.

Super Refractory Status Epilepticus

Patients who continue to seize for greater than 24 hours despite stepwise escalation of therapies qualify as SRSE. Evidence-based treatments of SRSE are limited to case reports and series (**Fig. 2**). Both those with known history of epilepsy and new-onset refractory status epilepticus (NORSE) require special consideration in their diagnostic evaluation. Combinations of mechanistically distinct ASDs may provide synergism. Ketogenic diet shifts neurons from glucose to lipid metabolism and has antiseizure effects. Data for use of ketogenic parenteral nutrition in SRSE are limited but present a promising area for future studies.[32] Inhaled anesthetics are an option when feasible.[33] Therapeutic hypothermia (32°C–34°C) for 24 hours decreased the incidence of EEG confirmed SE without benefit to 90-day mortality and had a higher incidence of adverse events.[34] Brain MRI or ictal single photon emission computed tomography may identify lesions amenable to surgery.[35] Empiric immune therapy for suspicion for autoimmune conditions is recommended. Treatment within 30 days of onset is associated with better functional status.[36] Options include high-dose corticosteroids, intravenous immunoglobulins, plasma exchange, rituximab, or cyclophosphamide.[37] Devices such as vagal nerve stimulators, responsive neurostimulation systems, transcranial magnetic stimulators, and electroconvulsive therapy have had some effect in case series but little randomized data.[38]

DIAGNOSTIC EVALUATION

Many acute and chronic medical conditions can cause SE. The initial diagnostic workup is broad and occurs in parallel with stabilization and ASD administration (**Fig. 1**). Patients with potential SE require continuous telemetry and pulse oximetry, as well as close serial airway assessments. Capillary blood glucose should be measured immediately and hypoglycemia corrected. Vascular access should be obtained urgently to facilitate administration of ASDs and obtain bloodwork. A comprehensive metabolic panel will identify common metabolic derangements. Urine toxicology for all and beta-hCG in women of childbearing age is standard. ASD levels may be drawn for concerns of nonadherence but should not delay treatment.

Physical examination should screen for findings suggestive of acute traumatic brain injury (TBI), stroke, or other intracranial cause of seizures. Urgent noncontrast head CT is pursued in all patients unless rapid return to baseline occurs in combination with a nonfocal examination and known history of epilepsy. CT angiography of the head and neck is considered for new focal neurologic deficits or persistent coma because acute ischemic stroke (AIS) may mimic or precipitate seizure.[39–41] Lumbar puncture is indicated when history suggests infection, or for new onset or unprovoked seizure. Cerebrospinal fluid (CSF) analysis of at minimum cell counts, glucose, protein, Gram stain and culture, and herpes simplex PCR assay is recommended. Additional CSF is often obtained for diagnosis of autoimmune, paraneoplastic or other viral encephalitides.[37] Antibiotics and antivirals should be administered without delay to avoid poor outcomes.[42] Finally, SE with obvious clinical manifestations often evolves into NCSE. Apparent resolution of clinical seizures in the absence of return to neurologic baseline should be treated as NCSE until proven otherwise with EEG monitoring.[43]

The need for more comprehensive diagnostic evaluation is guided by treatment responsiveness and presumed cause of seizures. For patients who return to baseline cognition after benzodiazepine administration and for whom history suggests a clear cause (eg, alcohol withdrawal seizures, epilepsy with ASD nonadherence, or hypoglycemia), routine bloodwork and telemetry monitoring may suffice.

When risk for SE is high, continuous EEG (cEEG) monitoring is preferred over intermittent EEG. cEEG reaches 95% sensitivity for seizure detection at 72 hours of monitoring, reduces time to diagnosis, and affords safe medication titration.[44–47] Initial characteristics of background and presence of epileptiform features may aid in triaging need for cEEG when resources are limited. Negative history of seizures and generalized slowing without epileptiform features are associated with low risk of seizures during extended monitoring. In contrast, epileptiform discharges or burst suppression on initial EEG have greater than 30% incidence of seizures on cEEG.[48]

SPECIFIC POPULATIONS
General Intensive Care Unit Patients

Patients with SE are at high risk for complications in the ICU due to prolonged critical illness, mechanical ventilation, seizure etiology, and ASD toxicities.[49,50] Immobility increases the incidence of decubitus ulcers, deep vein thrombosis, and nosocomial infections. Aggressive pulmonary toilet may mitigate atelectasis, mucous plugging, and pneumonia. Ileus is common and should be suspected in constipation and increased gastric residual volumes.[51] ASDs have numerous potential adverse effects. Drug–drug interactions can alter levels of ASDs or other medications; a single dose of a carbapenem may rapidly reduce VPA concentration to undetectable serum levels.[52] Optimal management of patients with RSE and SRSE is best achieved through a multidisciplinary team with neurocritical care and pharmacologic expertise.

SE may also result from general critical illness. Systemic inflammation in sepsis decreases seizure threshold and carries a seizure incidence of 10% to 20%.[53–55] Risk factors include severity of illness and past neurologic diagnosis.[56] Beta-lactam antibiotics competitively inhibit GABA receptors in a dose-dependent fashion, thus increasing seizure risk.[57] Although cefepime neurotoxicity is most reported, other cephalosporins with good central nervous system penetration such as ceftriaxone and ceftazidime also demonstrate neurotoxicity.[58] Evolving renal or hepatic injury may increase drug levels and exacerbate neurotoxicity.

STATUS EPILEPTICUS COMPLICATING ACQUIRED BRAIN INJURY
Ischemic and Hemorrhagic Strokes

Both hemorrhagic and ischemic strokes can be complicated by seizures. In intraparenchymal and subarachnoid hemorrhage, blood acts as a cortical irritant.[59] After AIS, metabolic failure, tissue hypoxia, and reperfusion injury can precipitate seizures. NCS are common, occurring in 3% in AIS to 13% in aneurysmal subarachnoid hemorrhage.[60,61] Seizure should be considered in stroke patients with unexpectedly poor (ie, out of proportion to imaging findings), fluctuating, or suddenly worsening neurologic examination.[62] Hemorrhagic conversion, rebleeding, and delayed cerebral ischemia/vasospasm are all potential causes of seizures and SE.

Traumatic Brain Injury

Severe TBI frequently leads to NCS and SE, with intracranial hemorrhage and penetrating injury significantly increasing seizure risk.[63] Seizures may precipitate metabolic and/or intracranial pressure crises in TBI patients, so cEEG monitoring is critical.[64]

Hypoxic Ischemic Brain Injury

Up to half of comatose postcardiac arrest patients have epileptiform EEG findings.[65,66] Incidence of seizures and SE maybe as high as 30% and 12%, respectively,[67,68] although variability in monitoring strategies and nomenclature exist.[45,47] EEG patterns that represent treatable epileptiform events versus secondary manifestations of severe brain injury are controversial. Burst suppression with identical bursts in time step lock with myoclonus meets criteria for electroclinical seizures, often does not respond to conventional ASDs, and is associated with diffuse cortical and subcortical necrosis on autopsy.[66,69] Treating seizures is recommended although aggressive treatment of periodic or rhythmic patterns that do not meet ACNS seizure criteria does not improve outcome.[70] Choice of ASD agent is driven by cardiac, hemodynamic, and other organ failure considerations.

Autoimmune Causes

Patients who present with SRSE, NORSE, or febrile infection-related epilepsy syndrome (seizure onset within 2 weeks of febrile illness, FIRES) warrant specific consideration of immunologic causes. Approximately 50% of NORSE or FIRES cases are autoimmune or paraneoplastic in etiology.[71] Early neurocritical care and neuroimmunology consultation is advised.[72] Whole-body cross-sectional imaging and transvaginal ultrasound may reveal immune active teratomas amenable to surgical resection or malignant source of paraneoplastic syndrome. Targeted immune therapies including anakinra and tocilizumab have been studied in small case series but no randomized controlled trials (RCTs) have been performed to date.[73,74] Patients with cancer often present with or develop altered mental status during hospitalization.[75] Although the differential is broad, SE is a potential cause. Checkpoint inhibitors and chimeric antigen receptor T cell therapy in particular are epileptogenic.[76,77]

Toxicologic

Seizures related to toxidromes may be overdose or withdrawal induced[78] from either abnormal excitation or loss of inhibition. Alcohol withdrawal is the most common toxicologic cause.[79] Consistent alcohol use modulates density of numerous neuronal ion channels, including upregulation of $GABA_a$ and glycine and inhibition of NMDA receptors.[80,81] Cessation of alcohol without medications or doses insufficient to maintain sufficient GABAergic tone results in excitotoxicity.

Clinical trials have focused on alcohol withdrawal syndrome and symptom management rather than seizures. A single RCT found PHT no better than placebo for seizure control.[82] Benzodiazepines are again recommended as initial therapy. Mechanistically, PHB and ketamine are attractive alternative agents for patients who fail initial benzodiazepine therapy or require escalating doses. In addition to GABAa agonism, PHB inhibits excitatory AMPA and Kainate receptors. Moreover, PHB's long half-life affords ease of titration and autotapering for prolonged control. Compared with benzodiazepines and barbiturates, ketamine binds to multiple sites of NMDA receptors that are inhibited in chronic alcoholism. Dexmedetomidine has gained popularity for autonomic symptom management but has no antiseizure properties.[83]

Bupropion is an antidepressant favored for being weight-neutral and aiding in smoking cessation. Chemically, bupropion decreases reuptake of dopamine and norepinephrine from synapses, which may cause uninhibited postsynaptic excitation.[84] Selective serotonin reuptake inhibitors and selective norepinephrine reuptake inhibitors have similar mechanisms and have minimal risk of seizures except in overdose situations.[85] Baclofen is a synthetic GABA agonist, and withdrawal or overdose may lead to seizure, the latter through presynaptic inhibition and subsequent postsynaptic disinhibition.[86,87] Baclofen toxicity must be considered in patients with in situ intrathecal drug delivery systems.[88] Pyridoxine is a cofactor critical for GABA synthesis, and deficiencies can occur with chronic isoniazid use or overdose,[89] malnutrition or marasmus,[90] Gyromitra esculenta ingestion,[91] and hydrazine exposure.[92] Early empiric pyridoxine is indicated when suspicion of deficiency exists. Apart from pyridoxine indications and thiamine administration in alcoholics, seizures related to intoxication or withdrawal is preferentially managed with GABAergic agents. Little data are available regarding second line agents in this population.[93]

Pediatrics

The initial treatment of pediatric patients presenting with SE is similar to that of adults. Benzodiazepines remain first-line treatment. In patients without intravenous access, intranasal MDZ is more efficacious than rectal DZP.[94] There is no clearly preferred second-line ASD in children. PHT and LEV were equally effective in 2 large RCTs.[95,96] In pediatric patients, no treatment arm was superior in the ESETT trial.[97] VPA is avoided in children with mitochondrial hepatopathies because a single dose can precipitate fulminant liver failure.[98] Pyridoxine-dependent epilepsy is rare but an important cause of pediatric SE; supplementation is recommended when second-line ASDs fail.[99] Propofol is avoided given risk of propofol infusion syndrome and potential fatal reactions in children. MDZ and PHB are preferred third-line ASDs. Ketamine is under active investigation but not yet guideline-recommended.[100,101]

Pregnancy

Preeclampsia is a syndrome of hypertension, proteinuria, and headache after 20-week gestation.[102] Eclampsia is the new onset of generalized seizure in the setting of preeclampsia, and the most common cause of SE in pregnancy.[103] It is a clinical diagnosis that has been reported up to 23 days postpartum.[104] IV magnesium is standard of care for prophylaxis and treatment of eclamptic seizures,[105–107] and neuroimaging is indicated in patients unresponsive to initial treatments. Eclamptic seizures may share pathogenesis with posterior reversible encephalopathy syndrome, where inflammation, hypertension, and deranged cerebrovascular autoregulation contribute to blood–brain barrier permeability, vasospasm, and vasogenic edema.[108,109]

Alterations in cardiac output, renal perfusion, volume of distribution, and serum protein levels in pregnancy affect ASD pharmacokinetics.[110] However, similar rates of breakthrough seizure are reported in pregnant versus nonpregnant patients with epilepsy.[111] Closer monitoring of serum drug levels is recommended.[112] Lamotrigine, LEV, and oxcarbazepine seem to have similar teratogenicity to controls, whereas carbamazepine and VPA at any dose are associated with congenital anomalies.[113] Apart from magnesium for eclampsia, there are no RCTs specific to SE in pregnancy. ASD choice is influenced by gestational age, prior ASD use, and potential adverse effects in consultation with epileptology and maternal and fetal medicine specialists.[114]

SUMMARY

SE is encountered as a presenting illness, complication of various primary brain injuries, and many seemingly nonneurological illnesses. Although expert consultation is recommended, all providers should be versed in the identification, evaluation, and early treatment of seizures to prevent time-dependent treatment resistance. A high index of suspicion, prompt diagnosis, and treatment targeted to specific causes contribute to improved outcomes in this complex disease.

CLINICS CARE POINTS

- Benzodiazepines are first-line treatment of status epilepticus. Subtherapeutic dosing of benzodiazepines is common and associated with treatment failure.
- Many second-line antiseizure drugs are available. Our practice is to administer the agent that is most rapidly available with secondary consideration of potential adverse effect profiles, drug–drug interactions, and past medical history.
- Antiseizure drugs have complex interactions with other antiseizure and commonly used drugs in the intensive care unit. Comanagement with a pharmacist with neurocritical care expertise is vital.
- Seizures refractory to first-line and second-line antiseizure drugs should prompt a broad diagnostic workup and expert consultation.

ACKNOWLEDGMENTS

Dr J. Elmer's research time is supported by the NIH through grant 5K23NS097629. Figures were created with BioRender.com.

DISCLOSURE

None.

REFERENCES

1. Fisher RS, et al. Operational classification of seizure types by the international League against epilepsy: Position Paper of the ILAE Commission for classification and Terminology. Epilepsia 2017;58:522–30.
2. Fountain NB. Status epilepticus: risk factors and complications. Epilepsia 2000; 41(Suppl 2):S23–30.
3. Lado FA, Moshé SL. How do seizures stop? Epilepsia 2008;49:1651–64.
4. Walker MC. Pathophysiology of status epilepticus. Neurosci Lett 2018;667: 84–91.
5. Mazarati AM, et al. Time-dependent decrease in the effectiveness of antiepileptic drugs during the course of self-sustaining status epilepticus. Brain Res 1998;814:179–85.
6. Alldredge BK, et al. A comparison of lorazepam, diazepam, and placebo for the treatment of out-of-hospital status epilepticus. N Engl J Med 2001;345:631–7.
7. Chin RF, et al. Treatment of community-onset, childhood convulsive status epilepticus: a prospective, population-based study. Lancet Neurol 2008;7:696–703.
8. Shinnar S, et al. How long do new-onset seizures in children last? Ann Neurol 2001;49:659–64.

9. Dingledine R, Varvel NH, Dudek FE. When and how do seizures kill neurons, and is cell death relevant to epileptogenesis? Adv Exp Med Biol 2014;813:109–22.

10. Trinka E, et al. A definition and classification of status epilepticus–report of the ILAE Task Force on classification of status epilepticus. Epilepsia 2015;56: 1515–23.

11. Brophy GM, et al. Guidelines for the evaluation and management of status epilepticus. Neurocrit Care 2012;17:3–23.

12. Hirsch LJ, et al. American clinical Neurophysiology Society's standardized critical care EEG Terminology: 2021 version. J Clin Neurophysiol 2021;38:1–29.

13. Dham BS, Hunter K, Rincon F. The epidemiology of status epilepticus in the United States. Neurocrit Care 2014;20:476–83.

14. Guterman EL, et al. Association between treatment progression, disease Refractoriness, and burden of illness among hospitalized patients with status epilepticus. JAMA Neurol 2021;78:588–95.

15. Penberthy LT, et al. Estimating the economic burden of status epilepticus to the health care system. Seizure 2005;14:46–51.

16. Neligan A, Shorvon SD. Frequency and prognosis of convulsive status epilepticus of different causes: a systematic review. Arch Neurol 2010;67:931–40.

17. Kantanen AM, et al. Predictors of hospital and one-year mortality in intensive care patients with refractory status epilepticus: a population-based study. Crit Care 2017;21:71.

18. Hawkes MA, et al. Causes of death in status epilepticus. Crit Care Med 2019;47: 1226–31.

19. Sculier C, et al. Long-term outcomes of status epilepticus: a critical assessment. Epilepsia 2018;59(Suppl 2):155–69.

20. Glauser T, et al. Evidence-based guideline: treatment of convulsive status epilepticus in children and adults: report of the guideline Committee of the American epilepsy Society. Epilepsy Curr 2016;16:48–61.

21. Treiman DM, et al. A comparison of four treatments for generalized convulsive status epilepticus. Veterans Affairs Status Epilepticus Cooperative Study Group. N Engl J Med 1998;339:792–8.

22. Silbergleit R, et al. Intramuscular versus intravenous therapy for prehospital status epilepticus. N Engl J Med 2012;366:591–600.

23. Rao SK, et al. Inadequate benzodiazepine dosing may result in progression to refractory and non-convulsive status epilepticus. Epileptic Disord 2018;20: 265–9.

24. Vasquez A, et al. First-line medication dosing in pediatric refractory status epilepticus. Neurology 2020;95:e2683–96.

25. Sathe AG, et al. Patterns of benzodiazepine underdosing in the established status epilepticus treatment trial. Epilepsia 2021;62:795–806.

26. Gaínza-Lein M, et al. Association of time to treatment with Short-term outcomes for pediatric patients with refractory convulsive status epilepticus. JAMA Neurol 2018;75:410–8.

27. Guterman EL, et al. Prehospital midazolam use and outcomes among patients with out-of-hospital status epilepticus. Neurology 2020;95:e3203–12.

28. Kapur J, et al. Randomized trial of three Anticonvulsant medications for status epilepticus. N Engl J Med 2019;381:2103–13.

29. Panda PK, et al. Efficacy of lacosamide and phenytoin in status epilepticus: a systematic review. Acta Neurol Scand 2021;144:366–74.

30. Sánchez Fernández I, et al. Meta-analysis and cost-effectiveness of second-line antiepileptic drugs for status epilepticus. Neurology 2019;92:e2339–48.

31. Vossler DG, et al. Treatment of refractory convulsive status epilepticus: a comprehensive review by the American epilepsy Society treatments Committee. Epilepsy Curr 2020;20:245–64.

32. Youngson NA, Morris MJ, Ballard JWO. The mechanisms mediating the antiepileptic effects of the ketogenic diet, and potential opportunities for improvement with metabolism-altering drugs. Seizure 2017;52:15–9.

33. Zeiler FA, et al. Modern inhalational anesthetics for refractory status epilepticus. Can J Neurol Sci 2015;42:106–15.

34. Legriel S, et al. Hypothermia for Neuroprotection in convulsive status epilepticus. N Engl J Med 2016;375:2457–67.

35. Basha MM, et al. Acute resective surgery for the treatment of refractory status epilepticus. Neurocrit Care 2017;27:370–80.

36. Nosadini M, et al. Use and safety of Immunotherapeutic management of N-Methyl-d-Aspartate receptor Antibody encephalitis: a meta-analysis. JAMA Neurol 2021;78:1333–44.

37. Abboud H, et al. Autoimmune encephalitis: proposed best practice recommendations for diagnosis and acute management. J Neurol Neurosurg Psychiatry 2021;92:757–68.

38. San-Juan D, et al. Neuromodulation techniques for status epilepticus: a review. Brain Stimul 2019;12:835–44.

39. Kim SJ, et al. Seizure in code stroke: stroke mimic and initial manifestation of stroke. Am J Emerg Med 2019;37:1871–5.

40. Brigo F, Lattanzi S. Poststroke seizures as stroke mimics: clinical assessment and management. Epilepsy Behav 2020;104:106297.

41. Saposnik G, Caplan LR. Convulsive-like movements in brainstem stroke. Arch Neurol 2001;58:654–7.

42. Køster-Rasmussen R, Korshin A, Meyer CN. Antibiotic treatment delay and outcome in acute bacterial meningitis. J Infect 2008;57:449–54.

43. Zehtabchi S, Silbergleit R, Chamberlain JM, Shinnar S, Elm JJ, Underwood E, Rosenthal ES, Bleck TP, Kapur J. Electroencephalographic Seizures in Emergency Department Patients After Treatment for Convulsive Status Epilepticus. J Clin Neurophysiol 2020. https://doi.org/10.1097/WNP.0000000000000800. Publish Ahead of Print.

44. Struck AF, et al. Time-dependent risk of seizures in critically ill patients on continuous electroencephalogram. Ann Neurol 2017;82:177–85.

45. Elmer J, et al. Sensitivity of continuous electroencephalography to detect ictal activity after cardiac arrest. JAMA Netw Open 2020;3:e203751.

46. Newey CR, et al. Continuous electroencephalography in the critically ill: clinical and continuous electroencephalography Markers for targeted monitoring. J Clin Neurophysiol 2018;35:325–31.

47. Rossetti AO, et al. Continuous vs routine electroencephalogram in critically ill adults with altered consciousness and No recent seizure: a Multicenter randomized clinical trial. JAMA Neurol 2020;77:1225–32.

48. Swisher CB, et al. Baseline EEG pattern on continuous ICU EEG monitoring and incidence of seizures. J Clin Neurophysiol 2015;32:147–51.

49. Baumann SM, et al. Frequency and implications of complications in the ICU after status epilepticus: No Calm after the Storm. Crit Care Med 2020;48:1779–89.

50. Hocker S. Systemic complications of status epilepticus–An update. Epilepsy Behav 2015;49:83–7.

51. Kim TJ, et al. Neostigmine for treating acute Colonic Pseudo-Obstruction in neurocritically ill patients. J Clin Neurol 2021;17:563–9.

52. Mori H, Takahashi K, Mizutani T. Interaction between valproic acid and carbapenem antibiotics. Drug Metab Rev 2007;39:647–57.
53. Singer BH, et al. Bacterial dissemination to the brain in sepsis. Am J Respir Crit Care Med 2018;197:747–56.
54. Tauber SC, et al. Sepsis-associated encephalopathy and septic encephalitis: an update. Expert Rev Anti Infect Ther 2021;19:215–31.
55. Semmler A, et al. Sepsis causes neuroinflammation and concomitant decrease of cerebral metabolism. J Neuroinflammation 2008;5:38.
56. Gilmore EJ, et al. Acute brain failure in severe sepsis: a prospective study in the medical intensive care unit utilizing continuous EEG monitoring. Intensive Care Med 2015;41:686–94.
57. Sutter R, Rüegg S, Tschudin-Sutter S. Seizures as adverse events of antibiotic drugs: a systematic review. Neurology 2015;85:1332–41.
58. Payne LE, et al. Cefepime-induced neurotoxicity: a systematic review. Crit Care 2017;21:276.
59. Kress GJ, Dineley KE, Reynolds IJ. The relationship between intracellular free iron and cell injury in cultured neurons, astrocytes, and oligodendrocytes. J Neurosci 2002;22:5848–55.
60. Belcastro V, et al. Non-convulsive status epilepticus after ischemic stroke: a hospital-based stroke cohort study. J Neurol 2014;261:2136–42.
61. Kondziella D, et al. Continuous EEG monitoring in aneurysmal subarachnoid hemorrhage: a systematic review. Neurocrit Care 2015;22:450–61.
62. Herman ST, et al. Consensus statement on continuous EEG in critically ill adults and children, part I: indications. J Clin Neurophysiol 2015;32:87–95.
63. Dhakar MB, et al. A retrospective cross-sectional study of the prevalence of generalized convulsive status epilepticus in traumatic brain injury: United States 2002-2010. Seizure 2015;32:16–22.
64. Vespa PM, et al. Nonconvulsive electrographic seizures after traumatic brain injury result in a delayed, prolonged increase in intracranial pressure and metabolic crisis. Crit Care Med 2007;35:2830–6.
65. Cloostermans MC, et al. Continuous electroencephalography monitoring for early prediction of neurological outcome in postanoxic patients after cardiac arrest: a prospective cohort study. Crit Care Med 2012;40:2867–75.
66. Solanki P, et al. Association of antiepileptic drugs with resolution of epileptiform activity after cardiac arrest. Resuscitation 2019;142:82–90.
67. Lybeck A, et al. Prognostic significance of clinical seizures after cardiac arrest and target temperature management. Resuscitation 2017;114:146–51.
68. Rittenberger JC, et al. Frequency and timing of nonconvulsive status epilepticus in comatose post-cardiac arrest subjects treated with hypothermia. Neurocrit Care 2012;16:114–22.
69. Endisch C, et al. Hypoxic-ischemic encephalopathy evaluated by brain autopsy and Neuroprognostication after cardiac arrest. JAMA Neurol 2020;77:1430–9.
70. Ruijter BJ, et al. Treating rhythmic and periodic EEG patterns in comatose survivors of cardiac arrest. N Engl J Med 2022;386:724–34.
71. Gaspard N, et al. New-onset refractory status epilepticus: etiology, clinical features, and outcome. Neurology 2015;85:1604–13.
72. Sculier C, Gaspard N. New onset refractory status epilepticus (NORSE). Seizure 2019;68:72–8.
73. Lai YC, et al. Anakinra usage in febrile infection related epilepsy syndrome: an international cohort. Ann Clin Transl Neurol 2020;7:2467–74.

74. Jun JS, et al. Tocilizumab treatment for new onset refractory status epilepticus. Ann Neurol 2018;84:940–5.
75. Tuma R, DeAngelis LM. Altered mental status in patients with cancer. Arch Neurol 2000;57:1727–31.
76. Nersesjan V, et al. Autoimmune encephalitis related to cancer treatment with immune Checkpoint inhibitors: a systematic review. Neurology 2021;97:e191–202.
77. Santomasso BD, et al. Clinical and Biological Correlates of neurotoxicity associated with CAR T-cell therapy in patients with B-cell acute Lymphoblastic Leukemia. Cancer Discov 2018;8:958–71.
78. Cock HR. Drug-induced status epilepticus. Epilepsy Behav 2015;49:76–82.
79. DeLorenzo RJ, et al. A prospective, population-based epidemiologic study of status epilepticus in Richmond, Virginia. Neurology 1996;46:1029–35.
80. Tran VT, et al. GABA receptors are increased in brains of alcoholics. Ann Neurol Official J Am Neurol Assoc Child Neurol Soc 1981;9:289–92.
81. Hoffman PL, et al. Ethanol and the NMDA receptor. Alcohol 1990;7:229–31.
82. Chance JF. Emergency department treatment of alcohol withdrawal seizures with phenytoin. Ann Emerg Med 1991;20:520–2.
83. Collier TE, et al. Effect of Adjunctive Dexmedetomidine in the treatment of alcohol withdrawal compared to benzodiazepine symptom-Triggered therapy in critically ill patients: the EvADE study. J Pharm Pract 2020. https://doi.org/10.1177/0897190020977755:897190020977755.
84. Landmark CJ, Henning O, Johannessen SI. Proconvulsant effects of antidepressants—what is the current evidence? Epilepsy Behav 2016;61:287–91.
85. Reichert C, et al. Seizures after single-agent overdose with pharmaceutical drugs: analysis of cases reported to a poison center. Clin Toxicol (Phila) 2014;52:629–34.
86. Zak R, et al. Baclofen-induced generalized nonconvulsive status epilepticus. Ann Neurol 1994;36:113–4.
87. Leung NY, Whyte IM, Isbister GK. Baclofen overdose: defining the spectrum of toxicity. Emerg Med Australas 2006;18:77–82.
88. Watve SV, et al. Management of acute overdose or withdrawal state in intrathecal baclofen therapy. Spinal Cord 2012;50:107–11.
89. Alvarez F, Guntupalli K. Isoniazid overdose: four case reports and review of the literature. Intensive Care Med 1995;21:641–4.
90. Spencer PS, Palmer VS. Interrelationships of undernutrition and neurotoxicity: food for thought and research attention. Neurotoxicology 2012;33:605–16.
91. Michelot D, Toth B. Poisoning by Gyromitra esculenta–a review. J Appl Toxicol 1991;11:235–43.
92. Nguyen HN, et al. The toxicity, pathophysiology, and treatment of acute hydrazine propellant exposure: a systematic review. Mil Med 2021;186:e319–26.
93. Fletcher ML, et al. A systematic review of second line therapies in toxic seizures. Clin Toxicol (Phila) 2021;59:451–6.
94. McMullan J, et al. Midazolam versus diazepam for the treatment of status epilepticus in children and young adults: a meta-analysis. Acad Emerg Med 2010;17:575–82.
95. Dalziel SR, et al. Levetiracetam versus phenytoin for second-line treatment of convulsive status epilepticus in children (ConSEPT): an open-label, multicentre, randomised controlled trial. Lancet 2019;393:2135–45.
96. Lyttle MD, et al. Levetiracetam versus phenytoin for second-line treatment of paediatric convulsive status epilepticus (EcLiPSE): a multicentre, open-label, randomised trial. Lancet 2019;393:2125–34.

97. Chamberlain JM, et al. Efficacy of levetiracetam, fosphenytoin, and valproate for established status epilepticus by age group (ESETT): a double-blind, responsive-adaptive, randomised controlled trial. Lancet 2020;395:1217–24.

98. Schwabe MJ, et al. Valproate-induced liver failure in one of two siblings with Alpers disease. Pediatr Neurol 1997;16:337–43.

99. Coughlin CR, et al. Consensus guidelines for the diagnosis and management of pyridoxine-dependent epilepsy due to α-aminoadipic semialdehyde dehydrogenase deficiency. J Inherit Metab Dis 2021;44:178–92.

100. Rosati A, et al. Efficacy and safety of ketamine in refractory status epilepticus in children. Neurology 2012;79:2355–8.

101. Conway JA, et al. Ketamine Use for Tracheal intubation in critically ill children is associated with a lower occurrence of adverse hemodynamic events. Crit Care Med 2020;48:e489–97.

102. Gestational hypertension and preeclampsia: ACOG practice Bulletin, Number 222. Obstet Gynecol 2020;135:e237–60.

103. Rajiv KR, Radhakrishnan A. Status epilepticus in pregnancy: etiology, management, and clinical outcomes. Epilepsy Behav 2017;76:114–9.

104. Sibai BM. Diagnosis, prevention, and management of eclampsia. Obstet Gynecol 2005;105:402–10.

105. Duley L, Henderson-Smart DJ, Chou D. Magnesium sulphate versus phenytoin for eclampsia. Cochrane Database Syst Rev 2010;Cd000128. https://doi.org/10.1002/14651858.CD000128.pub2.

106. Duley L, et al. Magnesium sulphate and other anticonvulsants for women with pre-eclampsia. Cochrane Database Syst Rev 2010;2010:Cd000025.

107. Duley L, et al. Magnesium sulphate versus diazepam for eclampsia. Cochrane Database Syst Rev 2010;2010:Cd000127.

108. Mahendra V, Clark SL, Suresh MS. Neuropathophysiology of preeclampsia and eclampsia: a review of cerebral hemodynamic principles in hypertensive disorders of pregnancy. Pregnancy Hypertens 2021;23:104–11.

109. Rana S, et al. Preeclampsia: pathophysiology, Challenges, and Perspectives. Circ Res 2019;124:1094–112.

110. Tomson T, Landmark CJ, Battino D. Antiepileptic drug treatment in pregnancy: changes in drug disposition and their clinical implications. Epilepsia 2013;54:405–14.

111. Pennell PB, et al. Changes in seizure frequency and antiepileptic therapy during pregnancy. N Engl J Med 2020;383:2547–56.

112. Harden CL, et al. Practice parameter update: management issues for women with epilepsy–focus on pregnancy (an evidence-based review): vitamin K, folic acid, blood levels, and breastfeeding: report of the Quality Standards Subcommittee and Therapeutics and Technology Assessment Subcommittee of the American Academy of Neurology and American Epilepsy Society. Neurology 2009;73:142–9.

113. Tomson T, et al. Comparative risk of major congenital malformations with eight different antiepileptic drugs: a prospective cohort study of the EURAP registry. Lancet Neurol 2018;17:530–8.

114. Rajiv KR, Radhakrishnan A. Status epilepticus in pregnancy - can we frame a uniform treatment protocol? Epilepsy Behav 2019;101:106376.

115. Claassen J, et al. Treatment of refractory status epilepticus with pentobarbital, propofol, or midazolam: a systematic review. Epilepsia 2002;43:146–53.

116. Shafer A. Complications of sedation with midazolam in the intensive care unit and a comparison with other sedative regimens. Crit Care Med 1998;26:947–56.

117. Alkhachroum A, et al. Ketamine to treat super-refractory status epilepticus. Neurology 2020;95:e2286–94.
118. Ehrnebo M. Pharmacokinetics and distribution properties of pentobarbital in humans following oral and intravenous administration. J Pharm Sci 1974;63:1114–8.
119. Stover J, Stocker R. Barbiturate coma may promote reversible bone marrow suppression in patients with severe isolated traumatic brain injury. Eur J Clin Pharmacol 1998;54:529–34.
120. Lander V, et al. Enteral feeding during barbiturate coma. Nutr Clin Pract 1987; 2:56–9.

Neurotrauma and Intracranial Pressure Management

Francis Bernard, MD, FRCPC, FNCS

KEYWORDS

- Intracranial pressure • Traumatic brain injury • Autoregulation
- Cerebral perfusion pressure • Lund therapy • Optimization of care
- Cerebral oxygenation • Multimodality monitoring

KEY POINTS

- Intracranial pressure (ICP) monitoring in traumatic brain injury (TBI) management has many limitations.
- Multimodality monitoring contributes to precision medicine in TBI.
- Understanding physiological mechanisms when managing ICP is critical to administer appropriate treatment.
- Neuroprotection and ICP management are best achieved by maintaining brain homeostasis.

Video content accompanies this article at http://www.criticalcare.theclinics. com.

INTRODUCTION

Historically, monitoring of severe traumatic brain injury (TBI) patients focused on intracranial pressure (ICP) and cerebral perfusion pressure (CPP) to prevent secondary brain injury. Indeed, elevated ICP (eICP) is associated with increase mortality, thus monitoring ICP is viewed as a measure of quality of care and compliance within various guidelines. ICP monitors represent the use of a bundle of care that is collaboratively managed by a multidisciplinary team rather than a simple measurement tool. ICP monitoring has been associated with decreased mortality[1–5] but its impact on functional outcome is less clear. The literature is biased by differences in methodologies, definitions, adjustment for important prognostic factors, and an absence of capacity to assess compliance to best treatment practices.[1] The relationship between ICP and outcome is summarized elsewhere.[1,6]

The author has nothing to disclose.
Critical Care, Department of Medicine, Hôpital du Sacré-Cœur de Montréal, University of Montréal, 5400 Boulevard Gouin Ouest, Montréal, Québec H4J 1C5, Canada
E-mail address: bernard.francis@gmail.com

Crit Care Clin 39 (2023) 103–121
https://doi.org/10.1016/j.ccc.2022.08.002
0749-0704/23/Crown Copyright © 2022 Published by Elsevier Inc. All rights reserved.

The only randomized controlled trial comparing ICP-driven versus clinical management based on imaging and physical examination (BEST-TRIP trial) did not show improved outcome with invasive monitoring.[7] This created confusion about the use of ICP that was addressed in a consensus statement.[8] In short, this RCT trial focused on how ICP monitoring was used in a particular setting and was a clear message to revise the "one size fits all" guideline approach. Patient-specific ICP thresholds need to be determined and new treatment methods and paradigms developed.[8] Some even advocate that the BEST-TRIP trial is a reason for more cerebral monitoring.[9]

Management of eICP is complex for many reasons (**Box 1**):

1. Indications and timing for ICP monitor insertion are debated.[1,10,11]
2. Underlying pathologic condition requiring ICP monitoring reflects disease heterogeneity.
3. Brain physiology leading to eICP differs between individuals and over time.

Consequently, refinement of therapeutic interventions through precision medicine may translate in improved TBI patient care.

This article highlights current concepts and controversies underlying management of eICP while providing a practical framework for management. It will explain current limitations of a guideline-based approach to ICP management and demonstrate how benefits of precision medicine with the aid of multimodality monitoring (MMM) can further inform eICP management.

BASIC PHYSIOLOGICAL CONCEPTS

Important physiologic concepts underlie ICP management. The Monro-Kellie doctrine relates volume changes to pressure changes in a fixed cranial space, so volume expansion from edema or a mass lesion results in an exponential increase in pressure

---

Box 1
Heterogeneity in TBI

Indications for ICP monitoring
1. Diffuse axonal injury
2. Cerebral contusions
3. After evacuation of a mass lesion
4. After secondary craniectomy

Altered physiology related to ICP
1. Interstitial edema
2. Cytotoxic edema
3. BBB permeability
4. Diffusion barrier
5. Altered limits of autoregulation
6. Loss of autoregulation
7. Vasospasm
8. Microcirculatory failure
9. Decrease cardiac output (heart-brain axis, polytrauma)
10. Altered venous return (jugular obstruction, thrombosis...)
11. Noncommunicating hydrocephalus
12. Communicating hydrocephalus
13. Increase resistance to cerebrospinal fluid (CSF) flow without franc hydrocephalus (small subarachnoid hemorrage (SAH), inflammation in CSF)
14. Seizures
15. Cortical spreading depolarization

once compensatory mechanisms are exhausted[12] (**Fig. 1**, red limb). In addition, changes in arterial diameter impacts ICP and has been used as a therapeutic tool[13] and a way to determine brain autoregulatory status.[14,15]

Changes in arterial diameter commonly occur because of changes in mean arterial pressure (MAP), which is the mechanism underlying cerebral autoregulation (**Fig. 2**A, black line). Many other mechanisms can alter arterial diameter (see **Fig. 1**), most notably variation in arterial pressure of CO_2 ($PaCO_2$). Regardless of cause, arterial diameter changes will affect cerebral blood flow (CBF) and eventually ICP if intracranial compliance is exhausted. Hyperventilation is used to urgently treat herniation but induces ischemia. Considering various causes of arterial diameter changes broadens possible reasons of eICP and management strategies.

Autoregulation drives the vasodilatory cascade and thus affects ICP management.[13] As MAP decreases, arteries vasodilate to maintain CBF increasing cerebral blood volume (CBV). In a noncompliant brain, increased CBV will increase ICP (see **Fig. 2**A, gray line). Naturally occurring oscillation in MAP will have vessels dilate and constrict once or twice a minute generating small oscillation in ICP at the same rate: the Lundberg B waves.[16,17] Observing Lundberg B waves at bedside means: (1) autoregulation is present and (2) the CPP at which it is observed probably represents the lower limit of autoregulation plateau. Finally, partial (**Fig. 2**B) or complete loss of autoregulation[18] (see **Fig. 2**A, B) occurs after TBI with an incidence of 20% to 87% (**Table 1**). Autoregulation alterations might last hours to days after TBI or be dynamic over a few hours because of transient physiological changes (eg, hypercapnia, sepsis, metabolic crisis) and can be altered regionally.[19–21] Prolonged absence of autoregulation is associated with poor prognosis.[21,22]

CPP is central to the prevention of secondary injuries. Measurement of CPP depends on MAP (CPP = MAP − ICP). MAP value in turn is dependent on transducer

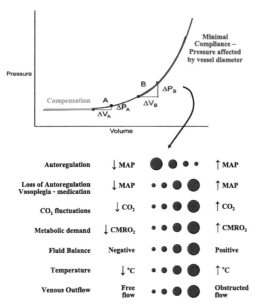

Fig. 1. Monro-Kellie curve and causes of vessel diameter change. Point (A) and (B) showing the influence of volume change (ΔV) on pressure (ΔP) according to compliance of intracranial volume. $CMRO_2$: cerebral metabolic rate of O_2, °C: degree Celsius.

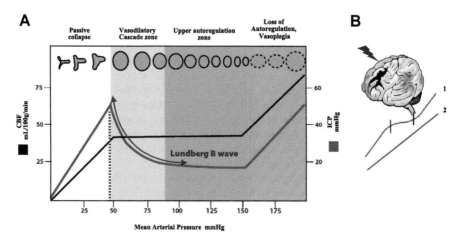

Fig. 2. (*A*) Relationship between autoregulation and ICP curves. See text for explanations. (*B*) In injury, the plateau of the autoregulation curve might be shortened (1), shifted to the right, partially (1) or completely (2) abolished over the entire range of MAP.

level (**Fig. 3**).[23] CPP measured with a transducer leveled at the heart will read a higher MAP (thus giving a higher CPP) than a transducer leveled at the ear. The height of the hydrostatic column between the 2 levels (depending on the degree of head of bed elevation) will determine the difference between the 2 readings. Clinically, maintaining a patient at 15° to 30° means an approximate difference of 10 to 15 mm Hg between readings. This is critical in interpreting literature regarding CPP targets.[24] For example, in the study describing the risk of ARDS with CPPs is greater than 70 mm Hg, the transducer was leveled at the ear.[25] If your institution levels the transducer at the heart, the "risk of ARDS" is present if "your" CPP is actually above 80 mm Hg. In contrast, the

Table 1
Incidence of Loss of Autoregulation

	Not Exhaustive List	
Year/Journal/First Author	Measure	Absence of Autoregulation (%)
1974 JNS, Overguaard	Angio Xe 133	61
1978 JNS, Enevoldsen	Angio Xe 133	85
1978 Acta Anest Scan, Cold	Angio Xe 133	83
1984 JNS, Muizelaar	Xe Scan	33
1989 JNS, Muizelaar	Xe Scan	41
1992 JNS, Bouma	Xe Scan	31
1996 Acta Neurochir, Sahuquillo	AVDO$_2$	57
1997 JNS, Junger	Doppler	28
2000 ICM, Mascia	Xe Scan	20
2001 JNS, Lee	Xe Scan-doppler	69
2002 JNS, Hlatky	Xe Scan-doppler	49–87
2003 JNNP, Lang	PRx-doppler	52
2005 Neurosurg, Hlatky	Doppler	57
2011 JNS, Rosenthal	Hemedex	47
2015 NCC, Dias	PRx	52

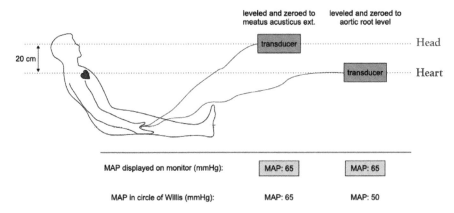

leveled and zeroed to meatus acusticus ext.

leveled and zeroed to aortic root level

transducer ·················· Head

20 cm

transducer ·················· Heart

MAP displayed on monitor (mmHg):   MAP: 65   MAP: 65

MAP in circle of Willis (mmHg):   MAP: 65   MAP: 50

Fig. 3. Effect of transducer level on MAP and CPP.

trial influencing the 2017 Brain Trauma Foundation (BTF) guideline[6] modification of CPP targets from 50 to 70 mm Hg to 60 to 70 mm Hg leveled the transducer at the heart.[26] Thus leveling MAP at the ear, means "your" target CPP should be 50 to 60 mm Hg. Further complicating things, some articles do not mention transducer level at all or use registries with multiple sites contributing data without uniformity in transducer leveling. Guidance from major societies regarding what transducer level to use and mandatory reporting of transducer level when publishing trials is urgently needed. Such an effort of standardization is underway in the United Kingdom since 2015.[27] It should be appreciated that the usual transducer level in critical care to management MAP in various clinical scenarios other than brain injury is at the phlebostatic level (heart).

INTRACRANIAL PRESSURE THRESHOLD

Recent BTF guidelines modified treatment ICP threshold from 20 to 22 mm Hg.[6] This new threshold originates from one monocentric trial using chi-square analysis of mean populational ICP (each patient's ICP being averaged from minute to minute) yielding the best mortality/functional outcome result.[26] Reducing the complexity of ICP changes over time for a given patient to a single number does not represent its true burden on the brain. A populational threshold originating from cohorts will not necessarily apply to an individual patient. It is known that herniation is possible from temporal mass lesion with ICP values less than 15 mm Hg[28] or from cerebral hypotension.[29] In 1965, Lundberg stated that *"no fixed limit between a tolerable and nontolerable intraventricular pressure can be established"* and regarded ICP between 15 and 40 to be abnormal but only *"values > 40 mm Hg should be regarded as potentially dangerous"*.[30]

Although eICP is associated with mortality, this association could be challenged as eICP might be subject to the self-fulfilling prophecy bias.[31–33] Exceeding a "dangerous" threshold may lead to nihilism despite reports of good outcome in up to 40% of patients exposed to sustained ICP greater than 25 mm Hg.[34,35] Finally, a substantial proportion of literature dates back to when bundles of care were drastically different (eg, hyperventilation, aggressive diuresis, and steroids use).

The relationship between ICP and CBF might be more informative about ICP threshold. Honda and colleagues[36] used Xenon and perfusion CT to measure the influence of ICP on flow. CBF was significantly decreased with ICP greater than 20 mm

Hg but the correlation was weak. Some patients had both eICP and elevated flow, which can be explained by the absence of autoregulation and/or hyperemia. Thus, appropriate ICP threshold should not be considered an *on/off* switch for treatment but rather part of a continuum that must be interpreted in a global context where intensity, duration, dose, and causes of eICP should be considered as well as information from other monitors.

There is a general consensus that ICP greater than 20 to 25 mm Hg should trigger actions to prevent secondary brain injuries and that ICP is refractory to treatment if it remains elevated for more than 30 minutes. **Box 2** highlights overarching principles guiding management of eICP. Treatment options should be organized in a tiered fashion, with more benign interventions attempted before more aggressive maneuvers. The Seattle International Severe Traumatic Brain Injury Consensus Conference (SIBICC) recently proposed an excellent management algorithm.[37] Key concepts will be presented to help guide appropriate, individualized interventions.

NEUROPROTECTION: KEEPING THE BRAIN HAPPY

Managing an injured brain should focus on maintaining normal homeostasis, which minimizes secondary injuries, edema formation, and improves outcome.[38] **Fig. 4** lists the 7 elements of the *"happy brain" concept*: EUthermia, EUglycemia, EUnatremia, EUvolemia, EUcapnia, normal oxygenation, and optimized CBF. These nEUroprotective elements are preventive steps in managing eICP (**Tier 0**).

1. **Glycemia.** Hyperglycemia can affect TBI outcome,[39,40] yet tight glycemic control should be avoided in TBI as cerebral hypoglycemia is also deleterious.[41–43] The suggested range in **Fig. 4** balances both options.[41]
2. **Temperature.** Hyperthermia has deleterious effects, yet all large hypothermia trials in TBI have failed.[44–46] Some facts about hypothermia are worth remembering:
   1. controlling temperature can help control ICP,[47]
   2. hypothermia improved outcomes in certain patient populations (hematoma particularly),[48,49]
   3. prophylactic and therapeutic hypothermia are different,
   4. temperatures lower than 35°C might decrease delivery of oxygen to the brain,[47,50]
   5. shivering induced by fever or treatment of fever may negatively impact brain oxygenation,[51,52] and
   6. lowering temperature affects $PaCO_2$ levels and can reduce CBF.[53]

   This evidence suggests an optimal range of temperature target between 35°C and 37°C. Lowering temperature might induce physiological derangements or complications that can negate the potential benefits of temperature control and should be used within a bundle of care in expert hands. On the other hand, fever can

---

Box 2
Principles of ICP management

Maintain homeostasis: neuroprotection

Figure ongoing and prevailing physiology affecting ICP

Use a tiered approach to treatment

Use MMM

Maintaining Normal Physiology: nEUroprotection

I.	EUthermia	Temperature between 35°C and 37°C
2.	Euglycemia	Glucose level 6–10 mmol/L
3.	Eunatremia	Na 140, no decrease >5 mEq/day
4.	Euvolemia	furosemide or volume expansion (measure cardiac index and PPV)
5.	Eucapnia	PaCO2 35-40 mmHg, maintain pH 7.35-7.45, correct for temp, use EtCO2
6.	PaO2	>90 mmHg (sat >96%) or titrate with the use PbtO2 (>20 mmHg)
7.	CPP (CBF)	> 60 mmHg initially, individual optimization, assess cardiac index

Fig. 4. Maintaining normal physiology: 7 elements of neuroprotection.

increase cardiac output, cause vasoplegia/loss of autoregulation and increase ICP through brain hyperemia.

3. **Serum sodium** (Na) level is central to brain water content management.[54–56] The physiological basis underlying Na management is the presence of an intact blood–brain barrier (BBB) impermeable to Na, and the brain's capacity to regulate its osmolality by producing (or removing) idiogenic osmoles.[54–56] The accumulation/deaccumulation of idiogenic osmoles is slow, occurring over 24 hours and reaching a steady state over 2 to 7 days.[54] Consequently, Na changes occurring more rapidly generates a flow of water according to an osmotic gradient: an increase in Na will make the brain shrink, a decrease will increase brain water content and volume, affecting ICP. For neuroprotection, the basic principles of Na management are as follows:
   1. avoid hyponatremia,
   2. avoid rapid decrease in Na,
   3. targeting higher Na levels is not beneficial,
   4. avoid Na greater than 155 mmol/L, and
   5. monitor fluid intake composition to maintain stable Na levels.
   Continuous infusion of hypertonic saline has no role in managing ICP apart from maintaining Na stability.[57]

4. **Fluid management** helps keep Na constant, regulates intravascular volume status, and maintains euvolemia.[58,59] The use of arterial pulse contour analysis technology may facilitate management of volume status by giving a continuous pulse pressure variation (PPV).[60] Changes in PPV may reflect hypovolemia or hypervolemia and provide useful real-time bedside information. Both hypovolemia and hypervolemia can be deleterious.[61,62] Hypovolemia or increasing MAP (afterload) with vasoconstricting agents in an under resuscitated patient may decrease cardiac index (CI) and CBF despite CPP being maintained.[63–65] Hypervolemia, however, can increase brain edema through a disrupted BBB and increases central venous pressure, which both increase the intracranial volume (brain and vascular).[66] Hypervolemia can also negatively affect lung function (pulmonary edema or ARDS), decreasing oxygenation. Furosemide can help maintain euvolemia and potentially decrease brain edema through direct effect on the brain.[67]

5. **PaCO2** regulates cerebral arteries diameter via its effect on local pH.[68] Hyperventilation induces cerebral ischemia[69–71] and should generally be avoided.[6] A small

1 mm Hg change of $PaCO_2$ alters CBF by 3%.[17] Spontaneous variation in ventilation/perfusion mismatch, minute ventilation, and VCO_2 can account for inadvertent hyperventilation.[72] Monitoring end-tidal CO_2 ($EtCO_2$) or cerebral oxygenation ($PbtO_2$) can help detect this. Although hyperventilation is useful if acute brain herniation occurs, using it to treat eICP should only be a short temporary measure since (1) vasoconstricting effect of low $PaCO_2$ only last for a few hours, (2) vessels regain their original diameter, (3) ICP increases again, and (4) a new $PaCO_2$ baseline is established (**Fig. 5**).[71,73] Moreover, deleterious effect on CBF might last longer than the positive effect on ICP.[74] Finally, hypocapnia can potentiate seizure.[71] If ICP allows, titrating $PaCO_2$ upward will likely increase CBF and provide a safety margin should an acute decrease occur, although in approximately 10% of patients,[17] an "inverse steal" might occur by diverting CBF toward normal brain as the injured area is already maximally vasodilated.[75] MMM with doppler flow velocity or $PbtO_2$ may detect this phenomenon.

6. ***Arterial oxygenation (PaO_2)*** plays a crucial role in oxygen delivery to the brain, more so than arterial hemoglobin saturation (Video 1). Once in the capillary, diffusion of oxygen from hemoglobin to the neuron is the rate-limiting step of oxygen delivery[76] and may be altered because of edema or microcirculatory failure.[76–78] PaO_2 is the force driving diffusion of oxygen to mitochondria.[79] The minimal PaO_2 required to overcome this diffusion barrier early after TBI is 94 mm Hg but may be as high as 300 mm Hg,[80] which equals to an arterial saturation value of 96.5%. Measurement of $PbtO_2$ allows titration of PaO_2, and various determinants of $PbtO_2$ must be considered before using ventilatory strategies (particularly increasing FiO_2) to increase PaO_2 (**Fig. 6**, bottom).[80] The brain oxygenation ratio (BOx ratio = $PbtO_2/PaO_2$) can help the clinician manage these determinants.[80]

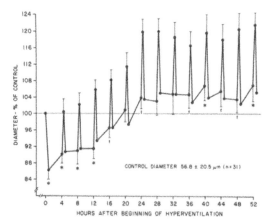

Progressive increase in vessel diameter despite hyperventilation

CONTROL DIAMETER 56.8 ± 20.5 μm (n=31)

DIAMETER - % OF CONTROL

HOURS AFTER BEGINNING OF HYPERVENTILATION

Fig. 5. Effect of CO_2 on pial vessel diameter. Graph showing the diameter at 30 minutes and at 4-hour intervals after the beginning of hyperventilation. Lower values were obtained at a $PaCO_2$ of 25 mm Hg, and peak values were taken during brief periods of normoventilation to a $PaCO_2$ of 38 mm Hg. (*From* Muizelaar JP, Poel HG van der, Li Z, Kontos HA, Levasseur JE. Pial arteriolar vessel diameter and CO2 reactivity during prolonged hyperventilation in the rabbit. J Neurosurg. 1988;69(6):923-927. https://doi.org/10.3171/jns.1988.69.6.0923; with permission.)

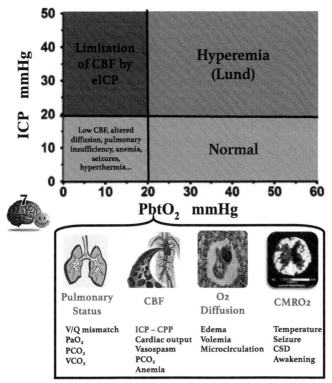

Fig. 6. (*Upper*) Four possible bedside scenarios of relationship between PbtO₂ and ICP. Threshold for ICP and PbtO₂ set at 20 mm Hg. (*Bottom*) Determinants of PbtO₂. Comprehensive list of various causes of variation in PbtO₂. Note that ICP and CPP are only one but many causes. (O2 Diffusion - Menon, David K. PhD et al., Diffusion limited oxygen delivery following head injury*. Critical Care Medicine: June 2004 - Volume 32 - Issue 6 - p 1384-1390 doi: 10.1097/01.CCM.0000127777.16609.08).

The BOOST-2 trial[81] compared an ICP alone to ICP-PbtO₂-guided strategy and showed a 43% reduction in interventions aimed at controlling eICP in the latter group, suggesting that secondary injuries and subsequent brain oedema were avoided.

7. **Optimized CBF.** Recent guidelines suggest a CPP target between 60 and 70 mm Hg,[6,82] with the comment that the minimal optimal level is unclear and may relate to the patient's autoregulation. It should be noted that more pressure does not necessarily mean more flow as resistance is part of the equation (Flow = ΔP/R). Measuring and augmenting CI might be necessary in certain situations such as (1) depressed CBF in acute TBI,[83] (2) if vasospasm is present,[83,84] (3) when heart failure from consequences of the brain–heart axis is present.[85,86] Dobutamine and milrinone have been used with success in some patients.[87,88]

Concerns exist for ARDS with CPP target greater than 70 mm Hg.[6,25] Multivariate analysis showed that ARDS was not related to CPP and actually occurred in more severe TBI receiving more fluid and given dopamine and epinephrine to maintain CPP.[25] Raising CPP itself may not be dangerous depending on the clinical context.

Fig. 7 summarizes the CPP targets, and Video 2 explains the bedside application of CPP optimization. Autoregulation plays a crucial role in determining optimal CPP and was the subject of a recent consensus.[89] Patients with intact autoregulation may tolerate wider variations in CPP because of intact BBB and vasoconstrictive power.[6,10,82] Decreasing CPP to 50 mm Hg and limiting edema formation through a leaking BBB is effective in selected cases.[90–95] Autoregulation reconciles 2 seemingly opposed treatment strategies: Rosner's vasodilatory cascade versus Lund therapy[96] **(Fig. 8).**[97] The treatment strategy should be tailored to autoregulatory status: if present apply the vasodilatory cascade theory, if absent use Lund therapy of lower CPP values to limit edema formation. This was demonstrated by Bouma and colleagues[98] in 1992: *"Artificially raising blood pressure, if necessary to maintain CPP, would only seem prudent when autoregulation is known to be intact."*

Autoregulation can be assessed at bedside by the following: (1) recognizing Lundberg B waves, (2) performing a MAP challenge as described elsewhere,[37] and (3) using the pressure reactivity index (PRx). PRx allows continuous bedside determination of the presence or absence of autoregulation in real time by correlating MAP and ICP. When autoregulation is present, changes in MAP and ICP occur in opposite directions and the correlation is negative (see **Figs. 2** and **7D,** *left*). PRx provides an estimation of optimal individualized CPP (CPPopt, **Fig. 7D,** *middle*).[14,15,99–101] Deviation from

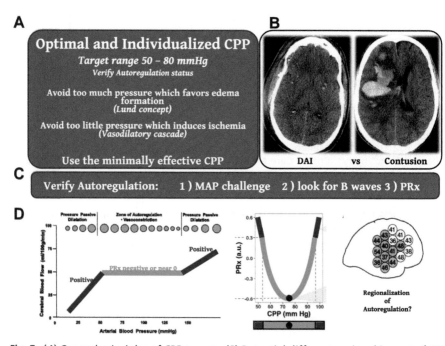

Fig. 7. (*A*) General principles of CPP targets. (*B*) Potential different regional impact of CPP on scan showing diffuse axonal injury (DAI) and contusion. (*C*) Means of verifying autoregulation at the bedside. (*D*) Pressure reactivity index (PRx). *Left,* PRx value according to the autoregulation curve. (*Middle*) - Middle, example of range of PRx over range of CPP with the determination of an optimal CPP (CPPopt). (From Donnelly J, Czosnyka M, Adams H, et al. Individualizing Thresholds of Cerebral Perfusion Pressure Using Estimated Limits of Autoregulation. Crit Care Med. 2017;45(9):1464-1471. doi:10.1097/ccm. 0000000000002575; with permission.)

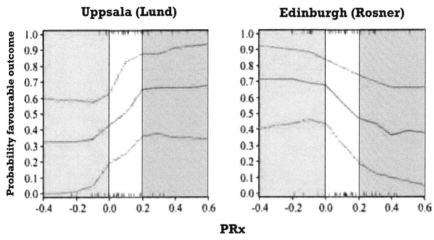

Fig. 8. Probability of favorable outcome according to center and autoregulation status. Uppsala center treated all patients according to Lund therapy. Edinburgh center treated all patients according to Rosner vasodilatory cascade. Green zone denotes the presence of autoregulation. Red zone denotes the absence of autoregulation. Ninety percent confidence intervals. (*Adapted from* Howells T, Elf K, Jones PA, et al. Pressure reactivity as a guide in the treatment of cerebral perfusion pressure in patients with brain trauma. J Neurosurg. 2005;102(2):311-317. https://doi.org/10.3171/jns.2005.102.2.0311; with permission.)

CPPopt, particularly below CPPopt, is associated with worse outcome.[99,101] Autoregulation might be defective regionally due to different injury patterns (see **Fig. 7**, scan and D, *left*).[20,21,102] Although attractive, uncertainty about PRx persists[89] but the concept supports efforts to individualize CPP targets.

LIMITATIONS OF INTRACRANIAL PRESSURE MANAGEMENT, CEREBRAL OXYGENATION MONITORING AND MULTIMODALITY MONITORING: EXPANDING OUR UNDERSTANDING OF BRAIN PHYSIOLOGY

The physiological rationale underlying ICP management is to preserve oxygen delivery to the brain, using CPP as a surrogate of CBF. This rationale has many limitations, and it has been shown that CBF is best approximated with MMM.[103] There are numerous reasons why brain oxygen delivery can be impaired despite normal ICP or CPP or why brain oxygen remains normal despite eICP (see **Fig. 6**).[80,104] Devices measuring $PbtO_2$ are available at bedside and algorithms of $PbtO_2$ management published.[80,81,105] Cerebral hypoxia is common, reversible, allows measurement of cerebral ischemic burden, and is independently associated with functional outcome.[81,104,106–109] Hyperemia is prevalent after TBI,[110,111] elevates ICP, and is managed through CBF reduction strategies. The use of $PbtO_2$ easily identifies hyperemia because luxury CBF increases oxygen delivery and facilitates ICP management decisions (see Video 2).

MMM was the object of a recent consensus conference.[112] Advance cerebral imaging, transcranial Doppler, continuous EEG, microdialysis, direct and continuous CBF monitor, depth electrodes, near infrared spectroscopy, and depth of sedation monitors are various options available to increase our capacity of deciphering brain physiology. MMM also includes systemic monitors that allow fine-tuning of systemic physiology affecting the brain such as continuous CI monitoring, continuous

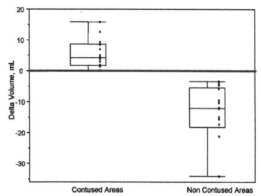

Fig. 9. Mean effect of hypertonic saline on the volume of contused and noncontused brain areas. Red line represents zero change in weight and volume. (*From* Lescot T, Degos V, Zouaoui A, Préteux F, Coriat P, Puybasset L. Opposed effects of hypertonic saline on contusions and noncontused brain tissue in patients with severe traumatic brain injury* Crit Care Med. 2006;34(12):3029-3033. https://doi.org/10.1097/01.ccm.0000243797.42346.64; with permission.)

temperature regulators, $EtCO_2$, respiratory pulmonary electrical impedance tomography, and advanced ventilator settings.

OSMOTHERAPY

Once considered the mainstay of eICP management, osmotherapy should now be used with circumspection.[113] Osmotherapy should be viewed as a temporizing measure such as hyperventilation. It should not be used prophylactically or on a regular basis. Osmotherapy works only in areas of the brain with an intact BBB, decreasing extracellular space volume in healthy brain. It does not reduce cerebral edema. In areas with BBB breakdown, osmoles will penetrate and remain in cerebral tissue creating a gradient favoring brain edema accumulation. This has been proven in an elegant CT scan study (**Fig. 9**).[114] Similarly, aggravation of cerebral edema with multiple doses of mannitol is well described.[115–117] Comparative efficacy of mannitol and hypertonic saline (HS) is beyond the scope of this article.[118] Both agents have potentially beneficial effects[113] but the main reason to choose one over the other should be its impact on volume status: mannitol will induce volume depletion through its diuretic effect, whereas HS is a volume expander well suited for resuscitation and CI augmentation.

SUMMARY

Monitoring only ICP is no longer sufficient for TBI management. MMM clearly improves our understanding of physiology and secondary injuries (see **Figs. 1** and **6**). It allows tailoring of therapy with better precision, minimizing the adverse effect of a one size fits all, general therapeutic strategy. The tier 0 *"happy brain"* concept of neuroprotection when applied with MMM (particularly $PbtO_2$) and combined with the search for physiological causes of eICP is so powerful that choosing the other tiers' interventions almost become obvious: sedation to decrease $CMRO_2$, neuromuscular blockade to reduce shivering, or improve ventilation (PaO_2 or PCO_2) and venous return to name a few. The future of eICP management resides in part in letting go of our historical attachment to ICP as the Holy Grail of TBI management.

CLINICS CARE POINTS

- Intracranial pressure (ICP) monitoring alone is insufficient to optimally manage severe traumatic brain injury and multimodality monitoring contributes to better interpretation of cerebral physiology necessary to provide individualized care.

- Neuroprotection and ICP management are best achieved by maintaining brain homeostasis summarized in 7 key components. MMM is necessary to achieve this homeostasis since ICP does not capture alterations of these components and the ensuing secondary injuries.

- Classic elevated ICP treatments such as hyperventilation or osmotherapy should be used with caution under multimodality monitoring (MMM) supervision.

- Interpretation of MMM and appropriate subsequent therapeutic interventions require significant knowledge integration that is best achieved with continuous education of a multidisciplinary team (nurses, respiratory nurses, intensivists, and neurosurgeons) committed to use a common standardized treatment algorithm.

SUPPLEMENTARY DATA

Supplementary data related to this article can be found online at https://doi.org/10.1016/j.ccc.2022.08.002.

REFERENCES

1. Chesnut R, Videtta W, Vespa P, et al. Intracranial pressure monitoring: fundamental considerations and rationale for monitoring. Neurocrit Care 2014; 21(Suppl 2):64–84.
2. Farahvar A, Gerber LM, Chiu YL, et al. Increased mortality in patients with severe traumatic brain injury treated without intracranial pressure monitoring. J Neurosurg 2012;117(4):729–34.
3. Talving P, Karamanos E, Teixeira PG, et al. Intracranial pressure monitoring in severe head injury: compliance with Brain Trauma Foundation guidelines and effect on outcomes: a prospective study. J Neurosurg 2013;119(5):1248–54.
4. Alali AS, Fowler RA, Mainprize TG, et al. Intracranial pressure monitoring in severe traumatic brain injury: results from the american college of surgeons trauma quality improvement program. J Neurotrauma 2013;30(20):1737–46.
5. Gerber LM, Chiu YL, Carney N, et al. Marked reduction in mortality in patients with severe traumatic brain injury. J Neurosurg 2013;119(6):1583–90.
6. Carney N, Totten AM, O'Reilly C, et al. Guidelines for the management of severe traumatic brain injury, Fourth Edition. Neurosurgery 2017;80(1):6–15.
7. Chesnut RM, Temkin N, Carney N, et al. A trial of intracranial-pressure monitoring in traumatic brain injury. N Engl J Med 2012;367(26):2471–81.
8. Chesnut RM, Bleck TP, Citerio G, et al. A consensus-based interpretation of the benchmark evidence from south american trials: treatment of intracranial pressure trial. J Neurotrauma 2015;32(22):1722–4.
9. Roux PL. Intracranial pressure after the BEST TRIP trial. Curr Opin Crit Care 2014;20(2):141–7.
10. Foundation BT, Surgeons AA of N, Surgeons C of N, et al. Guidelines for the management of severe traumatic brain injury. VI. Indications for intracranial pressure monitoring. J Neurotrauma 2007;24(supplement 1):S37–44.
11. Stocchetti N, Picetti E, Berardino M, et al. Clinical applications of intracranial pressure monitoring in traumatic brain injury. Acta Neurochir 2014;156(8): 1615–22.

12. Harary M, Dolmans RGF, Gormley WB. Intracranial pressure monitoring—review and avenues for development. Sensors Basel Switz 2018;18(2):465.

13. Rosner MJ, Rosner SD, Johnson AH. Cerebral perfusion pressure: management protocol and clinical results. J Neurosurg 1995;83(6):949–62.

14. Steiner LA, Czosnyka M, Piechnik SK, et al. Continuous monitoring of cerebro-vascular pressure reactivity allows determination of optimal cerebral perfusion pressure in patients with traumatic brain injury. Crit Care Med 2002;30(4):733–8.

15. Depreitere B, Güiza F, Berghe GV den, et al. Pressure autoregulation monitoring and cerebral perfusion pressure target recommendation in patients with severe traumatic brain injury based on minute-by-minute monitoring data. J Neurosurg 2014;120(6):1451–7.

16. Wijdicks EFM. Lundberg and his waves. Neurocrit Care 2019;31(3):546–9.

17. Cold GE. Cerebral blood flow in acute head injury. The regulation of cerebral blood flow and metabolism during the acute phase of head injury, and its significance for therapy. Acta Neurochir Suppl 1990;49:1–64.

18. Lang EW, Lagopoulos J, Griffith J, et al. Cerebral vasomotor reactivity testing in head injury: the link between pressure and flow. J Neurol Neurosurg Psychiatr 2003;74(8):1053.

19. Steiner LA, Johnston AJ, Chatfield DA, et al. The effects of large-dose propofol on cerebrovascular pressure autoregulation in head-injured patients. Anesth Analg 2003;97(2):572–6.

20. Schmidt EA, Czosnyka M, Steiner LA, et al. Asymmetry of pressure autoregulation after traumatic brain injury. J Neurosurg 2003;99(6):991–8.

21. Overgaard J, Tweed WA. Cerebral circulation after head injury: Part 1: cerebral blood flow and its regulation after closed head injury with emphasis on clinical correlations. J Neurosurg 1974;41(5):531–41.

22. Preiksaitis A, Krakauskaite S, Petkus V, et al. Association of severe traumatic brain injury patient outcomes with duration of cerebrovascular autoregulation impairment events. Neurosurgery 2016;79(1):75–82.

23. Saugel B, Kouz K, Meidert AS, et al. How to measure blood pressure using an arterial catheter: a systematic 5-step approach. Crit Care Lond Engl 2020; 24(1):172.

24. Depreitere B, Meyfroidt G, Güiza F. What do we mean by cerebral perfusion pressure? Acta Neurochir Suppl 2018;126:201–3.

25. Contant CF, Valadka AB, Gopinath SP, et al. Adult respiratory distress syndrome: a complication of induced hypertension after severe head injury. J Neurosurg 2001;95(4):560–8.

26. Sorrentino E, Diedler J, Kasprowicz M, et al. Critical thresholds for cerebrovascular reactivity after traumatic brain injury. Neurocrit Care 2012;16(2):258–66.

27. Thomas E, NACCS, Czosnyka M, Hutchinson P. SBNS. Calculation of cerebral perfusion pressure in the management of traumatic brain injury: joint position statement by the councils of the Neuroanaesthesia and Critical Care Society of Great Britain and Ireland (NACCS) and the Society of British Neurological Surgeons (SBNS). Br J Anaesth 2015;115(4):487–8.

28. Dahlqvist MB, Andres RH, Raabe A, et al. Brain herniation in a patient with apparently normal intracranial pressure: a case report. J Med Case Rep 2010;4(1):297.

29. Stiver SI. Complications of decompressive craniectomy for traumatic brain injury. Neurosurg Focus 2009;26(6):E7.

30. Lundberg N, Troupp H, Lorin H. Continuous recording of the ventricular-fluid pressure in patients with severe acute traumatic brain injury: a preliminary report. J Neurosurg 1965;22(6):581–90.
31. Turgeon AF, Lauzier F, Simard JF, et al. Mortality associated with withdrawal of life-sustaining therapy for patients with severe traumatic brain injury: a Canadian multicentre cohort study. Can Med Assoc J 2011;183(14):1581–8.
32. Souter MJ, Blissitt PA, Blosser S, et al. Recommendations for the critical care management of devastating brain injury: prognostication, psychosocial, and ethical management: a position statement for healthcare professionals from the neurocritical care society. Neurocrit Care 2015;23(1):4–13.
33. Harvey D, Butler J, Groves J, et al. Management of perceived devastating brain injury after hospital admission: a consensus statement from stakeholder professional organizations. Br J Anaesth 2018;120(1):138–45.
34. Resnick DK, Marion DW, Carlier P. Outcome analysis of patients with severe head injuries and prolonged intracranial hypertension. J Trauma Inj Infect Crit Care 1997;42(6):1108–11.
35. Young JS, Blow O, Turrentine F, et al. Is there an upper limit of intracranial pressure in patients with severe head injury if cerebral perfusion pressure is maintained? Neurosurg Focus 2003;15(6):1–7.
36. Honda M, Ichibayashi R, Suzuki G, et al. Consideration of the intracranial pressure threshold value for the initiation of traumatic brain injury treatment: a xenon CT and perfusion CT study. Neurocrit Care 2017;27(3):308–15.
37. Hawryluk GWJ, Aguilera S, Buki A, et al. A management algorithm for patients with intracranial pressure monitoring: the seattle international severe traumatic brain injury consensus conference (SIBICC). Intensive Care Med 2019;45(12):1783–94.
38. Patel HC, Menon DK, Tebbs S, et al. Specialist neurocritical care and outcome from head injury. Intensive Care Med 2002;28(5):547–53.
39. Lam AM, Winn HR, Cullen BF, et al. Hyperglycemia and neurological outcome in patients with head injury. J Neurosurg 1991;75(4):545–51.
40. Wettervik TS, Howells T, Ronne-Engström E, et al. High arterial glucose is associated with poor pressure autoregulation, high cerebral lactate/pyruvate ratio and poor outcome following traumatic brain injury. Neurocrit Care 2019;31(3):526–33.
41. Graffagnino C, Gurram AR, Kolls B, et al. Intensive insulin therapy in the neurocritical care setting is associated with poor clinical outcomes. Neurocrit Care 2010;13(3):307–12.
42. Finfer S, Chittock D, Li Y, et al. Intensive versus conventional glucose control in critically ill patients with traumatic brain injury: long-term follow-up of a subgroup of patients from the NICE-SUGAR study. Intensive Care Med 2015;41(6):1037–47.
43. Magnoni S, Tedesco C, Carbonara M, et al. Relationship between systemic glucose and cerebral glucose is preserved in patients with severe traumatic brain injury, but glucose delivery to the brain may become limited when oxidative metabolism is impaired. Crit Care Med 2012;40(6):1785–91.
44. Cooper DJ, Nichol AD, Bailey M, et al. Effect of early sustained prophylactic hypothermia on neurologic outcomes among patients with severe traumatic brain injury: the polar randomized clinical trial. JAMA 2018;320(21):2211.
45. Polderman KH. Induced hypothermia and fever control for prevention and treatment of neurological injuries. Lancet 2008;371(9628):1955–69.

46. Lewis SR, Evans DJ, Butler AR, et al. Hypothermia for traumatic brain injury. Cochrane Database Syst Rev 2017;9(9):CD001048.

47. Tokutomi T, Morimoto K, Miyagi T, et al. Optimal Temperature for the management of severe traumatic brain injury: effect of hypothermia on intracranial pressure, systemic and intracranial hemodynamics, and metabolism. Neurosurgery 2003;52(1):102.

48. Clifton GL, Valadka A, Zygun D, et al. Very early hypothermia induction in patients with severe brain injury (the National Acute Brain Injury Study: hypothermia II): a randomised trial. Lancet Neurol 2011;10(2):131–9.

49. Kollmar R, Staykov D, Dorfler A, et al. Hypothermia reduces perihemorrhagic edema after intracerebral hemorrhage. Stroke 2010;41(8):1684–9.

50. Gupta AK, Al-Rawi PG, Hutchinson PJ, et al. Effect of hypothermia on brain tissue oxygenation in patients with severe head injury. Br J Anaesth 2002;88(2): 188–92.

51. Oddo M, Frangos S, Maloney-Wilensky E, et al. Effect of shivering on brain tissue oxygenation during induced normothermia in patients with severe brain injury. Neurocrit Care 2010;12(1):10–6.

52. Badjatia N, Strongilis E, Gordon E, et al. Metabolic impact of shivering during therapeutic temperature modulation. Stroke 2008;39(12):3242–7.

53. Voicu S, Deye N, Malissin I, et al. Influence of α-Stat and pH-stat blood gas management strategies on cerebral blood flow and oxygenation in patients treated with therapeutic hypothermia after out-of-hospital cardiac arrest: a crossover study*. Crit Care Med 2014;42(8):1849–61.

54. Gullans SR, Verbalis JG. Control of brain volume during hyperosmolar and hypoosmolar conditions. Annu Rev Med 1993;44(1):289–301.

55. Adrogué HJ, Madias NE. Hypernatremia. N Engl J Med 2000;342(20):1493–9.

56. McDowell ME, Wolf AV, Steer A. Osmotic volumes of distribution; idiogenic changes in osmotic pressure associated with administration of hypertonic solutions. Am J Phys 1955;180(3):545–58.

57. Roquilly A, Moyer JD, Huet O, et al. Effect of continuous infusion of hypertonic saline vs standard care on 6-month neurological outcomes in patients with traumatic brain injury. JAMA 2021;325(20):2056–66.

58. Oddo M, Poole D, Helbok R, et al. Fluid therapy in neurointensive care patients: ESICM consensus and clinical practice recommendations. Intensive Care Med 2018;44(4):449–63.

59. Cook AM, Jones GM, Hawryluk GWJ, et al. Guidelines for the acute treatment of cerebral edema in neurocritical care patients. Neurocrit Care 2020;32(3): 647–66.

60. Lazaridis C. Advanced hemodynamic monitoring: principles and practice in neurocritical care. Neurocrit Care 2012;16(1):163–9.

61. Fletcher JJ, Bergman K, Blostein PA, et al. Fluid balance, complications, and brain tissue oxygen tension monitoring following severe traumatic brain injury. Neurocrit Care 2010;13(1):47–56.

62. Gantner D, Moore EM, Cooper DJ. Intravenous fluids in traumatic brain injury. Curr Opin Crit Care 2014;20(4):385–9.

63. Steiner LA, Coles JP, Johnston AJ, et al. Responses of posttraumatic pericontusional cerebral blood flow and blood volume to an increase in cerebral perfusion pressure. J Cereb Blood Flow Metab 2003;23(11):1371–7.

64. Dunn-Meynell AA, Hassanain M, Levin BE. Norepinephrine and traumatic brain injury: a possible role in post-traumatic edema. Brain Res 1998;800(2):245–52.

65. Brassard P, Seifert T, Secher NH. Is cerebral oxygenation negatively affected by infusion of norepinephrine in healthy subjects? Br J Anaesth 2009;102(6):800–5.
66. Pranevicius M, Pranevicius O. Cerebral venous steal: blood flow diversion with increased tissue pressure. Neurosurgery 2002;51(5):1267.
67. McManus ML, Strange K. Acute volume regulation of brain cells in response to hypertonic challenge. Anesthesiology 1993;78(6):1132–7.
68. Kontos HA, Raper AJ, Patterson JL. Analysis of vasoactivity of local pH, PCO2 and bicarbonate on pial vessels. Stroke 1977;8(3):358–60.
69. Coles JP, Minhas PS, Fryer TD, et al. Effect of hyperventilation on cerebral blood flow in traumatic head injury: clinical relevance and monitoring correlates. Crit Care Med 2002;30(9):1950–9.
70. Coles JP, Fryer TD, Coleman MR, et al. Hyperventilation following head injury: effect on ischemic burden and cerebral oxidative metabolism. Crit Care Med 2007;35(2):568–78.
71. Curley G, Kavanagh BP, Laffey JG. Hypocapnia and the injured brain: more harm than benefit. Crit Care Med 2010;38(5):1348–59.
72. Gagnon A, Laroche M, Williamson D, et al. Incidence and characteristics of cerebral hypoxia after craniectomy in brain-injured patients: a cohort study. J Neurosurg 2021;135(2):554–61.
73. Muizelaar JP, van der Poel HG, Li Z, et al. Pial arteriolar vessel diameter and CO2 reactivity during prolonged hyperventilation in the rabbit. J Neurosurg 1988;69(6):923–7.
74. Steiner LA, Balestreri M, Johnston AJ, et al. Sustained moderate reductions in arterial CO2 after brain trauma Time-course of cerebral blood flow velocity and intracranial pressure. Intensive Care Med 2004;30(12):2180–7.
75. Alexandrov AV, Sharma VK, Lao AY, et al. Reversed robin hood syndrome in acute ischemic stroke patients. Stroke 2007;38(11):3045–8.
76. Menon DK, Coles JP, Gupta AK, et al. Diffusion limited oxygen delivery following head injury*. Crit Care Med 2004;32(6):1384–90.
77. Veenith TV, Carter EL, Geeraerts T, et al. Pathophysiologic mechanisms of cerebral ischemia and diffusion hypoxia in traumatic brain injury. JAMA Neurol 2016; 73(5):542.
78. Kohler K, Nallapareddy S, Ercole A. In silico model of critical cerebral oxygenation after traumatic brain injury: implications for rescuing hypoxic tissue. J Neurotrauma 2019;36(13):2109–16.
79. Habler OP, Messmer KFW. The physiology of oxygen transport. Transfus Sci 1997;18(3):425–35.
80. Dellazizzo L, Demers SP, Charbonney E, et al. Minimal PaO2 threshold after traumatic brain injury and clinical utility of a novel brain oxygenation ratio. J Neurosurg 2019;131(5):1639–47.
81. Okonkwo DO, Shutter LA, Moore C, et al. Brain oxygen optimization in severe traumatic brain injury phase-II: a phase II randomized trial. Crit Care Med 2017;45(11):1907–14.
82. Geeraerts T, Velly L, Abdennour L, et al. Management of severe traumatic brain injury (first 24 hours). Anaesth Crit Care Pa 2018;37(2):171–86.
83. Martin NA, Patwardhan RV, Alexander MJ, et al. Characterization of cerebral hemodynamic phases following severe head trauma: hypoperfusion, hyperemia, and vasospasm. J Neurosurg 1997;87(1):9–19.
84. Oertel M, Boscardin WJ, Obrist WD, et al. Posttraumatic vasospasm: the epidemiology, severity, and time course of an underestimated phenomenon: a prospective study performed in 299 patients. J Neurosurg 2005;103(5):812–24.

85. Tahsili-Fahadan P, Geocadin RG. Heart–brain Axis. Circ Res 2017;120(3): 559–72.
86. Ibrahim MS, Samuel B, Mohamed W, et al. Cardiac dysfunction in neurocritical care: an autonomic perspective. Neurocrit Care 2019;30(3):508–21.
87. Lannes M, Zeiler F, Guichon C, et al. The use of milrinone in patients with delayed cerebral ischemia following subarachnoid hemorrhage: a systematic review. Can J Neurol Sci J Can Des Sci Neurologiques 2017;44(2):152–60.
88. Mutoh T, Ishikawa T, Suzuki A, et al. Continuous cardiac output and near-infrared spectroscopy monitoring to assist in management of symptomatic cerebral vasospasm after subarachnoid hemorrhage. Neurocrit Care 2010;13(3):331–8.
89. Depreitere B, Citerio G, Smith M, et al. Cerebrovascular autoregulation monitoring in the management of adult severe traumatic brain injury: a delphi consensus of clinicians. Neurocrit Care 2021;34(3):731–8.
90. Grände PO. Critical evaluation of the lund concept for treatment of severe traumatic head injury, 25 years after its introduction. Front Neurol 2017;8:315.
91. Huang SJ, Hong WC, Han YY, et al. Clinical outcome of severe head injury using three different ICP and CPP protocol-driven therapies. J Clin Neurosci 2006; 13(8):818–22.
92. Johnson U, Nilsson P, Ronne-Engström E, et al. Favorable outcome in traumatic brain injury patients with impaired cerebral pressure autoregulation when treated at low cerebral perfusion pressure levels. Neurosurgery 2011;68(3): 714–22.
93. Elf K, Nilsson P, Enblad P. Outcome after traumatic brain injury improved by an organized secondary insult program and standardized neurointensive care. Crit Care Med 2002;30(9):2129–34.
94. Nordström CH. Physiological and biochemical principles underlying volume-targeted therapy—the "lund concept. Neurocrit Care 2005;2(1):83–95.
95. Koskinen LOD, Olivecrona M, Grände PO. Severe traumatic brain injury management and clinical outcome using the Lund concept. Neuroscience 2014; 283:245–55.
96. Robertson CS. Management of cerebral perfusion pressure after traumatic brain injury. Anesthesiology 2001;95(6):1513–7.
97. Howells T, Elf K, Jones PA, et al. Pressure reactivity as a guide in the treatment of cerebral perfusion pressure in patients with brain trauma. J Neurosurg 2005; 102(2):311–7.
98. Bouma GJ, Muizelaar JP, Bandoh K, et al. Blood pressure and intracranial pressure-volume dynamics in severe head injury: relationship with cerebral blood flow. J Neurosurg 1992;77(1):15–9.
99. Aries MJH, Czosnyka M, Budohoski KP, et al. Continuous determination of optimal cerebral perfusion pressure in traumatic brain injury. Crit Care Med 2012;40(8):2456–63.
100. Donnelly J, Czosnyka M, Adams H, et al. Individualizing thresholds of cerebral perfusion pressure using estimated limits of autoregulation. Crit Care Med 2017; 45(9):1464–71.
101. Dias C, Silva MJ, Pereira E, et al. Optimal cerebral perfusion pressure management at bedside: a single-center pilot study. Neurocrit Care 2015;23(1):92–102.
102. Johnson U, Lewén A, Ronne-Engström E, et al. Should the neurointensive care management of traumatic brain injury patients be individualized according to autoregulation status and injury subtype? Neurocrit Care 2014;21(2):259–65.

103. Bouzat P, Marques-Vidal P, Zerlauth JB, et al. Accuracy of brain multimodal monitoring to detect cerebral hypoperfusion after traumatic brain injury*. Crit Care Med 2015;43(2):445–52.

104. Chang JJJ, Youn TS, Benson D, et al. Physiologic and functional outcome correlates of brain tissue hypoxia in traumatic brain injury*. Crit Care Med 2009; 37(1):283–90.

105. Chesnut R, Aguilera S, Buki A, et al. A management algorithm for adult patients with both brain oxygen and intracranial pressure monitoring: the Seattle International Severe Traumatic Brain Injury Consensus Conference (SIBICC). Intensive Care Med 2020;46(5):919–29.

106. Oddo M, Levine JM, Mackenzie L, et al. Brain hypoxia is associated with short-term outcome after severe traumatic brain injury independent of intracranial hypertension and low cerebral perfusion pressure. Neurosurgery 2011;69(5):1.

107. Maloney-Wilensky E, Gracias V, Itkin A, et al. Brain tissue oxygen and outcome after severe traumatic brain injury: a systematic review. Crit Care Med 2009; 37(6):2057–63.

108. Spiotta AM, Stiefel MF, Gracias VH, et al. Brain tissue oxygen–directed management and outcome in patients with severe traumatic brain injury: clinical article. J Neurosurg 2010;113(3):571–80.

109. Weiner GM, Lacey MR, Mackenzie L, et al. Decompressive craniectomy for elevated intracranial pressure and its effect on the cumulative ischemic burden and therapeutic intensity levels after severe traumatic brain injury. Neurosurgery 2010;66(6):1111–9.

110. Obrist WD, Langfitt TW, Jaggi JL, et al. Cerebral blood flow and metabolism in comatose patients with acute head injury. Relationship to intracranial hypertension. J Neurosurg 1984;61(2):241–53.

111. Bouma GJ, Muizelaar JP, Choi SC, et al. Cerebral circulation and metabolism after severe traumatic brain injury: the elusive role of ischemia. J Neurosurg 1991;75(5):685–93.

112. Roux PL, Menon DK, Citerio G, et al. Consensus summary statement of the international multidisciplinary consensus conference on multimodality monitoring in neurocritical care : a statement for healthcare professionals from the neurocritical care society and the European society of intensive care medicine. Intensive Care Med 2014;40(9):1189–209.

113. Ropper AH. Hyperosmolar therapy for raised intracranial pressure. N Engl J Med 2012;367(8):746–52.

114. Lescot T, Degos V, Zouaoui A, et al. Opposed effects of hypertonic saline on contusions and noncontused brain tissue in patients with severe traumatic brain injury&ast. Crit Care Med 2006;34(12):3029–33.

115. Cascino T, Baglivo J, Conti J, et al. Quantitative CT assessment of furosemide- and mannitol-induced changes in brain water content. Neurology 1983;33(7): 898–903.

116. Kaufmann AM, Cardoso ER. Aggravation of vasogenic cerebral edema by multiple-dose mannitol. J Neurosurg 1992;77(4):584–9.

117. McManus ML, Soriano SG. Rebound swelling of astroglial cells exposed to hypertonic mannitol. Anesthesiology 1998;88(6):1586–91.

118. Quintard H, Meyfroidt G, Citerio G. Hyperosmolar agents for TBI: all are equal, but some are more equal than others? Neurocrit Care 2020;33(2):613–4.

Neuromuscular Weakness in Intensive Care

Deepa Malaiyandi, MD[a],*, Elysia James, MD[a]

KEYWORDS

- Neuromuscular weakness • Neuromuscular respiratory failure
- Critical illness associated weakness • Intensive care unit acquired weakness
- Guillain-Barre syndrome • Myasthenic crisis • Acute myopathy

KEY POINTS

- Disorders of the peripheral nervous system causing weakness in the intensive care setting are not as readily recognized as those of the central nervous system.
- Failure to wean from mechanical ventilation may require an extensive evaluation of the nervous system. Evaluation is time-dependent, as potential for improvement increases with earlier intervention.
- The complex pathophysiology of critical illness can have deleterious effects throughout the neuroaxis, leading to intensive care unit-acquired weakness.
- Premorbid quality of life has important implications for outcomes of critical illness in this population and prognosis is often good.
- Peripheral neuromuscular dysfunction in intensive care is an area of active investigation into improved diagnosis and treatment.

INTRODUCTION

Neuromuscular weakness (NMW) in the intensive care unit (ICU) is a broad topic encompassing several disease processes. Important distinguishing features include localization and time course.[1] Primary neuromuscular diseases (NMD) such as myasthenia gravis (MG), Guillain-Barre Syndromes (GBS), amyotrophic lateral sclerosis (ALS), and others account for less than 0.5% of ICU admissions.[2] MG and GBS account for up to 35% and 15% of admissions for acute respiratory failure, respectively.[3] With increasing ICU survivorship, there is increased recognition of the impact of critical illness on the body. Accordingly, the incidence of ICU acquired weakness (ICUAW) is increasing with estimates of 30% to 50% and greater than 65% of survivors of critical illness and sepsis, respectively.[4] Other impactful forms of weakness acquired in the

a Division of Neurocritical Care, Department of Neurology, University of Toledo College of Medicine, UT/PPG Neurosciences Center, 2130 West Central Avenue, Suite 201, Room 2355, Toledo, OH 43606, USA
* Corresponding author.
E-mail address: Deepa.malaiyandi@utoledo.edu

Crit Care Clin 39 (2023) 123–138
https://doi.org/10.1016/j.ccc.2022.06.004
0749-0704/23/© 2022 Elsevier Inc. All rights reserved.
criticalcare.theclinics.com

ICU, that are not included in ICUAW are, disuse atrophy (DA), isolated diaphragm weakness (DW), pressure and/or traction palsies (PP), and postextubation dysphagia (PED).

EVALUATION/APPROACH

Despite prolonged ICU admission and respiratory support, within the spectrum of neurologic disorders, outcomes of ICU care for NMD are good.[5] Familiarity with an initial approach for the evaluation and management of NMW benefits all intensivists. A comprehensive differential diagnosis, organized by localization, is represented in **Fig. 1**. Important considerations for NMW in the ICU are addressed here per the following framework.

Decompensation, de novo presentation, and unmasking of chronic NMD
- Neuromuscular junction (NMJ) diseases
- Motor neuron diseases (MND)
- Muscular dystrophies (MD) and hereditary myopathies

Severe presentations of new-onset NMD
- Acute myopathies
- NMJ disorders

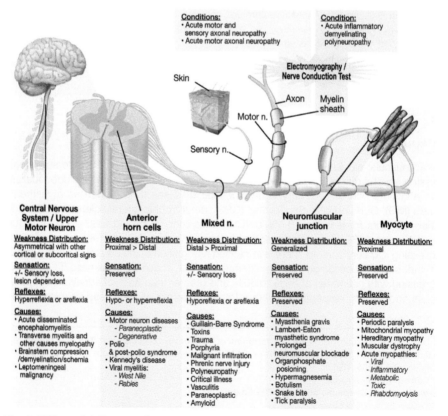

Fig. 1. Differential diagnosis for weakness encountered in intensive care with corresponding anatomic substrate throughout the neuroaxis.

- Neuropathies/radiculopathies
- Neuromuscular toxins
- Autoimmune (AI) and paraneoplastic neuromuscular presentations

Neuromuscular dysfunction that results from the maladaptive physiology of critical illness and consequent to ICU care.

- ICUAW
  - Critical illness polyneuropathy (CIP)
  - Critical illness myopathy (CIM)
  - Critical illness neuromyopathy (CINM)
- DA
- DW
- PP
- PED

Decompensation, de novo Presentation, and Unmasking of Chronic Neuromuscular Disease

Decompensation of chronic NMD occurs with disease progression. Acute physical stressors including infection, surgery, medication changes, endocrine disturbances, renal insufficiency, electrolyte derangements, or other illness are triggers.[1] NMD may also be diagnosed de novo during ICU admission. Manifestation is often of respiratory, cardiac, or hemodynamic complications.[6,7] Additionally, critical illness from multisystem organ failure can unmask latent NMD.

Chronic neuromuscular junction diseases

MG is a well-recognized NMJ disease typified by recurrent decompensation. NMJ transmission is interrupted by postsynaptic receptors autoantibodies diminishing myocyte response to acetylcholine.[8–10] Familiarity and testing for acetylcholine receptor and other MG autoantibodies informs epidemiology, evaluation, and specific treatments (**Table 1**).[8,10] Loss of voluntary muscle contraction produces ocular, bulbar, and generalized weakness patterns. During exacerbations, 10% to 15% of cases remain confined to the ocular muscles; however, progression to generalized weakness is typical, and respiratory failure occurs in severe cases.[8,10] Before the availability of immune therapies, "one-third of patients improved spontaneously, one-third declined, and one-third died."[8] With immunomodulation, mortality is less than 5%.[10] Predictors of prolonged ventilation include age, lower peak forced vital capacity in the first week, and elevated baseline bicarbonate level.[11] Outcomes improve with earlier treatment. Inpatient rehabilitation for respiratory muscle training, with psychological support may improve lung volumes, capacity, and quality of life, without increasing harm, particularly for moderate symptoms.[12]

Motor neuron disease

Chronic MNDs include genetic and sporadic conditions. ALS is the most common. Historically considered a devastating neurodegenerative disorder with a predilection for anterior horn cells, contemporary thinking is of dysfunctional programmed cell death, oxidative stress, mitochondrial pathologic condition, and impaired cell homeostasis that also affects nonmotor domains.[6,13,14] ALS is a truly multisystem disease with several contributing genetic mutations and associated disease complexes. Caution is warranted in de novo diagnoses of ALS in ICU as cervical myelopathy, infectious, postinfections, inflammatory, and paraneoplastic ALS mimics may represent treatable forms of MND.[15]

Investigation into survivorship and ICU utilization by ALS patients at a single-center during a 10-year period revealed an ICU mortality of 20% and median ICU stay of

Table 1
Autoantibodies in myasthenia gravis and their associated features

Antibody	Epidemiology	Clinical Pearls/Other Notes
Acetylcholine receptor (AchR-ab)	• Age <50 y/female predominance • Age >50 y/male predominance	• Assays for AChR-ab may be negative at onset and later become positive • AChR-ab level is not a marker of therapeutic response. Titers may increase as symptoms improve • Hyperplastic thymus glands
Muscle specific tyrosine kinase (MuSK-ab)	• Age < 40 y/female predominance	• Association with respiratory weakness • Poor response to cholinesterase inhibitors (ChEIs), can cause profuse fasciculations • Thymic changes are absent/minimal • Retrospective studies support rituximab
lipoprotein receptor-related protein 4 (LRP4-ab)	Age 30–50 y/female predominance	• Response to therapy is similar to AChR-ab • Early-onset disease, milder symptoms at onset • Not MG specific present in 23% of patients with amyotrophic lateral sclerosis
Antistriational muscle antibodies (StrAbs) 3 Epitopes: titin, ryanodine receptor, potassium channel	• Peak onset age 50 • Man/woman equal	• 75%–85% of patients with thymomatous myasthenia • High predictive value for thymoma • Less predictive of thymoma in age >60 y • Anti-titin ab coexists with moderate ACh-R ab titers
antiryanodine receptor	• Age >50 y/male predominance	• More severe, generalized, or predominantly bulbar weakness, with frequent myasthenic crisis
Antipotassium channel (Anti-Kv1.4 ab)	• N/A	• Bulbar involvement with frequent myasthenic crisis • QT prolongation and myocarditis
Double seronegative	• variable	• Management similarly to AChR-ab MG • Novel antibodies—anti-agrin, unknown clinical significance, may cluster with other antibodies

Data from J Neuroimmunol. 2005 Dec 30;170(1–2):141-9. https://doi.org/10.1016/j.jneuroim.2005.08.017. Epub 2005 Sep 22. Novel autoantibodies to a voltage-gated potassium channel Kv1.4 in a severe form of myasthenia gravis; Bodkin C, Pascuzzi RM. Update in the Management of Myasthenia Gravis and Lambert-Eaton Myasthenic Syndrome. Neurol Clin. 2021 Feb;39(1):133-146. https://doi.org/10.1016/j.ncl.2020.09.007. Epub 2020 Nov 7. PMID: 33223079; Damian MS, Srinivasan R. Neuromuscular problems in the ICU. Curr Opin Neurol. 2017 Oct;30(5):538-544. https://doi.org/10.1097/WCO.0000000000000480; and Guptill JT, Sanders DB. Disorders of neuromuscular transmission. In: Jankovic J, Mazziotta JC, Pomeroy SL, and Newman NJ, editors. Bradley and Daroff's Neurology in Clinical Practice, 8th Edition (Volume 2). London: Elsevier, 2022. p.1958-1977.e6.

4 days. In comparing survivors and nonsurvivors at 3-month, differences in age and degree of respiratory acidosis were significant. Sex, features of neurologic impairment, disease course, respiratory baseline, severity scores, duration, and mode of ventilation, were not significantly different.[13]

In terminal ALS disruption of the complex interplay between neurologic and pulmonary systems occurs.[6,13] Noninvasive positive pressure ventilation (NIPPV) is standard of care for improving quality of life.[6,16] Two drugs approved for ALS are riluzole and edaravone.[17,18] Edaravone likely protects motor neurons from free radical and oxidative stress.[18] Neither has been studied in patients with respiratory failure, and edaravone may cause respiratory decline.

Despite the success of diaphragmatic pacing (DP), outcomes in ALS are conflicting. One trial demonstrated increased survival and delayed need for mechanical ventilation (MV). Two others demonstrated increased mortality. DP in ALS is typically not recommended.[19–22]

Muscular dystrophy and hereditary myopathies
Some MD and hereditary myopathies may present with respiratory and/or cardiac failure despite still mild motor symptoms. Genetic testing identifies need for automatic implantable cardioversion defibrillators. Postoperative recovery can be complicated, particularly in Duchenne's. Intraoperative heart failure, inhaled anesthetic-related and succinylcholine-related rhabdomyolysis with hyperkalemia are possible.[5] More commonly, cardiopulmonary complications develop during late-stage disease when profound weakness may mask overt signs of respiratory failure.[5,23] A notable deviation is late-onset Pompe disease, the most common of these rare disorders to present to the ICU. It is characterized by early respiratory failure, preceding the nonambulatory stage. Enzyme replacement therapy exists.[5]

Further considerations of chronic neuromuscular disease in intensive care
Despite wide heterogeneity, chronic NMD share similar physiologic vulnerabilities evidenced by the coronavirus disease-19 (COVID-19) pandemic.[24] The French Rare Health Care for NMD Network guidance document warns of MG exacerbation with the use of hydroxychloroquine and azithromycin acutely and up to 29 days following treatment.[24] Hydroxychloroquine also increased the risk of fatal arrhythmias in Andersen Syndrome, a multisystem channelopathy.[24] The authors detail the impact of overestimation of frailty scales in determining prognosis and share pathologies that may have a better prognosis than predicted, including MG, muscle channelopathies, and neuropathies.[24] Suggested criteria for resuscitation account for cardiopulmonary function, and physical autonomy and social engagement.[24] Importantly, advances in home ventilation technology alleviate the need to acutely consider the potential likelihood of successful liberation from MV. An individualized approach to advance critical care support is necessary.

Severe Presentation of New-Onset Neuromuscular Weakness

Despite dramatic presentations of severe weakness and debility, and protracted ICU and rehabilitation stays, prognosis is generally good in new onset NMW.[23]

Acute myopathies
Acute inflammatory myopathies are classified by clinical-serological findings of myositis-associated antibodies. Necrotizing acute myositis is most likely to present with rapidly progressing weakness requiring ICU admission. Association with signal recognition peptide antibody indicates need for immunosuppression with rituximab or tacrolimus over steroids alone.[23]

Acute neuromuscular junction disorders

Acute NMJ dysfunction in the ICU is commonly due to prolonged neuromuscular blockade (NMB). Rarely, organophosphate poisoning, hypermagnesemia, botulism, tick paralysis, and snake bites occur. MG, discussed above, can also present as acute NMJ failure when crisis is the first manifestation of disease.

Lambert-Eaton myasthenic syndrome (LEMS) presents a contrast to generalized MG. Antibodies target the NMJ presynaptic P/Q type voltage-gated calcium channel.[25] LEMS characteristically does not cause the fatigable weakness, respiratory insufficiency, and bulbar dysfunction that typifies MG.[11,25] Instead, LEMS is heralded by potentiation with repetition, gait disturbance, lower extremity weakness, and autonomic dysfunction.[25,26] Respiratory failure is rare but seen in advanced disease, from pulmonary malignancy, and exposure to muscle relaxants and other medications. LEMS is most often associated with an underlying malignancy but an AI type exists in younger patients with female predominance.[25,26] Treatment includes the voltage-gated potassium channel antagonist 3,4 diaminopyridine, addressing the underlying malignancy, and immunotherapy for rare refractory cases.[11,25,26]

Neuropathies/radiculopathies

Many causes of radiculopathy, neuropathy, and radiculoneuropathy may warrant ICU admission (**Fig. 1**). Of these, GBS accounts for a large portion of ICU admission for neuromuscular respiratory failure. It is an umbrella of diseases including acute inflammatory demyelinating polyneuropathy (AIDP), Miller Fisher syndrome, acute motor axonal neuropathy, and acute motor and sensory axonal neuropathy.[11] In addition to crippling neurologic dysfunction from acute demyelination, there may be long-standing complications from cytoarchitectural disruption of peripheral nerve/Schwann cell complex.[27] AIDP is best known for acute ascending flaccid paralysis culminating in hemodynamic lability and respiratory failure.[11] The Miller-Fischer triad of ophthalmoplegia, areflexia and ataxia and may be missed before generalized weakness.[11,28] Due to extensive involvement of the autonomic system, frank hemodynamic instability is well described but could be misattributed to sepsis.[3,23] Additional complications include adynamic ileus, urinary retention, sodium imbalance, and ICUAW.[11] Treatment includes intravenous immunoglobulins (IVIG) and plasma exchange/pheresis. IVIG maybe more effective in GM1, GM1b, or GalNac-GD1a subtypes.[23] In GBS, albuminocytological dissociation may be negative in the first week, despite severe presentation or rapid progression. If diagnostic uncertainty exists, repeat lumbar puncture may be informative. The mortality associated with the need for MV is ~20%. For the 80% who survive, 75% are ambulatory at 6 months, and inability to wean from MV is rare.[23]

Neuromuscular toxins/drugs

Poisoning and heavy metal toxicities readily come to mind when considering neuromuscular toxins. However, iatrogenic toxicity is more common. Cyclosporine, amiodarone, zidovudine, statins, corticosteroids, hydroxychloroquine/chloroquine, and even labetalol are known causes.[29] Immune checkpoint inhibitors allow the immune system to treat cancer cells as infectious antigens.[30] These medications can disrupt neuromuscular transmission resembling NMJ disorders or unmasking previously occult NMD.[26] The pathophysiology is ill-defined. The postsynaptic NMJ is affected, producing a spectrum of clinical presentations including ocular, bulbar, and limb-girdle weakness.[25,26,29] Treatment depends on symptom grade as per the American College of Clinical Oncology guideline.[29] Discontinuation of the medication is insufficient and MG evaluation is indicated.[25,29]

Further considerations for severe presentations of new onset neuromuscular weakness
For all severe presentations and rapidly progressive forms of AI or paraneoplastic processes, cerebrospinal fluid (CSF) along with serum should be submitted for antibody panel testing. For mild symptoms, or slow progression, CSF can be banked for later testing if serum is negative. Another important consideration in these presentations is that titers are not reflective of disease severity. Low-positive titers, within the appropriate clinical context, should be treated as positive.

Weakness Acquired in the ICU

Weakness that develops secondary to critical illness and intensive care includes ICUAW, disuse atrophy, DW, PP, and PED. These are entertained after complication of primary injury, new central nervous system (CNS) insult, and endocrinological or electrolyte derangements have been excluded. Failure to wean from MV and/or decreased limb movements are common presentations, and in patients with severe acute brain injury or spinal cord injury, an unexplained decline, or lack of improvement in neurologic function, further evaluation is warranted. Unrecognized, this weakness may mislead physicians to assume a poor prognosis for patients with primary CNS injury.

Intensive care unit acquired weakness
ICUAW exists as 3 subtypes, CIP, CIM, and combined CINM. These may present as either a diffuse symmetric weakness with relative sparing of the cranial nerves, failure to wean from MV secondary to diaphragmatic and/or phrenic nerve involvement, or both. Disuse atrophy is considered a separate entity that is diagnosed in the absence of abnormality on electromyography/nerve conduction studies (EMG/NCS).

The premise of intensive care causing weakness is that the pathophysiology of critical illness encompasses a variety of maladaptive processes that have a deleterious effect on neurons, nerves, NMJs, muscles, or combinations of these in the following ways:

- The catabolic state, immobilization, and inflammatory response associated with critical illness contribute to myonecrosis, fat infiltration, fibrosis, and severe muscle atrophy.
- Membrane and ion channel dysfunction occur such that the sodium channel inactivation may contribute to rapid, reversible hypoexcitability of nerves and muscles, and altered intracellular calcium homeostasis may alter nerve-muscle coupling and attenuate the response to NMB within the NMJ, necessitating higher doses to achieve adequate paralysis.
- Altered cholinergic transmission in the NMJ can result from a combination of increased cholinesterase activity and a decreased number, or spreading of acetylcholine receptors.
- Microcirculatory impairment and resulting hypoperfusion have been suggested as a potential inciting factor for neuronal injury, depolarization of terminal motor axon membranes, and axonal degeneration.
- Relative insufficiency of autophagy fails to address damaged mitochondria, which result from hyperglycemia, free radicals, stress, and inflammation. Accumulation of these damaged organelles contributes to impaired oxygen utilization and further injury to both neurons and myocytes.
- Peripheral edema, which is common in the immobilized critically ill, may cause muscle and nerve injury by compression.

- A CNS role is theorized, whereby a lack of coordinated repetitive depolarization of the motor neuron may precede failure at the NMJ, impairing nerve-muscle coupling, including altering gene expression within myocytes.
- Prolonged immobilization and many ICU treatments contribute to weakness.[2,31]

The evidence for many independent modifiable and nonmodifiable risk factors is established yet some remain inconclusive (**Table 2**). Conflicting data exists for both exposure to corticosteroids and NMB. Meta-analyses evaluating steroid use as a ICUAW risk factor combined studies with variable statistical control for hyperglycemia as a confounding factor.[32] One study that did control for hyperglycemia found steroid use to have a protective effect against ICUAW, whereas another demonstrated increased risk when combined with NMB.[33] Similarly, risk related to NMB is being refined. Specifically, use greater than 48 hours in combination with deep sedation or steroids may negatively affect neuromuscular function. Interestingly, premorbid obesity is associated with a protective effect against muscle weakness and atrophy during critical illness.[2,34]

The short-term and long-term consequences for NMW that develop in the ICU are many (**Box 1**).[2,34–37] Therefore, optimizing all modifiable risk factors is critical to improving outcomes.

Within the context of limited data, 2 single-center observational studies revealed vastly different estimates for incidence of ICUAW in severe COVID-19 disease. One study using EMG/NCS found a 4% to 10% incidence. In contrast, the study using minimum criteria without EMG/NCS, reported an incidence as high as 72%. Although local differences in screening practices may account for this difference, overdiagnosis in the absence of EMG/NCS is one possibility. Without EMG/NCS, diseases that may be treatable, as discussed above, may be misdiagnosed as ICUAW.[38] Accurate diagnosis of ICUAW and subtype is clinically relevant (**Table 3**).[4] CIM carries a better prognosis for full recovery with a shorter recovery period than CIP or CINM.[4]

Table 2	
Established risk factors for intensive care unit-acquired weakness	
Risk Factors Not Modifiable During Treatment	**Risk Factors Modifiable During Treatment**
Illness severity	Higher degree of hyperglycemia
Presence of multiorgan failure	Exposure to parenteral nutrition
Duration of mechanical ventilation	Dose and duration of vasoactive medications ■ Beta agonists increased risk vs alpha agonists
Duration of intensive care admission	Exposure to vancomycin or aminoglycosides
Higher lactate level	Deeper and longer duration of sedation
Older age	Longer duration of immobilization
Female sex	[a] Steroids
Premorbid disability/frailty	[a] Neuromuscular blocking agents

[a] Inconclusive evidence of risk but overall data trend toward increasing risk of ICU-acquired weakness.

Data from Vanhorebeek I, Latronico N, Van den Berghe G. ICU-acquired weakness. Intensive Care Med (2020) 46:637–653.https://doi.org/10.1007/s00134-020-05944-4; Wilcox SR. Corticosteroids and neuromuscular blockers in development of critical illness neuromuscular abnormalities: A historical review. J Crit Care. 2017 Feb;37:149-155. https://doi.org/10.1016/j.jcrc.2016.09.018. Epub 2016 Sep 26. PMID: 27736708; and Hermans G, Wilmer A, Meersseman W, Milants I, Wouters PJ, Bobbaers H, Bruyninckx F, Van den Berghe G (2007) Impact of intensive insulin therapy on neuromuscular complications and ventilator dependency in the medical intensive care unit. Am J Respir Crit Care Med 175:480–489

Box 1
Impact of intensive care unit acquired weakness on outcomes

Short-term (in-hospital)
  Increases ICU and hospital mortality
  Prolongs mechanical ventilation
  Increases rates of extubation failure
  Contributes to ICU and postextubation dysphagia
  Impairs adequate cough contributing to need for reintubation and aspiration pneumonia
  Increases hospital costs
  Increases discharge to facility versus home

Long-term (1–5 years posthospital discharge)
  Severity and duration dependent increase in 1-year mortality
  Severity and duration dependent increase in 1-year mortality
  Increases 1-year mortality even with mild weakness on ICU-day 8, decrease in CMAP amplitude OR low MIP
  Decreases 5-year survival when MRC sum score less than 55, abnormal CMAP at ICU discharge
  Decreases 5-year survival when MRC sum score less than 48 at hospital discharge
  Increases varying degrees of weakness (lower hand grip force, 6-MWD, physical quality of life) 5-years post-ICU discharge

Abbreviations: 6-MWD, 6-min walking distance; ADL, activities of daily living; CMAP, compound muscle action potential; ICU, intensive care unit; MIP, Maximal inspiratory pressures; MRC, Medical Research Council (MRC sum score defines relevant weakness as < 48 and severe weakness as < 36)

Data from Vanhorebeek I, Latronico N, Van den Berghe G. ICU-acquired weakness. *Intensive Care Med* (2020) 46:637–653.https://doi.org/10.1007/s00134-020-05944-4

Beyond prognostic utility, there are treatment implications. Systematic reviews of onxandrolone, an anabolic steroid, growth hormone, propranolol, IVIG, and glutamine therapy for treatment of ICUAW are disappointing.[2] However, a deeper understanding of the individual pathophysiology of CIM versus CIP, has led to the pursuit of subtype-specific therapeutics and biomarkers. Access to inpatient EMG/NCS is often limited. Investigation into alternate reliable, readily available testing methods is underway. Stimulus electrodiagnosis test (SET), performed with a simple universal pulse generator allows for point-of-care screening in neuromuscular dysfunction to triage cases that require EMG/NCS studies.[39] Other areas of interest include biomarkers and high-resolution ultrasound (US).[40]

Until then, early mobilization, exercise, and neuromuscular electrical stimulation (NMES) are promising for prevention and recovery in ICUAW. Early mobilization and exercise preserve muscle fiber cross-section, decreased incidence of ICUAW, ICU length of stay, and MV days, as well as improve short-term and long-term functional outcomes but not ICU, hospital, or 28-day mortality.[4,41] Early NMES can prevent ICUAW and improve quality of life by enhancing muscle strength and shortening the duration of MV and ICU and hospital length of stay. It does not affect inpatient functional status or mortality.[42] However, protocols have varied and are typically determined based on normal muscle excitability thresholds. Preliminary work suggests significant impedance develops during critical illness from muscle edema, fat infiltration, and necrosis. This impedance results in significant increase in muscle excitability thresholds including requiring both an increased duration and current of stimulation for muscle contraction.[39] Screening with SET also yields information on the stimulation threshold in individuals. Further investigation of impact on effectiveness of SET-guided NMES is needed.[4,39]

Table 3
Summary of distinguishing features for critical illness polyneuropathy, critical illness myopathy, and critical illness neuromyopathy

	CIP	CIM	CINM

Examination:
Weakness
Spares
Sensory
Reflexes
	Distal > proximal
	Involves lower > upper limbs
	+/− phrenic nerve
	Ocular and facial muscles
	Affected
	Reduced or absent
		Proximal > distal
		Generalized
		+/− diaphragm
		Ocular and facial
		    muscles
		Spared
		Preserved
			Proximal = distal
			Generalized
			+/− phrenic nerve
			    and diaphragm
			Ocular and facial muscles
			Affected
			Reduced

NCS
CMAP
SNAP
Velocity
RNS
EMG
	Reduced/absent
	Reduced/absent
	Normal/slightly reduced
	Normal
	Normal
	- Decreased recruitment of
	    polyphasic MUAPs
	- Decreased recruitment high
	    amplitude, long MUAPs
		Reduced and
		    Prolonged
		Normal
		Normal
		Normal
		Early recruitment
		    of small
		    amplitude,
		    short MUAPs
			Reduced
			Reduced
			Normal/slightly reduced
			Normal
			Early recruitment of small
			    amplitude, short MUAPs

Biopsy
Nerve
Muscle
	Axonal neuropathy
	Denervation atrophy
	    of Type 1 and 2 fibers
		Normal
		Selective loss of
		    myosin filaments
		Necrosis
			Features of
			    CIP and CIM

Prognosis	50%–75% persistent
	    severe weakness at 1 y
		Near complete
		    recovery by 1 y
			Worst

Abbreviations: CIM, critical illness myopathy; CINM, critical illness neuromyopathy; CIP, critical illness polyneuropathy; CMAP, compound muscle action potential; EMG, electromyography; MUAP, motor unit action potential; NCS, nerve conduction study; RNS, repetitive nerve stimulation; SNAP, sensory nerve action potential.

Data from Vanhorebeek I, Latronico N, Van den Berghe G. ICU-acquired weakness. Intensive Care Med (2020) 46:637–653 https://doi.org/10.1007/s00134-020-05944-4; and Singh TD, Wijdicks EFM. Neuromuscular Respiratory Failure. Neurol Clin. 2021;39(2):333-353. https://doi.org/10.1016/j.ncl.2021.01.010

Diaphragm weakness

DW constitutes both a reduced thickness and force-generating capacity in mechanically ventilated patients. It is unclear if it is simply ICUAW affecting the diaphragm and/or phrenic nerve, a variation along a similar spectrum, or its own entity. However, it warrants separate consideration here because it is twice as common as ICUAW and there is poor correlation between the degree of proximal upper extremity weakness in ICUAW and that of the diaphragm.[43] Moreover, unlike ICUAW of other muscle groups, a specific form of disuse atrophy of the diaphragm from MV, or ventilator-induced diaphragm dysfunction (VIDD), exists that is thought to be completely reversible with resumption of spontaneous breathing and minimization of sedation.[7]

Several techniques for bedside evaluation of diaphragm dysfunction have been summarized by Supinski *and colleagues.*[7] Quantitative assessment using bedside US techniques has been shown in observational studies to predict extubation success and is itself a major determinant of MV days and ICU mortality. In fact, its effect on ICU mortality is greater than the degree of organ failure, severity of lung dysfunction, and even age.[7] Currently, a trial comparing temporary transvenous diaphragmatic pacing to standard of care for weaning from MV in the ICU (RESCUE 3) is underway. It follows the RESCUE 2 feasibility trial, for which preliminary results demonstrated a 308%

increase in maximal inspiratory pressure (MIP) and 167% increase in the rapid shallow breathing index (RSBI) with transvenous temporary diaphragmatic pacing compared with standard care.[44] Notably, both trials exclude patients with neurologic causes of DW. Other active research is ongoing with preclinical trials for 2 groups of pharmacologic agents, one aimed at inhibiting proteolysis and the other at enhancing protein synthesis with a goal-preserving strength and endurance.[7] It is hopeful that one of these interventions, alone or in combination, will eventually lead to greater ventilator-free days for ICU patients with weakness.

Pressure and traction nerve palsies

The recent COVID-19 crisis highlights the importance of assessing for mechanical peripheral nerve injuries in critically ill patient, as literature suggests that 14% to 16% of severe COVID-19 patients experience mechanical nerve injury.[38] The brachial plexus and median, ulnar, radial, sciatic, and fibular nerves are commonly affected.[45] Prone positioning can cause stretch injury to the brachial plexus. This position also contributes to compression on the ulnar nerve at the cubital tunnel and the fibular nerve at the fibular head if not appropriately positioned and protected. Frequent and prolonged cycling of automated blood pressure cuffs and positioning for other standard ICU procedures and care are thought to contribute to radial, median, and sciatic nerve palsies. extracorporeal membrane oxygenation (ECMO) specifically, with femoral cannulation, contributes to the injury of the femoral nerve from the weight of bulky cannulas. If compartment syndrome complicates therapy, sural, tibial, and fibular injury ipsilateral to cannulation are possible.[38] No specific features have been identified in ICUAW from COVID compared with other causes of ICUAW. It is reasonable to expect that patients who require prolonged proning or ECMO for other diseases are likely to be at the same risk for peripheral nerve injury. A combination of EMG/NCS, US, and MRI modalities has been successfully used to accurately diagnose such injuries in complex cases with multiple confounders.[38] Peripheral nerve injuries can contribute to long-term poor outcomes and functional limitations, which often persist despite significant improvement in comorbid ICUAW. Identifying this additional impairment presents a significant challenge because they are likely to go unrecognized without careful neurologic examinations for subtle focal deficits superimposed on diffuse weakness.

Postextubation dysphagia

PED is another form of weakness acquired in the ICU. Its estimated incidence is 15% in a mixed ICU population and up to 62% following cardiac surgery or acute ischemic stroke. The pathophysiological mechanisms responsible for PED are unclear when known CNS insult or direct trauma to the oropharyngeal and laryngeal structures is absent. However, it is an independent predictor of 28-day and 80-day mortality and may persist for many years, affecting the quality of life in survivors. Future focus in this area is needed.[45]

COMPLICATIONS AND CONCERNS
Failure to Wean from Mechanical Ventilation

There is good potential for the treatment of many of these conditions.[7] If not already involved, consultation with a neuromuscular disease expert is indicated. Despite a lack of patient participation, many important details can be elicited by a neurologist. These patients are not well served by telehealth consultation. Initial evaluation of NMD requires examination components that are not possible with currently available telehealth platforms and transfer to a center with on-site neurologic, and preferably neuromuscular expertise is recommended.[46]

This category of patients is not just "difficult to wean" due to their underlying illness but the dearth of evidence regarding an approach to weaning.[11] Although the diaphragm is a key component of respiratory mechanics, in neuromuscular compromise, oropharyngeal weakness may be grossly underestimated. These are more fully appreciated in CNS pathologic condition.[11] Here useful markers of respiratory function such as RSBI, MIP, and others will fall short without adequate consideration of oropharyngeal dysfunction. A recent single-center study investigating correlation between increased gastric residuals and oropharyngeal dysfunction used fiberoptic endoscopic evaluation of swallow to score the degree of oropharyngeal dysfunction.[47] More research is needed in this area to inform and guide management.

Strategies for weaning from mechanical ventilation
Specialized ventilator modes present another potential tool in managing difficult to wean patients. Advances in this area include the development of neurally adjusted ventilator assist and proportional assist ventilation modes. Each is intended to address VIDD.[48] Optimized variables include decreased patient-ventilator dyssynchrony and potential decrease in overassistance or underloading of the diaphragm by the ventilator, leading to decreased MV days. Potential obstacles to widespread use include nascent settings still under investigation for patient personalization, monitor displacement, provider unfamiliarity, and resource limitation.[48,49] Current studies have not evaluated protocols for this specific population, and no studies have evaluated their use in NMD patients.[48,50]

Noninvasive ventilation in palliative care
There have been changes in the approach to palliative care for patients with end stage NMW. The hallmark pathologic condition in this area is ALS. Supplementation with NIPPV improves quality at end-of-life and aids in the administration of full comfort measures.[16] Due to the nature of respiratory system dysfunction, and the chronicity of use, withdrawal of NIPPV during transition to comfort measures may produce the opposite effect of comfort.[16] Pursuing a patient-centered approach inclusive of modalities previously not considered comfort measures is in evolution in this patient population.

FUTURE DIRECTIONS

The past decade has seen significant advancements in understanding of the pathophysiology of NMW in the ICU. Laboratory studies and genetic evaluations continue to advance the field leading to comprehensive and definitive diagnosis including the expansion of gene panels and early study of potential biomarkers.[1] Accordingly, efforts are underway to develop therapeutic options that target key pathways not only for a particular disorder but also for specific disease subtypes. However, access to advanced diagnostic modalities such as EMG/NCS remains limited to tertiary and quaternary medical facilities, often in high-resource regions of the world. Advances in electrodiagnostic technology in the form of more user-friendly, portable, and lower cost technology could improve global access. Future focus on noninvasive, inexpensive, and less time-consuming tests is essential for consistent accurate diagnosis. This will be key for timely enrollment in future clinical trials and for broader application of trial results to patients without access to such centers. In this respect, the identification of reliable biomarkers and the development of widely available assays need active research. Finally, despite operator-dependent variation and potential inaccuracies, US is a widely available technology in many ICUs and is ideal for point-of-care testing. Much research has already been done in this area and greater dissemination of this knowledge and necessary skills has potential to hasten time-to-diagnosis and treatment to improve outcomes.

SUMMARY

NMW in the ICU affects both short-term and long-term morbidity and mortality. This is irrespective of the underlying cause, be it chronic disease, severe presentations of acute to subacute processes, or deranged pathophysiology and side effects of treatments for critical illness. Although some presentations are considerably more common than others, the differential diagnosis remains extensive. With treatment options available for symptom control and, in some cases, reversal or delay in disease progression, accurate diagnosis is critical. A systematic approach to evaluation based on localization and chronology is key. A thorough neurologic history and examination are fundamental to this approach. Close coordination of care between intensivists and neurologists to optimize care is crucial in achieving good outcomes, which can be realized by most patients with NMW in the ICU.

CLINICS CARE POINTS

- Identification of the various MG autoantibodies when present is useful for treatment and prognosis.
- Caution is warranted in de novo diagnoses of ALS in ICU as cervical myelopathy, infectious, postinfectious, inflammatory, and paraneoplastic MNDs represent treatable forms of illness with severe consequences if missed.
- In GBS, albuminocytological dissociation maybe negative initially, despite severe presentation and rapid progression. Repeat lumbar puncture maybe informative.
- IVIG may be more effective in GM1, GM1b, or GalNac-GD1a immunologic subtypes.
- Early mobilization, exercise, and NMES have shown promise for prevention and recovery in ICUAW.
- Quantitative bedside US assessment of DW may predict extubation success, MV days, and ICU mortality.
- In neuromuscular respiratory compromise, typical weaning parameters fall short without adequate consideration of oropharyngeal dysfunction.

DISCLOSURE

D. Malaiyandi and E. James have no disclosures.

REFERENCES

1. Pasnoor M, Dimachkie MM. Approach to muscle and neuromuscular junction disorders. Continuum (Minneap Minn) 2019;25(6):1536–63.
2. Vanhorebeek I, Latronico N, Van den Berghe G. ICU-acquired weakness. Intensive Care Med 2020;46(4):637–53.
3. Birch TB. Neuromuscular disorders in the intensive care Unit. Continuum (Minneap Minn) 2021;27(5):1344–64.
4. Cheung K, Rathbone A, Melanson M, et al. Pathophysiology and management of critical illness polyneuropathy and myopathy. J Appl Physiol (1985) 2021;130(5): 1479–89.

5. Damian MS, Wijdicks EFM. The clinical management of neuromuscular disorders in intensive care. Neuromuscul Disord 2019;29(2):85–96.

6. Niedermeyer S, Murn M, Choi PJ. Respiratory failure in amyotrophic lateral sclerosis. Chest 2019;155(2):401–8.

7. Supinski GS, Morris PE, Dhar S, et al. Diaphragm dysfunction in critical illness. Chest 2018;153(4):1040–51.

8. Guptill JT, Sanders DB. Disorders of neuromuscular transmission. In: Jankovic J, Mazziotta JC, Pomeroy SL, et al, editors. Bradley and Daroff's Neurology in clinical practice, vol. 2, 8th edition. London: Elsevier; 2022. p. 1958–77.e6.

9. Guptill JT, Sanders DB. Proximal, distal and generalized weakness. In: Daroff RB, Fenichel GM, Janovik J, Mazziota JC, editors. Bradley and Daroff's Neurology in clinical practice. 6th edition. London: Elsevier; 2012. p. 279–95.

10. Ciafaloni E. Myasthenia gravis and Congenital myasthenic syndromes. Continuum (Minneap Minn) 2019;25(6):1767–84.

11. Singh TD, Wijdicks EFM. Neuromuscular respiratory failure. Neurol Clin 2021; 39(2):333–53.

12. Corrado B, Giardulli B, Costa M. Evidence-based practice in rehabilitation of myasthenia gravis. A systematic review of the literature. J Funct Morphol Kinesiol 2020;5(4):71.

13. Mayaux J, Lambert J, Morélot-Panzini C, et al. Survival of amyotrophic lateral sclerosis patients after admission to the intensive care unit for acute respiratory failure: an observational cohort study. J Crit Care 2019;50:54–8.

14. Moujalled D, Strasser A, Liddell JR. Molecular mechanisms of cell death in neurological diseases. Cell Death Differ 2021;28(7):2029–44.

15. Mélé N, Berzero G, Maisonobe T, et al. Motor neuron disease of paraneoplastic origin: a rare but treatable condition. J Neurol 2018;265(7):1590–9.

16. Gifford AH. Noninvasive ventilation as a palliative measure. Curr Opin Support Palliat Care 2014;8(3):218–24.

17. Jaiswal MK. Riluzole and edaravone: a tale of two amyotrophic lateral sclerosis drugs. Med Res Rev 2019;39(2):733–48.

18. Shefner J, Heiman-Patterson T, Pioro EP, et al. Long-term edaravone efficacy in amyotrophic lateral sclerosis: post-hoc analyses of Study 19 (MCI186-19). Muscle Nerve 2020;61(2):218–21.

19. Onders RP, Elmo M, Khansarinia S, et al. Complete worldwide operative experience in laparoscopic diaphragm pacing: results and differences in spinal cord injured patients and amyotrophic lateral sclerosis patients. Surg Endosc 2009; 23(7):1433–40.

20. Onders RP, Elmo M, Kaplan C, et al. Final analysis of the pilot trial of diaphragm pacing in amyotrophic lateral sclerosis with long-term follow-up: diaphragm pacing positively affects diaphragm respiration. Am J Surg 2014;207(3):393–7.

21. DiPALS Writing Committee; DiPALS Study Group Collaborators. Safety and efficacy of diaphragm pacing in patients with respiratory insufficiency due to amyotrophic lateral sclerosis (DiPALS): a multicentre, open-label, randomised controlled trial. Lancet Neurol 2015;14(9):883–92.

22. Gonzalez-Bermejo J, Morélot-Panzini C, Tanguy ML, et al. Early diaphragm pacing in patients with amyotrophic lateral sclerosis (RespiStimALS): a randomised controlled triple-blind trial. Lancet Neurol 2016;15(12):1217–27 [published correction appears in Lancet Neurol. 2016 Dec;15(13):1301].

23. Damian MS, Srinivasan R. Neuromuscular problems in the ICU. Curr Opin Neurol 2017;30(5):538–44.

24. Solé G, Salort-Campana E, Pereon Y, et al. Guidance for the care of neuromuscular patients during the COVID-19 pandemic outbreak from the French rare health care for neuromuscular diseases Network. Rev Neurol (Paris) 2020; 176(6):507–15.

25. Guidon AC. Lambert-eaton myasthenic syndrome, botulism, and immune checkpoint Inhibitor-related myasthenia gravis. Continuum (Minneap Minn) 2019;25(6): 1785–806.

26. Bodkin C, Pascuzzi RM. Update in the management of myasthenia gravis and Lambert-Eaton myasthenic syndrome. Neurol Clin 2021;39(1):133–46.

27. Moss KR, Bopp TS, Johnson AE, et al. New evidence for secondary axonal degeneration in demyelinating neuropathies. Neurosci Lett 2021;221:744, 135595.

28. Sheikh KA. Guillain-barré syndrome. Continuum (Minneap Minn) 2020;26(5): 1184–204.

29. Janecek J, Kushlaf H. Toxin-induced channelopathies, neuromuscular junction disorders, and myopathy. Neurol Clin 2020;38(4):765–80.

30. Lentz RW, Colton MD, Mitra SS, et al. Innate immune checkpoint inhibitors: the Next Breakthrough in medical Oncology? Mol Cancer Ther 2021;20(6):961–74.

31. Camdessanché JP. End-plate disorders in intensive care Unit. J Clin Neurophysiol 2020;37(3):211–3.

32. Sánchez Solana L, Goñi Bilbao I, Ruiz García P, et al. Acquired neuromuscular dysfunction in the intensive care unit. Disfunción neuromuscular adquirida en la unidad de cuidados intensivos. Enferm Intensiva (Engl Ed) 2018;29(3):128–37.

33. Hermans G, Wilmer A, Meersseman W, et al. Impact of intensive insulin therapy on neuromuscular complications and ventilator dependency in the medical intensive care unit. Am J Respir Crit Care Med 2007;175(5):480–9.

34. Yang T, Li Z, Jiang L, et al. Hyperlactacidemia as a risk factor for intensive care unit-acquired weakness in critically ill adult patients. Muscle Nerve 2021;64(1): 77–82.

35. Van Aerde N, Meersseman P, Debaveye Y, et al. Five-year impact of ICU-acquired neuromuscular complications: a prospective, observational study. Intensive Care Med 2020;46(6):1184–93.

36. Yang T, Li Z, Jiang L, et al. Risk factors for intensive care unit-acquired weakness: a systematic review and meta-analysis. Acta Neurol Scand 2018;138(2):104–14.

37. Wilcox SR. Corticosteroids and neuromuscular blockers in development of critical illness neuromuscular abnormalities: a historical review. J Crit Care 2017;37: 149–55.

38. Hokkoku K, Erra C, Cuccagna C, et al. Intensive care unit-acquired weakness and positioning-related peripheral nerve injuries in COVID-19: a case Series of three patients and the latest literature review. Brain Sci 2021;11(9):1177.

39. Silva PE, Maldaner V, Vieira L, et al. Neuromuscular electrophysiological disorders and muscle atrophy in mechanically-ventilated traumatic brain injury patients: new insights from a prospective observational study. J Crit Care 2018; 44:87–94 [published correction appears in J Crit Care. 2018 Nov 28;:].

40. Witteveen E, Sommers J, Wieske L, et al. Diagnostic accuracy of quantitative neuromuscular ultrasound for the diagnosis of intensive care unit-acquired weakness: a cross-sectional observational study. Ann Intensive Care 2017;7(1):40.

41. Trethewey SP, Brown N, Gao F, et al. Interventions for the management and prevention of sarcopenia in the critically ill: a systematic review. J Crit Care 2019;50: 287–95.

42. Liu M, Luo J, Zhou J, et al. Intervention effect of neuromuscular electrical stimulation on ICU acquired weakness: a meta-analysis. Int J Nurs Sci 2020;7(2): 228–37.

43. Piva S, Fagoni N, Latronico N. Intensive care unit-acquired weakness: unanswered questions and targets for future research. F1000Res 2019;8:F1000. Faculty Rev-508.

44. Dres M, Gama De Abreu M, Similowski T. Late Breaking Abstract - temporary transvenous diaphragm Neurostimulation in difficult-to-wean mechanically ventilated patients - results of the RESCUE 2 randomized controlled trial. Eur Respir J 2020;56:4352.

45. Perren A, Zürcher P, Schefold JC. Clinical Approaches to assess post-extubation dysphagia (PED) in the critically ill. Dysphagia 2019;34(4):475–86.

46. Garibaldi M, Siciliano G, Antonini G. Telemedicine for neuromuscular disorders during the COVID-19 outbreak. J Neurol 2021;268(1):1–4.

47. Muhle P, Konert K, Suntrup-Krueger S, et al. Oropharyngeal dysphagia and impaired Motility of the upper Gastrointestinal Tract-is there a clinical Link in neurocritical care? Nutrients 2021;13(11):3879.

48. Jonkman AH, Rauseo M, Carteaux G, et al. Proportional modes of ventilation: technology to assist physiology. Intensive Care Med 2020;46(12):2301–13.

49. Akoumianaki E, Prinianakis G, Kondili E, et al. Physiologic comparison of neurally adjusted ventilator assist, proportional assist and pressure support ventilation in critically ill patients. Respir Physiol Neurobiol 2014;203:82–9.

50. Vasconcelos RS, Sales RP, Melo LHP, et al. Influences of duration of inspiratory effort, respiratory mechanics, and ventilator type on Asynchrony with pressure support and proportional assist ventilation. Respir Care 2017;62(5):550–7.

Neuroprognostication

Victoria Fleming, BA[a],
Susanne Muehlschlegel, MD, MPH, FNCS, FCCM, FAAN[a,b,c,*]

KEYWORDS

- Prognostication • Neurocritical care • Uncertainty • Surrogate decision-makers
- Prognosis • Shared decision-making

KEY POINTS

- There are no guidelines to assist clinicians in the formulation or communication of prognostication in the neurocritical care setting; hence, prognostication is highly variable, potentially biased, and often premature.
- Uncertainty is unavoidable in prognostication; families ask for frank acknowledgment of its presence and forthright disclosure of uncertainty by clinicians during prognostication.
- The prognostic communication in the neurologic intensive care unit may be strengthened by focusing on patient- or surrogate-centeredness to foster trust, manage overly optimistic bias, and help surrogate decision-makers arrive at decisions that patients would choose for themselves.

INTRODUCTION

"Prognosis" stems from the Greek words "pro" meaning "before" and "gnosis" meaning "knowledge."[1] Prognosis therefore means *"knowing something beforehand,"* which is unrealistic in the context of helping families understand a future outlook for their loved one admitted to an intensive care unit (ICU), simply because clinicians cannot predict the future with certainty to claim "knowledge" of the future. On the other hand, "prognostication" stems from the Greek word "prognōstikos," which means "foretelling," which is exactly what clinicians attempt to do. The undertaking of "prognostication" is using signs, symptoms, or various diagnostic modalities (eg, imaging) to foretell the future.[1] The term "neuroprognostication" relates to prognostication specific to the setting of neurologic illness. Patients with severe acute brain injuries (SABIs), including those with severe acute ischemic strokes, intracerebral hemorrhage, traumatic brain injury (TBI), or hypoxic-ischemic encephalopathy, are

 ^a Department of Neurology, University of Massachusetts Chan Medical School, 55 Lake Avenue North, S-5, Worcester, MA 01655, USA; ^b Department of Anesthesiology/Critical Care, University of Massachusetts Chan Medical School, 55 Lake Avenue North, S-5, Worcester, MA 01655, USA; ^c Department of Surgery, University of Massachusetts Chan Medical School, 55 Lake Avenue North, S-5, Worcester, MA 01655, USA
* Corresponding author.
E-mail address: susanne.muehlschlegel@umassmed.edu

Crit Care Clin 39 (2023) 139–152
https://doi.org/10.1016/j.ccc.2022.06.005
0749-0704/23/© 2022 Elsevier Inc. All rights reserved.
criticalcare.theclinics.com

usually comatose, sedated or encephalopathic and, hence, incapacitated for decision-making. This places the burden of decision-making onto the shoulders of surrogate decision-makers, often family members. As these families grapple with the sudden onset of severe illness, they yearn for prognostication to prepare for the future and decide on treatments or care paths that are best for the patient. Physicians and other care providers also use prognostication to triage, decide on what treatments to offer, and how to communicate with families.

SABIs are extremely common across the globe, with millions of deaths and an even larger number of resulting lifelong disabilities worldwide.[2] Owing to an aging population and increased survival after SABI attributable to advances in medical care, the incidence and prevalence of SABIs have even further increased over the past 30 years.[2] Patients with SABI necessitate rapid treatments to prevent or ameliorate worsening brain injury and irreversible illness. Life-or-death treatment decisions, such as intubation, craniotomy, craniectomy, or other interventions, must be made swiftly to preserve brain function or prevent death.[2] Most patients with SABI survive the first 5 to 10 days in the ICU. To reach the next stage of recovery, SABI patients often need airway and artificial nutrition support, with care by others for their most basic needs for the initial weeks to months, or even years. Thus, while considering the patient's potential for long-term disability and diminished quality of life, surrogates must make the difficult decision about continuation or withdrawal of life-sustaining therapies (WLSTs). Survival following acute injury may be accompanied by higher or lower levels of disability, but at a minimum with a large degree of uncertainty about the degree of recovery. Because of this, it is especially important for neurocritical care providers to prognosticate as accurately as possible while also communicating all possible outcomes and their associated risks as well as the existing uncertainty about the prognosis and uncertainty about recovery to surrogate decision-makers.

CURRENT APPROACHES TO PROGNOSTICATION

Prognostication can be dissected into two components: (1) clinicians' knowledge of the type and severity of the neurologic injury and its anticipated long-term sequalae and (2) communication and disclosure of these aspects to the patient or their surrogate decision-makers. There are limited studies that have examined how clinicians formulate their prognostication for SABI. In a prospective five-center study of intracerebral hemorrhage, researchers qualitatively examined the factors considered by physicians when prognosticating. Physicians described using a wide range of the types and combination of factors, such as age, clinical examination severity, radiological findings, preexisting cognitive impairment, the presence of social support, and etiology of the injury to form their prognosis.[3] A recent study of neurologic prognostication after cardiac arrest used semi-structured interviews with disease experts and general physicians and applied the innovative approach of "mental models" to summarize the cognitive approaches physicians take for neuroprognostication.[4] This study found that all participating physicians, regardless of expert or general physician status, used a similar iterative process of assessment and data collection to continuously formulate their prognoses.[4] For the first time, this study shed light on the cognitive process of how physicians derive their prognostication. Participating physicians formed an initial prognosis and then modified it after considering test results, medical imaging findings, patient age, patient frailty, patient premorbid state, hospital resource availability, and their own optimistic or pessimistic leanings.[4] This study showed the complexity of the cognitive approach to prognostication after one type of SABI (cardiac arrest), although this approach is likely representative for prognostication after all types of SABI.

Regarding the second aspect of neuroprognostication, its communication to families, very little research has been conducted in SABI or the neuroICU. One recent pilot mixed-methods study of clinician communication in the neuroICUs at seven centers found significant variability between clinicians and specialties regarding clinician approach to prognostication.[5] However, further validation of these findings is necessary in a larger study.

This current state of neuroprognostication has often been described by many researchers as an "art."[6–8] Others, however, have in turn criticized that neuroprognostication should not be an "art," as this implies that individualism and variability by the clinicians formulating the prognostication is acceptable and welcome. Instead, researchers have suggested that neuroprognostication should be performed as "scientifically" as possible.[7] This may include a combination of more precise data with longer outcome assessment periods and the addition of machine learning to allow the inclusion of more variables and an individualized prognostication that also includes the ICU course and trajectory.[9] Additional research into how physicians cognitively derive the prognosis and how to communicate it effectively is certainly necessary to change the current perception of neuroprognostication from being an "art" to it being a "science."

Because prognostication is so important for patients and their surrogates, formalized guidelines have been suggested to guide clinicians and introduce some form of standardization with the hope of ameliorating variability.[10] Recently, a joint guideline on "Disorders of Consciousness" was published by the American Academy of Neurology, American Congress of Rehabilitation Medicine, and the National Institute on Disability, Independent Living and Rehabilitation Research.[11] This document provided guidance on what NOT to do when prognosticating for patients with disorders of consciousness.[11] A strong recommendation was made, stating *"When discussing prognosis with caregivers of patients with a disorder of consciousness during the first 28 days postinjury, clinicians must avoid statements that suggest these patients have a universally poor prognosis."*[11] The American Heart Association has published a scientific statement on the "Standards for Studies of Neurologic Prognostication in Comatose Survivors of Cardiac Arrest" concluding that the "overall quality of existing neurologic prognostication studies is low."[12] This scientific statement provided suggestions to improve the quality of research studies in neuroprognostication, but this document does not, nor was it intended to, fulfill the role of a clinical practice guideline on how to "best" prognosticate.[10–12] With this goal in mind, a clinical guideline examining current published literature is currently underway by the Neurocritical Care Society and German Society for Neurointensive Medicine (Deutsche Gesellschaft für Neurointensivmedizin).[13] Preliminary results have been presented at a recent conference (ANIM 2022[13]) with an anticipated publication year of 2022.

BIAS, HEURISTICS, AND THE SELF-FULFILLING PROPHECY

Clinicians in the neuroICU must make quick medical decisions for their patients as a routine part of clinical practice. Substantial discoveries in psychology have described human judgments, including those for prognostication, are based on either "System-One processes" (fast, automatic, heuristic) or "System-Two processes" (slow, deliberate, analytical)[14] (**Fig. 1**). In medical decision-making, particularly in fast-paced environments such as the emergency department or ICU, System-One processes using heuristics commonly underpin decision-making.[15] Here, clinicians generate solutions to complex problems through pattern recognition and simplifying assumptions.[16]

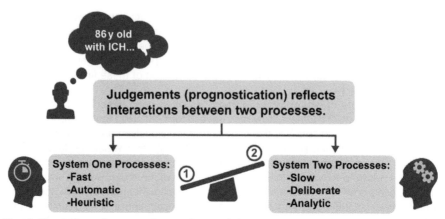

Fig. 1. The balance between System-One and System-Two processes in decision-making. Prognostication requires balancing System-One though processes with System-Two thought processes. System-One processes are fast, automatic, stereotyped, emotional, unconscious, and heuristic. System-Two processes are slow, deliberate, analytical, effortful, conscious, and infrequent. In the presence of uncertainty, heuristics help the clinician generate solutions to complex problems through pattern recognition based on previously acquired knowledge and experience.

Heuristics may be practical using "mental shortcuts," particularly in the presence of uncertainty; however, when poorly calibrated, clinicians make "bad" decisions based on biases that may result in worse patient outcomes.[17–19] This has been shown in a randomized-controlled trial of emergency room triage of trauma patients and in a systematic review of physician cognitive biases, which found that cognitive biases were associated with diagnostic inaccuracies and medical management errors.[15–18]

Heuristics and clinician bias may potentially also play a role in the known high variability of death from WLST.[20,21] WLST is the leading cause of death after SABI and varies widely by center, with reports ranging from 0% to 96% in stroke and 45% to 87% in severe TBI.[2,20,21,22] Variability persists even after adjusting for epidemiologic patient, surrogate, or provider characteristics.[23] Previous studies have also shown that WLST is more likely when the acute neurologic insult is deemed "more severe" by the clinician.[24–26] This is problematic because several studies have suggested that some clinicians may be overly pessimistic regarding prognosis, leading to clinical nihilism, an "inappropriately pessimistic view of a patient's outcome and the ability of a patient to benefit from aggressive care."[24,25,27,28] This in turn can result in a self-fulfilling prophecy of poor prognosis (**Fig. 2**).[19,29,30]

In the case of prognostication, the self-fulfilling prophecy involves WLST for a subset of individuals who suffered from a devastating neurologic injury, but a subset of WLST patients might have survived otherwise. The resulting mortality of that neurologic injury seems higher than it should.[22] The self-fulfilling prophecy affects prognostic statistical models; poor prognosis leads to WLST and subsequent fatality, which then contributes to poor outcome in the models.[19,22] In an effort to mitigate clinician bias and premature WLST, experts in neurocritical care currently recommend at least a 72-h treatment period before any WLST decisions, although it is uncertain whether this would truly solve the problem of self-fulfilling prophecy.[31] Only studies that do not allow any WLST and follow the trajectory of patients out until at least 1 year after SABI may provide insights into true long-term outcomes of patients.

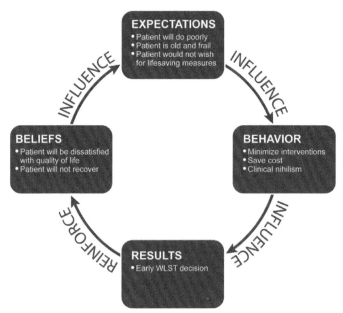

Fig. 2. The self-fulfilling prophecy. This figure demonstrates the cycle of the self-fulfilling prophecy: beliefs and expectations influence clinicians' behavior and results, which in turn reinforce beliefs. For example, a clinician might have biases about a patient's age, pre-existing code status, or prognosis. This contributes to the clinician's prognostication and recommended treatments.

Recently, a study from South Korea, a country where WLST is not permitted by law, showed that in their cohort of greater than 1000 cardiac arrest survivors followed for 6 months or longer, awakening occurred in 42% at a median of 30 hours after rewarming, with the longest awakening time at 1415 hours (nearly 59 days).[32] Late awakening (>72 hour after rewarming from therapeutic temperature management) was common and occurred in nearly a quarter (24.3%) of all patients who awakened.[32] Good neurologic outcomes (cerebral performance scale 1–2) occurred in the vast majority (84.5%) of patients who awakened.[32] Insight into the true outcome of patients, when WLST is not permitted, is unique, and repeating such studies for other neurologic emergencies is valuable.

WHAT SURROGATES NEED

Surrogates find prognostication by a physician an important and necessary step in communication with the clinical team.[33,34] Empirical research in general critical care has shown that surrogates use clinicians' prognostication in some part to inform their clinical decisions.[35] Despite this, prognostication only forms a small part of what goes into a surrogate's perception of the patient's prognosis. Only 2% of surrogates reported that they relied on clinician prognostication alone when considering the overall prognosis of a patient.[36] Other factors, including the patient's will to live, physical appearance, and prior medical history, were often coupled with clinician's prognostic input to inform surrogate prognostic impression.[36] Surrogates may be skeptical of the clinicians' ability to prognosticate reliably. In one qualitative study using semi-structured interviews with 50 surrogate decision-makers of critically ill patients without

SABI, 88% of surrogates expressed doubt in the clinicians' ability to prognosticate.[35] Reasons for this were beliefs that God affected the disease course, foretelling the future is inherently inaccurate, prior experiences with inaccurate prognostication, and ongoing experiences with prognostication during the current ICU admission.[35] Nonetheless, hearing the clinician's prognostication was important to all surrogates in this study before making decisions.[35]

Several studies have shown that most surrogates would rather receive exact numeric estimates when discussing prognosis despite clinician reluctance to provide them. In a multicenter qualitative study of surrogate decision-makers of moderate–severe TBI patients and their physicians from across the United States, most surrogates (82%) preferred receiving exact numeric estimates from physicians when discussing their loved one's prognosis, and very few (18%) were satisfied with qualitative prediction statements such as "highly likely" or "unlikely."[34] Although outcome prediction models are available and can produce numerical estimates, many clinicians report mistrust of the statistical derivation data used to produce percentage values, worry about giving false hope, or believe that those models are inappropriate to use on individual patients.[34,37] Clinician reluctance to use quantitative terms when prognosticating may be attributed to lack of training on prognostic communication, reluctance to predict the future, and uncertainty about their own prognostic estimates.[38,39] Experts in risk communication recommend clinicians communicate prognosis with population-based outcome language.[40] For example, instead of saying "there is a very poor prognosis," or "there is a 10% chance of survival," clinicians should say, "If there were 100 patients in your mother's condition, roughly 90 would not survive and 10 would survive."[40]

In addition to quantitative prognostic estimates, surrogates also ask for prognostic information delivered to them quickly, accurately, and without false hope.[41,42] They prefer to receive consistent prognostic estimates from multiple providers to minimize confusion or ideally to meet consistently with the same provider.[35,42,43] Surrogates responded favorably to thorough explanations regarding their loved one's care and treatment options, and they appreciated when clinicians took time to answer questions using simple-to-understand language.[43] Surrogates report feeling that it is the clinicians' duty to prognosticate realistically, but to do so empathetically and with emotional support when the news is bad.[33,41,42]

UNCERTAINTY

For all prognostication, especially in SABI, uncertainty is inherently present and unavoidable. Research shows that both clinicians and surrogates are frustrated by the presence of prognostic uncertainty.[33,34,43,44] Uncertainty can take a psychological toll on surrogates; in one qualitative study in severe TBI, surrogates acknowledged feeling unprepared for uncertainty during prognostication meetings and struggled to come to terms with it for months after the meeting.[34] This was made worse when quantitative estimates were withheld, and some surrogates confessed to feeling suspicious of providers who refused to give numeric estimates.[34] A more dated study from 1998 found that the most of the physicians (92%) were uncomfortable communicating uncertainty to patients and were reluctant to prognosticate at all when faced with uncertainty.[39] Surrogates, however, found that more information provided by the clinician lessened their own feelings of uncertainty even when uncertainty was explicitly discussed.[43]

Clinicians sometimes attempt to resolve uncertainty by generating and analyzing more data, often in the form of additional imaging and tests.[4,45] Although surrogates find these helpful, these cannot totally eliminate uncertainty from prognostication.[45] Prognostication for SABI patients occurs in the critical care setting, usually just days after injury and often too early for the outcome to be accurately predicted.[25,46] Clinicians must extrapolate their prognoses from variables studied in a much smaller subset of the general population.[45] Certain clinical or radiographic findings have been identified as markers of poor prognosis (eg, intracerebral hemorrhage: hematoma volume >60 mL, hydrocephalus, and intraventricular hemorrhage[25]), but patients with many of those findings have been known to survive with a spectrum of residual disability.[25] Clinicians might avoid mentioning uncertainty at all due to concerns about being wrong, undermining their own authority as a doctor, the fear of causing false hope in families, or emotionally disturbing families with the uncertainty.[34,37,43,47] Finally, some clinicians might be ambiguous about uncertainty or avoid talking about it altogether.[43,45,48] Surrogates report that uncertainty affects their decision-making, causing them to err on the side of giving the patient more time before deciding.[43] The "wait and see" approach can occasionally lead to the resolution of uncertainty, but it also might waste valuable time or prolong the dying process.[45]

How should uncertainty be approached in the neuroICU? **Box 1** summarizes recommendations for prognosticating for SABI in the presence of uncertainty. Some clinicians choose to approach uncertainty by projecting absolute certainty to avoid giving false hope; although this removes the uncertainty from the conversation, it has the effect of increasing the optimistic bias surrogates have regarding patient prognosis and forging mistrust and suspicion regarding the clinician's prognosticating capabilities.[43,44,49] Clinicians and surrogates in a multicenter qualitative study in critically ill TBI patients both found that acknowledging uncertainty explicitly reduced frustration.[43] In the same cohort, surrogates reported an unfulfilled need for clinicians to acknowledge the association between uncertainty, hope, and optimism.[48] Offering a time-limited trial during a challenging medical decision can help reduce uncertainty for family members[50]; here, the clinician and surrogates decide together to continue treatment for a defined period of time to explore if the patient improves or worsens. This option has several advantages: it preserves hope that a patient might respond to treatment, allows family members to remain involved with treatment decisions, and reduces conflict between the clinical team and family.[50]

Box 1
Summary of recommendations for prognosticating for severe acute brain injuries

This box shows recommendations for practicing family- and patient-centered prognostication in the presence of uncertainty.
Suggestions for Neuroprognostication
- Acknowledge uncertainty when prognosticating
- Give numeric estimates if possible and use population-based language
- Avoid using prognostic scales for individual prognostication
- Practice prompt and consistent communication with families and surrogate decision-makers; use shared decision-making; elicit and include patient values and preferences
- Include expert knowledge from the entire clinical team (neurocritical care plus neurosurgery, neurology, oncology, and so forth)
- Offer emotional and family support to surrogates at all times, but particularly after "bad" news has been shared; continue to support families even after WLST
- Provide at least a 72-h treatment period before WLST decisions
- Use a time-limited trial in instances where uncertainty is high

STATISTICAL PREDICTION MODELS FOR PROGNOSTICATION

Many statistical prediction models derived from large patient populations have been developed to aid prognostication for SABI. These established and usually validated outcome prediction models, which are often scale-based, are simple to apply, disease-specific, and can offer quantitative outcome predictions based on variables pertaining to the individual patient. Despite these tempting advantages, many clinicians are hesitant to use such prediction scales because of the lack of specificity for individual patients, never including all individual detail about a patient, concern about their accuracy because they have been derived from large populations and ignore outliers, and fear of creating "false hope" when using numerical estimations.[34,37] Some have suggested that quantitative models should supersede "eyeballing" prognosis in the clinical setting because clinician judgment is subject to bias and error.[7] Although few studies have examined how outcome prediction models compare against clinician judgment in the clinical setting, one 5-center study in intracerebral hemorrhage found clinician judgment (attending physician and ICU nurses) to be more accurate than the statistical models in predicting outcome 3 months after the insult.[30] Outcome prediction scales also carry other disadvantages that make them unsuitable for use in individual patients in a clinical setting. In TBI, for example, the IMPACT model only uses admission information to estimate outcomes and does not factor in the patient's clinical course after ICU admission, which is often prolonged.[37] In the case of stroke outcome prediction models, many were formulated before reperfusion therapies were widely used, were calibrated specifically on Western populations, and may not reflect a wider population or the efficacy of more recent advances in medicine.[7] Many investigators of prediction models caution against their use in a clinical setting for decision-making, especially around WLST, in individual patients.[51–53]

BARRIERS TO COMMUNICATION

Poor communication during prognostication was shown to exacerbate psychological distress and led to value-discordant care and prolonged the dying process.[54–56] One earlier study found that 50% of the families of ICU patients experienced breakdowns in communication with physicians.[56] Families report finding the surrogate decision-making process intense, difficult, and traumatic, and the resulting psychological distress was found to persist for months or even years in up to one-third of surrogates.[57] Poor communication also hindered the surrogates' understanding of the diagnosis, prognosis, and treatment options for a patient and also caused mistrust and conflict between the surrogate and the clinical team.[56] **Fig. 3** outlines the downstream effects from the breakdowns in communication in the ICU, especially related to prognostication.

Although timely and effective communication is critical to prognostication, there are barriers to prognostication that affect the quality of communication offered. Clinicians must find the time and space to hold a detailed and complex conversation about the patient's medical status and prognosis which must be translated into language the patient's family can understand. If there are language barriers, translators must be found and used. Cross-cultural communication requires additional skill and training to manage sensitively. If multiple providers are involved with care, they should discuss their opinions regarding prognosis with each other in advance and agree on a unified message to share with the family. Whenever possible, representatives from all teams should be present during family meetings. Finally, the circumstances surrounding a family meeting are often stressful, as is the process of surrogate decision-making,

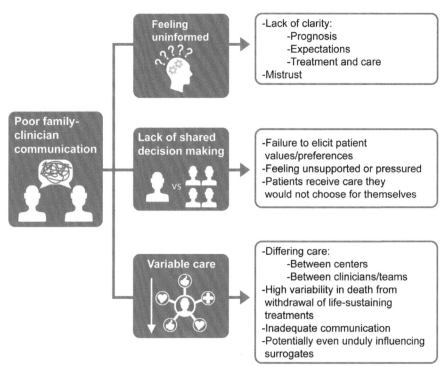

Fig. 3. Breakdowns in communication are very common in ICUs and have important downstream effects. The downstream effects of poor family-clinician communication, particularly about prognosis, are detrimental. The most important downstream effects include families feel unformed, lack of shared decision-making, and variability of care and decisions that are not related to patient or family values.

which can hinder the family's ability to understand and react to the information being provided by the clinicians.[58] Ongoing research in the developing field of neurocritical care continues to study and improve clinician-family communication in the neuro-ICU.

SHARED DECISION-MAKING AND PROGNOSTICATION

The American College of Critical Care Medicine and American Thoracic Society recommend using shared decision-making (SDM) as a guide for communication with all critically ill patients and their surrogates.[59,60] Ideally, the surrogate and clinicians work together under the SDM paradigm, which is a collaborative effort between the clinical team and patient's family to arrive at a decision that reflects the patient's values. Professional critical care societies strongly recommend SDM as it enables the surrogate to make informed decisions together with the clinician[60]. Research has shown that when SDM does not occur, it can result in value-discordant care for the patient and detrimental psychological impacts for surrogate decision-makers.[61,62] Studies of audio-recorded meetings in primarily non-neuro-ICUs have provided valuable insight about ways prognostication might be improved during family meetings. These studies have shown that family conferences generally do not meet criteria for comprehensive SDM in goals of care decisions, and sometimes do not even include discussions of long-term survival prognosis.[63–66]

SUMMARY

Owing to the devastating nature of SABI, patients are left incapacitated, placing the immense burden of decision-making on their surrogate decision-makers. Currently, there are no formally published guidelines for how prognostication should occur in the setting of neurocritical care. As a result, neuroprognostication is still considered an "art" with too much room for individual clinician interpretation and biases.[7,10,22] Further research is needed to move from art to science to uncover effective strategies of neuroprognostication in the neuroICU. If the goal of neuroprognostication is to provide patient- and surrogate-centered care, then it is important to consider what surrogates want and need from clinicians. This would include honest, concrete, consistent, and compassionate prognostication that leaves room for hope.[33–35,41,43] Although surrogates desire quantitative language from clinicians, statistical prediction models should be used judiciously when applied to individual patients and explained with population-based language and a frank acknowledgment of residual uncertainty.[7,53] Formalized guidelines may help clinicians limit bias and uncertainty during prognostication in the future.

CLINICS CARE POINTS

- Patients and their surrogates rely on clinicians for accurate prognostication. Clinicians have a duty to provide accurate and sensitive information regarding prognosis to their patient and surrogates to facilitate shared decision-making regarding goals of care decisions.
- Clinicians should refrain from prognostication for at least a 72-hour treatment period to mitigate the influence of bias and heuristics.
- Early neuroprognostication within the first 28 days following neurological injury should avoid statements that suggest patients have a universally poor prognosis.
- When possible, using numeric estimates and population-based outcome language is more patient-and surrogate-centric than qualitative prediction statements.
- All communication with SABI patients and their surrogates should utilize shared decision-making. Failure to utilize SDM leads to value-discordant care and negative psychological impacts for surrogate decision makers.

DISCLOSURE

Susanne Muehlschlegel has received research funding from the National Institutes of Health (R21NR020231, U01NS119647 and U01NS099046) and honoraria from the American Academy of Neurology as a speaker. Dr. Muehlschlegel has no conflict of interest.. Ms V. Fleming has been supported by the University of Massachusetts Chan Medical School's Chancellor's Scholarship.

REFERENCES

1. Prognosis Definition & meaning - Merriam-Webster. Available at: https://www.merriam-webster.com/dictionary/prognosis#note-1. Accessed January 18, 2022.
2. Feigin VL, Vos T, Nichols E, et al. The global burden of neurological disorders: translating evidence into policy. Lancet Neurol 2020;19(3):255–65.
3. Hwang DY, Chu SY, Dell CA, et al. Factors considered by clinicians when prognosticating intracerebral hemorrhage outcomes. Neurocrit Care 2017;27(3):316–25.

4. Steinberg A, Grayek E, Arnold RM, et al. Physicians' cognitive approach to prognostication after cardiac arrest. Resuscitation 2022. https://doi.org/10.1016/J.RESUSCITATION.2022.01.001.

5. Ge C, Goss AL, Crawford S, et al. Variability of Prognostic Communication in Critically Ill Neurologic Patients: A Pilot Multicenter Mixed-Methods Study. Crit Care Explor 2022;4:e0640

6. Rabinstein AA, Hemphill JC. Prognosticating after severe acute brain disease: science, art, and biases. Neurology 2010;74(14):1086–7.

7. Gao MM, Wang J, Saposnik G. The art and science of stroke outcome prognostication. Stroke 2020;1358–60.

8. Maciel CB. Neurologic outcome prediction in the intensive care Unit. Continuum (Minneapolis, Minn) 2021;27(5):1405–29.

9. Fidali BC, Stevens RD, Claassen J. Novel approaches to prediction in severe brain injury. Curr Opin Neurol 2020;33(6):669.

10. Johnston SC. Prognostication matters. Muscle & Nerve 2000;23(6):839–42.

11. Giacino JT, Katz DI, Schiff ND, et al. Practice guideline update recommendations summary: disorders of consciousness: report of the guideline Development, Dissemination, and Implementation Subcommittee of the American Academy of neurology; the American Congress of Rehabilitation medicine; and the national Institute on disability, Independent living, and Rehabilitation research. Neurology 2018;91(10):450.

12. Geocadin RG, Callaway CW, Fink EL, et al. Standards for studies of neurological prognostication in comatose survivors of cardiac arrest: a scientific statement from the American Heart association. Circulation 2019;140(9):E517–42.

13. Muehlschlegel S, Wartenberg K, Alexander S, et al. Neuroprognostication guideline - a collaboration of neurocritical care society (NCS)and Deutsche Gesellschaft fuer Neurointensivmedizin (DGNI). ANIM 2022.

14. Kahneman D. Thinking, Fast and Slow. Farrar, Straus and Giroux; 2011.

15. Mohan D, Farris C, Fischhoff B, et al. Efficacy of educational video game versus traditional educational apps at improving physician decision making in trauma triage: randomized controlled trial. BMJ 2017;359.

16. Tversky A, Kahneman D. Judgment under uncertainty: heuristics and biases. Science 1974;185(4157):1124–31.

17. Marewski JN, Gigerenzer G. Heuristic decision making in medicine. Dialogues Clin Neurosci 2012;14(1):77.

18. Saposnik G, Redelmeier D, Ruff CC, et al. Cognitive biases associated with medical decisions: a systematic review. BMC Med Inform Decis Making 2016;16(1):1–14.

19. Becker KJ, Baxter AB, Cohen WA, et al. Withdrawal of support in intracerebral hemorrhage may lead to self-fulfilling prophecies. Neurology 2001;56(6):766–72.

20. Turgeon AF, Lauzier F, Simard JF, et al. Mortality associated with withdrawal of life-sustaining therapy for patients with severe traumatic brain injury: a Canadian multicentre cohort study. CMAJ 2011;183(14):1581–8.

21. Creutzfeldt CJ, Longstreth WT, Holloway RG. Predicting decline and survival in severe acute brain injury: the fourth trajectory. BMJ (Clinical research ed) 2015;351. https://doi.org/10.1136/BMJ.H3904.

22. Hemphill JC, White DB. Clinical nihilism in Neuroemergencies. Emerg Med Clin North America 2009;27(1):27–37.

23. Williamson T, Ryser MD, Ubel PA, et al. Withdrawal of life-supporting treatment in severe traumatic brain injury. JAMA Surg 2020;155(8):723.

24. Holloway RG, Benesch CG, Burgin WS, et al. Prognosis and decision making in severe stroke. JAMA 2005;294(6):725–33.

25. Graham M. Burying our mistakes: Dealing with prognostic uncertainty after severe brain injury. Bioethics 2020;34(6):612.

26. Zahuranec DB, Fagerlin A, Sánchez BN, et al. Variability in physician prognosis and recommendations after intracerebral hemorrhage. Neurology 2016;86(20):1864.

27. Hirschi R, Rommel C, Hawryluk GWJ. Should we have a guard against therapeutic nihilism for patients with severe traumatic brain injury? Neural Regen Res 2017;12(11):1801.

28. Moore NA, Brennan PM, Baillie JK. Wide variation and systematic bias in expert clinicians' perceptions of prognosis following brain injury. Br J Neurosurg 2013;27(3):340–3.

29. Geocadin RG, Peberdy MA, Lazar RM. Poor survival after cardiac arrest resuscitation: a self-fulfilling prophecy or biologic destiny? Crit Care Med 2012;40(3):979–80.

30. Izzy S, Compton R, Carandang R, Hall W, Muehlschlegel S. Self-fulfilling prophecies through withdrawal of care: do they exist in traumatic brain injury, too? Neurocrit Care 2013;19:347-63.

31. Souter MJ, Blissitt PA, Blosser S, et al. Recommendations for the critical care management of devastating brain injury: prognostication, Psychosocial, and ethical management: a Position statement for Healthcare Professionals from the neurocritical care society. Neurocrit Care 2015;23(1):4–13.

32. Lee DH, Cho YS, Lee BK, et al. Late awakening is common in settings without withdrawal of life-sustaining therapy in out-of-hospital cardiac arrest survivors who Undergo Targeted temperature management. Crit Care Med 2022;50(2):235–44.

33. Schenker Y, White DB, Crowley-Matoka M, et al. It Hurts to Know and it helps": Exploring how surrogates in the ICU Cope with prognostic information. J. Palliat Med 2013;16(3):243–9. Available at: https://home.liebertpub.com/jpm.

34. Quinn T, Moskowitz J, Khan MW, et al. What families need and physicians deliver: Contrasting communication preferences between surrogate decision-makers and physicians during outcome prognostication in critically ill TBI patients. Neurocrit Care 2017;27(2):154–62.

35. Zier LS, Burack JH, Micco G, et al. Doubt and belief in physicians' ability to prognosticate during critical illness: the perspective of surrogate decision makers. Crit Care Med 2008;36(8):2341.

36. Boyd EA, Lo B, Evans LR, et al. It's not just what the doctor tells me:" Factors that influence surrogate decision-makers' perceptions of prognosis. Crit Care Med 2010;38(5):1270.

37. Moskowitz J, Quinn T, Khan MW, et al. Should We Use the IMPACT-model for the outcome prognostication of TBI patients? A qualitative study assessing physicians' perceptions. MDM Pol Pract 2018;3(1). 2381468318757987.

38. Creutzfeldt CJ, Holloway RG, Curtis JR. Palliative care: a Core Competency for stroke Neurologists. Stroke 2015;46(9):2714–9.

39. Christakis NA, Iwashyna TJ. Attitude and self-reported practice regarding prognostication in a national sample of internists. Arch Intern Med 1998;158(21):2389–95.

40. White DB, Engelberg RA, Wenrich MD, et al. The language of prognostication in intensive care Units. Med Decis making : Int J Soc Med Decis Making 2010;30(1):76.

41. Apatira L, Boyd EA, Malvar G, et al. Hope, Truth, and preparing for death: Perspectives of surrogate decision makers. Ann Intern Med 2008;149(12):861.
42. Muehlschlegel S, Perman SM, Elmer J, et al. The Experiences and Needs of Families of Comatose Patients After Cardiac Arrest and Severe Neurotrauma: The Perspectives of National Key Stakeholders During a National Institutes of Health-Funded Workshop. Crit Care Explor 2022;4:e0648
43. Jones K, Quinn T, Mazor KM, et al. Prognostic uncertainty in critically ill patients with traumatic brain injury: a Multicenter qualitative study. Neurocrit Care 2021; 35(2):311–21.
44. Evans LR, Boyd EA, Malvar G, et al. Surrogate decision-makers' Perspectives on discussing prognosis in the Face of uncertainty. Am J Respir Crit Care Med 2009; 179(1):48.
45. Smith AK, White DB, Arnold RM. Uncertainty: the other side of prognosis. N Engl J Med 2013;368(26):2448.
46. Lazaridis C. Withdrawal of life-sustaining treatments in Perceived devastating brain injury: the Key role of uncertainty. Neurocrit Care 2019;30(1):33–41.
47. Smith AK, Williams BA, Lo B. Discussing overall prognosis with the very Elderly. N Engl J Med 2011;365(23):2149.
48. Schutz REC, Coats HL, Engelberg RA, et al. Is there hope? Is She there? How families and clinicians experience severe acute brain injury. J Palliat Med 2017; 20(2):170–6.
49. Zier LS, Sottile PD, Hong SY, et al. Surrogate decision makers' interpretation of prognostic information: a mixed-methods study. Ann Intern Med 2012;156(5): 360–6.
50. Quill TE, Holloway R. Time-limited trials near the end of life. JAMA - J Am Med Assoc 2011;306(13):1483–4.
51. Hemphill JC, Farrant M, Neill TA. Prospective validation of the ICH Score for 12-month functional outcome. Neurology 2009;73(14):1088.
52. Hwang DY, Dell CA, Sparks MJ, et al. Clinician judgment vs formal scales for predicting intracerebral hemorrhage outcomes. Neurology 2016;86(2):126–33.
53. Dijkland SA, Foks KA, Polinder S, et al. Prognosis in moderate and severe traumatic brain injury: a systematic review of contemporary models and validation studies. J Neurotrauma 2020;37(1):1–13.
54. Pochard F, Azoulay E, Chevret S, et al. Symptoms of anxiety and depression in family members of intensive care unit patients: ethical hypothesis regarding decision-making capacity. Crit Care Med 2001;29(10):1893–7.
55. Curtis JR, Engelberg RA, Wenrich MD, et al. Missed Opportunities during family conferences about end-of-life care in the intensive care Unit. Am J Respir Crit Care Med 2012;171(8):844–9.
56. Azoulay E, Chevret S, Leleu G, et al. Half the families of intensive care unit patients experience inadequate communication with physicians. Crit Care Med 2000;28(8). Available at: https://journals.lww.com/ccmjournal/Fulltext/2000/08000/Half_the_families_of_intensive_care_unit_patients.61.aspx.
57. Wendler D, Rid A. Systematic review: the effect on surrogates of making treatment decisions for others. Ann Intern Med 2011;154(5):336–46.
58. Gay EB, Pronovost PJ, Bassett RD, et al. The intensive care unit family meeting: making it happen. J Crit Care 2009;24(4):629.e1.
59. Kon AA, Davidson JE, Morrison W, et al. Shared decision making in intensive care Units: an American College of critical care medicine and American Thoracic society policy statement. Crit Care Med 2016;44(1):188.

60. Azoulay E. The end-of-life family conference. Am J Respir Crit Care Med 2012; 171(8):803–4.
61. Khan MW, Muehlschlegel S. Shared decision-making in neurocritical care. Neurol Clin 2017;35(4):825.
62. Heyland DK, Heyland R, Dodek P, et al. Discordance between patients' stated values and treatment preferences for end-of-life care: results of a multicentre survey. BMJ Support Palliat Care 2017;7(3):292–9.
63. Bouniols N, Leclère B, Moret L. Evaluating the quality of shared decision making during the patient-carer encounter: a systematic review of tools. BMC Res Notes 2016;9(1). https://doi.org/10.1186/S13104-016-2164-6.
64. White DB, Engelberg RA, Wenrich MD, et al. Prognostication during physician-family discussions about limiting life support in intensive care units. Crit Care Med 2007;35(2):442–8.
65. White DB, Braddock CH, Bereknyei S, et al. Toward shared decision making at the end of life in intensive care Units: Opportunities for Improvement. Arch Intern Med 2007;167(5):461–7.
66. White DB, Malvar G, Karr J, et al. Expanding the paradigm of the physician's role in surrogate decision-making: an empirically derived framework. Crit Care Med 2010;38(3):743–50.

Neurocritical Care in the General Intensive Care Unit

Firas Abdulmajeed, MD[a],*, Mohanad Hamandi, MD[b], Deepa Malaiyandi, MD[c], Lori Shutter, MD[a]

KEYWORDS

- Postcardiac arrest • AMS • HE • PRES • Neurologic complications • Neurotoxicity

KEY POINTS

- Neurologic conditions are common in intensive care units, and early identification and management may improve outcomes.
- Good neurologic recovery is possible after cardiac arrest. Developing an institutional postcardiac arrest protocol that follows national guidelines based on local hospital capabilities is encouraged.
- Altered mental status can be due to multiple etiologies. A thorough investigation will help identify treatable causes.

INTRODUCTION

Neurologic care in the general intensive care units (ICU) has become an integral part of comprehensive critical care. Management of postcardiac arrest, a general approach to altered mental status, delirium, hepatic encephalopathy, immune effector cell-associated neurotoxicity syndrome, beta-lactam toxicity, posterior reversible encephalopathy syndrome, CNS infections, and other neurologic complications of medical conditions are discussed in this review as a practical guide for the practitioner in the general ICU.

DISCUSSION
Postcardiac Arrest Care

Cardiac arrest (CA) can result from many different diseases, however, the hypoxemia, ischemia, and reperfusion that occur during and after resuscitation may all cause

[a] Department of Critical Care Medicine, University of Pittsburgh School of Medicine, 3550 Terrace Street, Scaife Hall Suite 600, Pittsburgh, PA, 15261, USA; [b] Department of Medicine, University of Pittsburgh School of Medicine, 3550 Terrace Street, 1218 Scaife Hall, Pittsburgh, PA, 15261, USA; [c] Division of Neurocritical Care, Department of Neurology, University of Toledo College of Medicine, 2130 West Central Avenue, Suite 201, Room 2355, UT/PPG Neurosciences Center, Toledo, OH 43606, USA
* Corresponding author. Department of Critical Care Medicine, University of Pittsburgh School of Medicine, 3550 Terrace Street, Scaife Hall, Suite 600, PA 15261, USA.
E-mail address: Abdulmajeedfn2@upmc.edu

Crit Care Clin 39 (2023) 153–169
https://doi.org/10.1016/j.ccc.2022.08.003
0749-0704/23/© 2022 Elsevier Inc. All rights reserved.
criticalcare.theclinics.com

multi-organ damage with variable severity.[1] Return of spontaneous circulation (ROSC) and long-term survival with favorable neurologic outcomes are the most important outcomes and continue to improve over time. Early priority is effective post-CA care to identify and treat the precipitating cause of arrest, and to prevent rearrest.[1] The flow chart (**Fig. 1**) summarizes our approach to post-CA management.[1–26]

Patients who achieve ROSC should be rapidly evaluated for coronary intervention and targeted temperature management (TTM) to prevent secondary brain injury. Reducing core body temperature decreases cerebral oxygen demand and attenuates multiple cellular pathways involved in ongoing brain injury in the hours and days after the arrest.[27] There is not an abundant body of evidence investigating TTM at 33°C versus 36°C and its effect on neurologic outcomes in isolation. There are several recent observational studies demonstrating both statistically significant decreases and trends toward decreased survival among patients receiving TTM at 36C versus 33C when there is severe post-CA illness.[19,22] There is a randomized controlled clinical trial suggesting improved survival with a favorable neurologic outcome with TTM at 33C compared with therapeutic normothermia at 37C with severe disease.[21] The Neurocritical Care Society recommends implementing TTM at a target temperature between 32 and 36 °C.[28] TTM is strongly recommended for patients with an out of hospital CA of suspected cardiac origin.[27] Data on patients with CA from other causes and in the hospital setting are mixed. Patients with initial asystole or pulseless electrical activity may also derive some benefit from TTM. Induction of TTM should be implemented rapidly with chilled crystalloids, ice packing, surface or intravascular cooling devices. This should be maintained for 24 hours. During that time, shivering should be controlled using a consistent shivering protocol (see **Fig. 1**). Thus, far rewarming is to be started 24 hours after cooling with the targeted rewarming rate of 0.2 to 0.5°C/hour until normothermia is achieved. The ongoing ICECAP study will hopefully provide additional insight on the optimal duration for cooling.[29]

Providers should aim for balancing cerebral perfusion pressure by targeting a MAP of 80 to 100 mm Hg and cardiac protection, against the effects of fluid resuscitation with isotonic crystalloid, vasopressors, inotropes, and possibly mechanical circulatory support on other organ systems.

Coronary revascularization is indicated for post-CA patients with electrocardiogram (ECG) findings of ST-elevation myocardial infarction (STEMI), new left bundle branch block, hemodynamic instability due to cardiogenic shock, rising troponin levels, or evidence of focal wall-motion abnormalities on echocardiogram. These patients might also qualify for mechanical circulatory support.

Accurate neurologic prognostication after CA is challenging. In the first 72 h after CA, no specific sign, symptom, or combination of findings, short of brain death, precludes favorable recovery. The incidence of nonconvulsive status epilepticus (NCSE) ranges from 12% to 24% in postarrest patients.[27,30] Seizures may directly worsen brain injury and should be treated. In patients who are comatose or have limited neurologic examinations, continuous EEG is recommended to detect subclinical seizure activity and should start 6 to 12 hours after TTM initiation and continue for at least 24 hours after rewarming. Some EEG patterns are associated with poor prognosis and reduced hospital survival, these are termed malignant and include NCSE, convulsive status epilepticus (SE), myoclonic SE, and rhythmic and periodic epileptiform discharges. Malignant epileptiform patterns are less common in patients with early, diffuse cerebral edema; these patients tend to have burst suppression or complete suppression as their primary EEG pattern, which is associated with worse prognosis. Premature withdrawal of life-sustaining therapy based on perceived neurologic prognosis has been linked to high incidence of preventable deaths after CA.[31] Therefore,

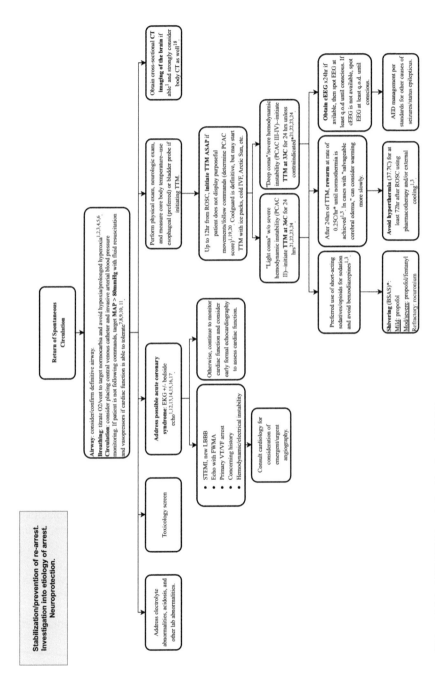

Fig. 1. Postcardiac arrest management flowchart.

*Relative contraindications to TTM at 33C include coagulopathy and signs of nonsurvivable brain injury.

early aggressive care should not be limited or withheld based only on perceived poor neurologic prognosis. Diffusion-weighted magnetic resonance imaging can be used to estimate the degree of brain injury after CA. Apparent diffusion coefficient (ADC) seems to be predictive of outcomes. Hirsch and colleagues showed that an ADC less than 650×10^{-6} mm^2/s in greater than 10% of brain tissue in an MRI obtained by postarrest day 7 is highly specific for poor outcomes in comatose patients after CA.[32]

Approach to Altered Mental Status

Altered mental status (AMS) is common in ICUs and can be caused by systemic illness, intoxication, isolated organ system dysfunction, trauma, delirium, or neurologic disease. A systematic approach involves an initial assessment of the level of consciousness. Evaluation of the following immediate threats is key:

- Airway: assessment for airway protection
- Breathing: adequate oxygenation and ventilation or depressed respiratory status
- Circulation: includes checking pulses, blood pressure, heart rate, and rhythm, warm or cool to touch
- Disability: comprehensive neurologic examination including Glasgow Coma Score or Full Outline of Unresponsiveness Scale and postictal signs.[33] Spine protection should be performed if there is any suspicion of trauma
- Check blood glucose, liver function test, lipase, urine drug screen (hypoglycemia and opioid overdose), serum chemistries, ammonia level, thyroid function tests, and blood gas analysis
- Emergent cranial computed tomography (CT) and CT angiography (CTA), when appropriate to determine whether AMS etiology is structural or vascular
- Consider brain MRI for focal neurologic deficits, suspicion of neuroinflammatory disease, seizures, strokes, intracranial bleeds, head trauma, suspected tumor, posterior reversible encephalopathy syndrome (PRES), and reversible cerebral vasoconstriction syndrome.
- Consider lumbar puncture (LP) when suspecting CNS infection, suspicion for subarachnoid hemorrhage is high but CT scan is negative, CNS malignancies, autoimmune encephalitis, and central or peripheral demyelinating diseases.
- EEG to rule out subclinical or nonconvulsive seizure, assess patients with fluctuating mental status, or confirm certain pathologies with characteristic EEG pattern

In patients who are comatose, additional measures are needed for initial evaluation such as brain stem reflexes, respiratory pattern, and motor function (weakness, tone, reflexes including assessing for clonus, and evaluating symmetry).

- Visual threat response
- Pupillary response: pinpoint pupils raise concern of pontine damage, whereas large, unreactive pupils suggest midbrain damage or 3rd nerve compression
- Corneal reflex
- Eye movements: spontaneous, oculocephalic reflex (Doll's Eyes) horizontal and vertical, vestibulo-ocular reflex (cold caloric testing)
- Cough and gag reflexes

The following breathing patterns may have localization value (**Fig. 2**)

- Neurogenic hyperventilation: midbrain and pons
- Cluster breathing: pons

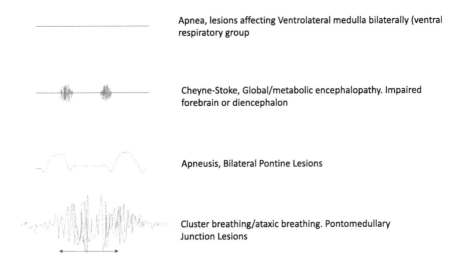

Apnea, lesions affecting Ventrolateral medulla bilaterally (ventral respiratory group

Cheyne-Stoke, Global/metabolic encephalopathy. Impaired forebrain or diencephalon

Apneusis, Bilateral Pontine Lesions

Cluster breathing/ataxic breathing. Pontomedullary Junction Lesions

Fig. 2. Breathing pattern in patients with altered mental status.

- Ataxic breathing: medulla

Key findings on the neurologic examination of comatose patients can identify abnormalities suggestive of toxic syndromes that can lead to the rapid treatment of coma (**Table 1**). In patients with coma out of proportion to imaging findings or metabolic derangements, suspect basilar thrombosis as early identification and revascularization are key to improve outcome. Elevated intracranial pressure (ICP) can occur in a variety of processes and cannot be excluded by imaging alone.

There are a variety of noninvasive devices that have been studied to assess ICP, but most have not demonstrated reproducible clinical success or been studied in large clinical trials. Transcranial doppler (TCD) is a poor predictor of ICP, although, in trauma patients, TCD finding may correlate with outcomes at 6 months.[34,35] Tissue resonance analysis (TRA), is an ultrasound-based method that has shown some promise in measuring ICP.[36] Similarly, ocular sonography can provide a noninvasive measure of optic nerve sheath diameter, which has been found to correlate with ICP as many studies have found that diameters of 5 to 6 mm have the ability to discriminate

Table 1	
Toxins that may contribute to altered mental status	
Alcohols	Hallucinogenic (e.g., LSD, mushrooms)
Alpha-2 Adrenergic agonists	Heavy metals
Anticholinergics	Hydrogen sulfide
Antidepressants,	Hypoglycemic agents
Antihistamines	Inert gases
Antipsychotics	Lithium
Antiseizure medications	Methemoglobinemia
Barbiturates	Muscle relaxants
Belladonna alkaloids	Organophosphates
Benzodiazepines	Opiates
Carbamates	Phenothiazines
Carbon mono- and dioxide	Salicylates
Cyanide	Sedative-hypnotics
Gamma-hydroxybutyrate	Volatile inhalants

between normal and elevated ICP in patients with intracranial hemorrhage and traumatic brain injury (TBI), moreover intraocular pressure can be assessed by ultrasonic handheld optic tonometer.[37–39]

Delirium

Delirium is a syndrome reflecting acute cerebral dysfunction typified by fluctuations in mental status including the level of consciousness, attention, thought process, and content. It commonly occurs during hospital admission and particularly in the ICU setting. It has long been known that delirium is associated with increased, morbidity, mortality, length of stay, as well as the risk of institutionalization and dementia.[40–43]

Owing to the significant impact of delirium on the functional outcome of ICU survivors, the Society of Critical Care Medicine maintains a clinical practice guideline, most recently updated in 2018, on pain, agitation/sedation, delirium, immobility, and sleep (PADIS) for adult ICU patients.[44] However, the studies guiding the recommendations represent the general medical, surgical, and cardiothoracic patient population, and considerations specific to patients critically ill from neurologic failure, are lacking due to an overall paucity of literature in this focused area of delirium research.

Delirium may complicate any number of disease states, of these, neurologic disorders are an independent risk factor among a myriad of others. Delirium is estimated to complicate 25% to 30% of strokes, and 50% to 75% of TBI.[45–47] The PADIS guidelines recommend consistent delirium screening in all ICU patients. Common screening tools such as the Confusion Assessment Method for the Intensive Care Unit (CAM-ICU) and Intensive Care Delirium Screening Checklist (ICDSC) are well validated in the general ICU population. Only recently has their validity been assessed in the neurocritical ill. A qualitative synthesis of a small number of studies estimates the sensitivity, specificity, positive and negative predictive values for CAM-ICU at 62% to 76%, 74% to 98%, 63% to 91%, and 70% to 94%, respectively. For ICDSC the values were 64%, 79%, 74%, and 69%, respectively.[48] The DSM-V criteria were applied as the reference standard. The authors suggest these findings are reassuring and that it is reasonable to use these tools to screen for delirium in the Neuro ICU population. Despite the high incidence of delirium reported in ischemic stroke, hemorrhagic stroke, and TBI using these screening methods, recent work by Reznik and colleagues, suggests that limitations in available screening tools maybe contributing to a significant underdiagnosis of delirium in the stroke population when compared with expert assessment combining neurologic examination and Richmond Agitation Scale Score data. Interestingly they noted a higher sensitivity and specificity for the ICDSC for patients with aphasia (77% & 97%, area under the receiver operating curve 0.87) over CAM-ICU (41% & 88%, area under the receiver operating curve 0.64).[49]

Delirium can be subcategorized into hyper-, normo-, hypoactive, and mixed subtypes. Subcategorization is clinically relevant for management and the hyperactive subtype is typically associated with a better prognosis. Literature guiding pharmacologic management of delirium in any ICU population is sparse, and even more so for the neurocritical ill. Notably, data guiding pharmacologic interventions for hypoactive delirium in those with neurologic failure can be difficult to isolate from disorders of consciousness, and the use of neurostimulants in both populations is a nascent field of study. The pathophysiology of delirium is complex involving several inter-related and somewhat opposing pathways with respect to hyperactivity versus impaired arousal. However, the hypothesis that an imbalance of serotoninergic, GABAergic, dopaminergic, noradrenergic, and cholinergic transmission has predominated current pharmacologic treatment strategies. To date, studies are limited to direct comparison of single drug interventions to one another or to placebo. Given the complex interplay of the multiple neurotransmitter systems involved, it seems reasonable that future studies should focus on multidrug combination therapies that address all targets instead of a select few.

Hyperactive delirium can be challenging to differentiate from agitation related to structural brain injury. For those with symptoms that pose a threat to themselves or members of the care team, it is reasonable to try a combination of medications used for either of these indications. Aside from the long list of medications that are commonly used, phenobarbital, owing to its broad neurochemistry, may present an underrecognized/underutilized resource in managing agitation related to hyperactive delirium in the Neurocritical Care population. One case report outlines its success in managing severe refractory poststroke hyperactive delirium when nearly all other medication classes failed to provide adequate symptom control including dexmedetomidine and ketamine infusions.[50]

One area of agreement is that benzodiazepines are an independent risk factor for delirium and the PADIS guidelines recommend avoiding their use. Benzodiazepines are particularly problematic in patients with both acute and chronic underlying central nervous system (CNS) pathology who are at particular risk for delirium and alternative medication strategies should be used whenever feasible.[44]

Alcohol withdrawal delirium is a unique case in which benzodiazepines continue to be used as a first-line agent. The common benzodiazepine-based protocol, Clinical Institute of Withdrawal from Alcohol Revised (CIWA-Ar), has not been validated in the ICU population whereby wide variation in scoring can result from subjective interpretation of clinical features that are common to both alcohol withdrawal and critical illness. This is exaggerated in those with neurologic injury whose underlying insult may add additional confounding manifestations. Mounting evidence supports the use of phenobarbital as a safe and effective alternative for this indication.[51] Both prophylactic regimens that weigh the risk of withdrawal versus the risk of sedation or airway compromise, and acute treatment protocols are available and are recommended to be used over benzodiazepine-based protocols.

Hepatic Encephalopathy

Hepatic encephalopathy (HE) is a spectrum of neuropsychiatric abnormalities associated with liver dysfunction or the presence of a portosystemic shunt. It occurs in up to 45% of patients with liver cirrhosis and up to 50% of those with portosystemic shunt.[52,53] HE can be categorized based on the underlying disease, severity of the manifestation, time course, and precipitating factors.[54]

Symptoms can range from subtle deficits to overt findings, with impairments in attention and working memory. In patients with acute liver failure, HE can rapidly progress to coma and cerebral herniation. Whereas in patients with cirrhosis, it can exhibit a slow onset with cognitive and motor deficits.[55] HE in patients with cirrhosis is associated with 42% and 23% survival rates at 1-year and 3-year, respectively.[56]

The 2014 AASLD-EASL Practice Guideline on HE recommends treatment mainly for persons with overt symptoms.[57] Patients with severe HE require hospital admission, typically to an ICU. Management of HE in the ICU setting is aimed at the correction of precipitating factors along with supportive strategies to reduce intestinal ammonia production and absorption. Precipitating factors include gastrointestinal bleeding, infections (including spontaneous bacterial peritonitis), hypokalemia, renal failure, hypovolemia, hypoglycemia, constipation or the use of sedatives or tranquilizers.[58] Most patients with HE respond within the first 48 hours of treatment. Prolonged symptoms beyond 72 hours of treatment should prompt further investigation for other causes of AMS. Nonabsorbable disaccharides, such as lactulose decrease the absorption of ammonia and are considered a first-line treatment of HE.[59] Lactulose is converted to Lactic acid and acetic acid, resulting in the acidification of gut lumen and facilitating conversion of NH_3^+ to NH_4^+, which is less absorbable.[60] Ammonia-lowering antibiotics such as rifaximin, and neomycin are FDA approved for patients with HE. Plasma ammonia-lowering devices (eg, renal replacement therapy, molecular adsorbent recirculating systems) and nonpharmacological interventions are increasingly used in HE management. L-ornithine-L-aspartate use can lower the blood concentration of ammonia and potentially improve HE. Use of L-ornithine-L-aspartate for 7 days has been associated with improved psychometric testing and lower postprandial levels of ammonia.[61] Zinc is a cofactor for urea cycle enzymes, and it is an important cofactor in ammonia detoxification. A randomized, open-label trial suggested possible benefits of zinc supplementation in persons with HE.[62]

The 2014 AASLD-EASL Practice Guideline states that overt HE by itself is not an indication for liver transplantation, unless associated with hepatic failure. However, patients with severe HE refractory to maximal therapy can be considered for liver transplant referral.[57]

Immune Effector Cell-associated Neurotoxicity Syndrome (ICANS)

Chimeric antigen receptor-modified T (CAR T) cell therapy is a treatment of hematological malignancies and recently is being investigated in neurologic malignancies.[63–65] A complication of CAR T-cell therapy is the immune effector cell-associated neurotoxicity syndrome (ICANS), which has also been called CAR T-cell-related Therapy Encephalopathy Syndrome. ICANS has been attributed to endothelial activation and blood–brain barrier disruption with passive cytokine diffusion along with increased levels of IL-5, IL-6, excitatory NMDA receptor agonists, glutamate, quinolinic acid, and myeloid cells other than activated T cells.[63–66] Effects can be progressive and may include aphasia, altered level of consciousness and cognition, tremor, motor weakness, seizures (convulsive and nonconvulsive), and cerebral edema. The incidence and severity of ICANS vary based on the CAR T-cell product and underlying disease, and it has a median onset of 4 to 5 days after the initiation of CAR T-cell therapy with a duration of usually 14 to 17 days. ICANS is often preceded by Cytokine Release Syndrome (CRS), so evidence of CRS should raise concern for the development of neurologic symptoms. Assessment should use the standardized immune effector cell-associated encephalopathy (ICE) score (**Table 2**).[66]

The severity of ICANS is graded based on the most severe neurotoxicity finding not attributable to any other cause; for example, a patient with an ICE score of 3 who has a generalized seizure is classified as grade 3 ICANS (**Table 3**).[67] Head CTs are usually normal but can exclude other conditions to explain symptoms. Findings on MRI may include nonspecific T2/FLAIR signal changes involving subcortical structures, vasogenic edema, microhemorrhages, and leptomeningeal enhancement.[63] EEG generally shows generalized or focal slowing, frontal intermittent rhythmic delta activity, and generalized periodic discharges with triphasic waves, although epileptiform discharges and seizure activity may occur with higher ICANS grades.[63] Management of ICANS is primarily supportive, based on the grade, and focuses on the attenuation of the immune system, often using corticosteroids. Patients at ICANS grade 2 should be considered for ICU monitoring, and ICANS grade 3 and higher should be in the ICU. Care in the ICU should focus seizure control, airway assessment, frequent monitoring for signs of cerebral edema, and management of elevated ICP.

Beta-Lactam Toxicity

Beta-lactam antibiotics are commonly prescribed in the ICU setting, and while they are generally safe, neurotoxicity has been reported as the earliest use of penicillin,

Table 2		
Immune effector cell-associated encephalopathy (ICE) score		
Domain	**Assessment**	**Point Value**
Orientation	Orientation to: Year, Month, City, Hospital	1 point each, maximum = 4
Naming	Ability to name 3 objects (eg, pen, flashlight, phone)	1 point each, maximum = 3
Following Commands	Able to follow simple commands (eg, show 2 fingers, stick out your tongue)	1 point
Writing	Ability to write a standard sentence. Use the same sentence every time.	1 point
Attention	Count backward from 100 by 10s (must complete to 0)	1 point
Total Score		Maximum = 11

with recent incidence reported at 10% to 23% of ICU patients.[68,69] Awareness of risk factors and recognition of symptoms allows for early identification and minimizes the adverse effects of these agents. Risk factors for neurotoxicity include renal impairment, older age, existing CNS conditions (eg, epilepsy, dementia, structural lesions), disruption of the blood–brain barrier (eg, sepsis, uremia, CNS infections, trauma), and high beta-lactam trough levels (**Table 4**). Clinical symptoms include AMS, delirium, myoclonus, ataxia, and seizures (convulsive and nonconvulsive). EEG can assist in diagnosis when abnormalities such as lateralized or generalized periodic discharges with a triphasic morphology, brief ictal rhythmic discharges, sharp waves, spike discharges, or slow waves are present. Treatment should focus on the discontinuation of the offending drug, management of seizures, and supportive care. Ongoing efforts exist to define optimal dosing regimens based on pharmacokinetic targets.

Posterior Reversible Encephalopathy Syndrome

Posterior reversible encephalopathy syndrome (PRES) originally derived its name from characteristic findings in neuroimaging studies. Disordered cerebral autoregulation and endothelial dysfunction seem to be the likely pathophysiology.[70,71] Uremia and sepsis can affect the function of the vascular endothelium and therefore could also be implicated in certain clinical settings.[72] PRES typically involves the subcortical white matter in the posterior cerebral hemispheres. The most common cause is systemic hypertension and more specifically wide systemic blood pressure fluctuations.[73] It can present with headache, AMS, seizures, or visual changes. Neuroimaging can reveal white matter edema which is typically found in both posterior cerebral hemispheres. Involvement of the cerebellum and brainstem is common. Characteristic MRI finding is focal or confluent areas of increased signal on T2-weighted images. Diffusion-weighted imaging shows vasogenic edema and adds considerable diagnostic and prognostic information.[74] Treatment recommendations are based on observational data. In general, gradual blood pressure lowering is recommended. In patients with malignant hypertension, the initial drop in blood pressure should not exceed 25% of the presenting value.[75] However, in moderate hypertension, it is recommended to lower the blood pressure in 10 to 25% increments of the mean arterial blood pressure (MAP).[76] Furthermore, antiseizure medications are used in patients with PRES and seizure.[77] In cases of PRES in patients with immunosuppressive drugs, a dose reduction or removal of the cytotoxic drug is usually recommended and is often

Table 3
ICANS grading for adults based on ASTCT consensus incorporating pupillometer

Neurotoxicity Domain	Grade 1	Grade 2	Grade 3	Grade 4
ICE score	7–9	3–6	0–2	0 (patient is unarousable, unable to perform ICE)
Depressed level of consciousness	Awakens spontaneously	Awakens to voice	Awakens only to tactile stimulus	Unarousable or requires vigorous or repetitive tactile stimuli to arouse. Stupor or coma
Seizure	N/A	N/A	Clinical seizure (focal or generalized) with rapid resolution or nonconvulsive seizures on EEG that resolve with therapy	Prolonged seizure (>5 min); or repetitive clinical or electrical seizures without return to baseline in between
Motor findings	N/A	N/A	N/A	Focal motor weakness, for example, hemiparesis or paraparesis
Elevated ICP/cerebral edema	Pupillometer NPI > 4	Pupillometer NPI > 3	Focal/local edema on neuroimaging; Pupillometer NPI < 3, or LP OP < 20 mm Hg	Any of the following: diffuse cerebral edema on neuroimaging, flexor or extensor posturing, cranial nerve VI palsy, papilledema, Pupillometer NPI < 2; LP OP > 20 mm Hg, Cushing's triad

Abbreviations: ASTCT, American Society of Transplant and Cell Therapy, ICE, immune effector cell-associated encephalopathy, LP, lumbar puncture, NPI, Neurologic Pupil Index, OP, Opening pressure.

Data from Maggs L, Cattaneo G, Dal AE, Moghaddam AS, Ferrone S. CAR T Cell-Based Immunotherapy for the Treatment of Glioblastoma. Front Neurosci. 2021;15:662064.

Table 4
Beta-lactam trough level concentrations associated with neurotoxicity

Beta-Lactam	Trough Concentration
Cefepime	>20 mg/L
Meropenem	64 mg/L
Flucloxacillin	125 mg/L
Piperacillin (without tazobactam)	360 mg/L

Data from Roger C, Louart B. Beta-Lactams Toxicity in the Intensive Care Unit: An Underestimated Collateral Damage? Microorganisms. 2021;9(7):1505.

associated with clinical improvement.[78] If promptly recognized and treated, the clinical syndrome usually resolves within a week, and the changes seen in magnetic resonance imaging (MRI) resolve over days to weeks.

Central Nervous System Infections

Patients with meningitis or encephalitis are often critically ill and cared for in the ICU setting. Clinical symptoms include headache, fever, AMS, and seizures. Early identification and treatment are needed to minimize long-term deficits. A head CT should be conducted before LP in the presence of particular risk factors (**Box 1**).[79] The LP should be performed in the lateral decubitus position to allow measurement of the opening pressure (OP). Cerebrospinal fluid (CSF) should be collected in 4 tubes (**Table 5**), with both tubes 1 and 4 being sent for red and white blood cell (RBC; WBC) counts to assess for a traumatic tap. If the OP was elevated, the needle stylet should be replaced after CSF collection and empiric treatment of elevated ICP with mannitol or hypertonic saline should be considered.[80] The initial management of CNS infections should be similar to that recommended for patients with sepsis and septic shock, including fluid resuscitation to maintain a MAP above 65 mm Hg, rapid initiation of antibiotics, and close neurologic and hemodynamic monitoring. Guidelines recommend that empiric dexamethasone (10 mg every 6 hours for 2–4 days) be given 10 to 20 minutes before or simultaneously with the first dose of antibiotics.[79] The initial antibiotic regimen should include Vancomycin, Ceftriaxone, and Acyclovir, with Ampicillin in elderly (> age 50) or immunocompromised patients (includes diabetics and pregnant patients). The regimen is narrowed based on CSF results.[80]

Box 1
Risk factors for the presence of CT abnormality in patients with CNS infections

- >/ = 60 y of age
- History of CNS disease (eg, mass lesion, stroke, focal infection)
- Immunocompromised state (eg, HIV infection, immunosuppressive therapy, or transplantation)
- Seizure within 1 wk before presentation
- Altered level of consciousness
- Focal neurologic deficit

Table 5 CSF studies in CNS infections	
Tube 1	Cell count (RBC and WBC)
Tube 2	Protein, glucose, lactic acid
Tube 3	Gram stain, culture, antigens, India ink, herpes PCR
Tube 4	Cell count (RBC and WBC)

Abbreviations: PCR, polymerase chain reaction; RBC, red blood cells; WBC, white blood cells.

Neurologic Complications of Medical Conditions

A full discussion of neurologic complications of medical conditions is beyond the scope of this article, but 2 items do warrant some discussion. Multiple neurologic symptoms have been reported in COVID-19, including encephalopathy (49%), coma (17%), stroke (3%), seizure and/or status epilepticus (1%), and CNS infection (<1%). The presence of any neurologic symptom is associated with higher mortality.[81] Both systemic and primary CNS factors may contribute to the development of COVID-19 encephalopathy, and clinical findings include AMS, delirium, and coma. Diagnostic work-up of COVID-19 encephalopathy includes a thorough neurologic examination, general metabolic and infectious laboratory testing, neuroimaging, EEG, and LP for CSF studies including SARS-CoV-2 and antiviral antibodies. Management should include neuromonitoring including EEG, avoidance of secondary brain injury, control of temperature, blood pressure, and seizures. Depending on the clinical scenario consideration should be given to the use of corticosteroids, plasma exchange, IVIG, or tocilizumab.[82]

Extracorporeal membrane oxygenation (ECMO) provides life support to patients with refractory cardiac and respiratory failure. This life-saving therapy is associated with neurologic complications related to either thrombus formation or hemorrhage. The incidence of complications differs based on the type of ECMO therapy, veno-venous (VV) or veno-arterial (VA) (**Table 6**).[83] Management of ECMO-related neurologic symptoms generally aligns with standard treatments. Intracranial hemorrhage requires stopping anticoagulation and strict blood pressure control. Thrombolytic therapy for an acute ischemic stroke is not recommended, but mechanical thrombectomy may be considered in the setting of large vessel occlusion. Seizure management should rely on EEG monitoring and antiseizure medications, which requires monitoring of serum levels due to altered pharmacokinetics. Cerebral edema and elevated ICP should be managed aggressively based on published guidelines.[84] In the event of brain death, a clinical examination with apnea testing can be performed if sweep speeds can be adjusted adequately to allow the required rise in $Paco_2$. Due to the frequency of neurologic complications, patients on ECMO should have frequent

Table 6 Incidence of neurologic complications of ECMO		
Complication	VV ECMO	VA ECMO
Intracranial hemorrhage	3.6%	1.8%
Brain death	2%	7.9%
Ischemic stroke	1.7%	3.6%
Seizure	1.2%	1.8%

neurologic assessments, minimization of sedatives, and use of neuromonitoring tools (eg, pupillometer, EEG, transcranial Doppler, imaging) whenever possible.

SUMMARY

Neurologic symptoms are frequently encountered in the ICU setting and may have a variety of causes. Early recognition allows for timely management and may lessen long-term neurologic effects.

CLINICS CARE POINTS

- Adequate CPR with minimal interruption is a key component in improving postarrest outcomes. Identifying the etiology of the arrest is a key to preventing rearrest
- A target MAP of greater than 80 should allow adequate cerebral perfusion pressure in the event of elevated intracranial pressure
- Limitations in available delirium screening tools may contribute to significant underdiagnosis of delirium in patients with neurologic conditions in the ICU
- Critically elevated ammonia levels can lead to brain edema and increased intracranial pressure. In patients with an ammonia level that is 3 or more folds times higher than the normal value and is refractory to conventional therapy, hemodialysis should be considered.

DISCLOSURE

The authors have nothing to disclose.

REFERENCES

1. Callaway CW, Donnino MW, Fink EL, et al. Part 8: post-cardiac arrest care: 2015 American heart association guidelines update for cardiopulmonary resuscitation and Emergency Cardiovascular care. Circulation 2015;132(18_suppl_2):S465–82.
2. Sunde K, Pytte M, Jacobsen D, et al. Implementation of a standardised treatment protocol for post resuscitation care after out-of-hospital cardiac arrest. Resuscitation 2007;73(1):29–39.
3. Nolan JP, Sandroni C, Böttiger BW, et al. European resuscitation Council and European Society of intensive care medicine guidelines 2021: post-resuscitation care. Intensive Care Med 2021;47(4):369–421.
4. McKenzie N, Williams TA, Tohira H, et al. A systematic review and meta-analysis of the association between arterial carbon dioxide tension and outcomes after cardiac arrest. Resuscitation 2017;111:116–26.
5. Callaway CW, Soar J, Aibiki M, et al. Part 4: Advanced life support: 2015 International Consensus on cardiopulmonary resuscitation and Emergency Cardiovascular care Science with treatment recommendations. Circulation 2015;132(16 Suppl 1):S84–145.
6. Wang CH, Chang WT, Huang CH, et al. The effect of hyperoxia on survival following adult cardiac arrest: a systematic review and meta-analysis of observational studies. Resuscitation 2014;85(9):1142–8.
7. Russo JJ, Di Santo P, Simard T, et al. Optimal mean arterial pressure in comatose survivors of out-of-hospital cardiac arrest: an analysis of area below blood pressure thresholds. Resuscitation 2018;128:175–80.
8. Beylin ME, Perman SM, Abella BS, et al. Higher mean arterial pressure with or without vasoactive agents is associated with increased survival and better

neurological outcomes in comatose survivors of cardiac arrest. Intensive Care Med 2013;39(11):1981–8.

9. Roberts BW, Kilgannon JH, Hunter BR, et al. Association between elevated mean arterial blood pressure and neurologic outcome after resuscitation from cardiac arrest: results from a Multicenter prospective cohort study. Crit Care Med 2019; 47(1):93–100.

10. Ameloot K, Meex I, Genbrugge C, et al. Hemodynamic targets during therapeutic hypothermia after cardiac arrest: a prospective observational study. Resuscitation 2015;91:56–62.

11. Ameloot K, De Deyne C, Eertmans W, et al. Early goal-directed haemodynamic optimization of cerebral oxygenation in comatose survivors after cardiac arrest: the Neuroprotect post-cardiac arrest trial. Eur Heart J 2019;40(22):1804–14.

12. Reynolds JC, Callaway CW, El Khoudary SR, et al. Coronary angiography predicts improved outcome following cardiac arrest: propensity-adjusted analysis. J Intensive Care Med 2009;24(3):179–86.

13. Camuglia AC, Randhawa VK, Lavi S, et al. Cardiac catheterization is associated with superior outcomes for survivors of out of hospital cardiac arrest: review and meta-analysis. Resuscitation 2014;85(11):1533–40.

14. Redfors B, Råmunddal T, Angerås O, et al. Angiographic findings and survival in patients undergoing coronary angiography due to sudden cardiac arrest in western Sweden. Resuscitation 2015;90:13–20.

15. Millin MG, Comer AC, Nable JV, et al. Patients without ST elevation after return of spontaneous circulation may benefit from emergent percutaneous intervention: a systematic review and meta-analysis. Resuscitation 2016;108:54–60.

16. Elfwén L, Lagedal R, James S, et al. Coronary angiography in out-of-hospital cardiac arrest without ST elevation on ECG-Short- and long-term survival. Am Heart J 2018;200:90–5.

17. Harhash AA, Huang JJ, Howe CL, et al. Coronary angiography and percutaneous coronary intervention in cardiac arrest survivors with non-shockable rhythms and no STEMI: a systematic review. Resuscitation 2019;143:106–13.

18. Branch KRH, Strote J, Gunn M, et al. Early head-to-pelvis computed tomography in out-of-hospital circulatory arrest without obvious etiology. Acad Emerg Med 2021;28(4):394–403.

19. Rittenberger JC, Tisherman SA, Holm MB, et al. An early, novel illness severity score to predict outcome after cardiac arrest. Resuscitation 2011;82(11): 1399–404.

20. Coppler PJ, Elmer J, Calderon L, et al. Validation of the Pittsburgh cardiac arrest category illness severity score. Resuscitation 2015;89:86–92.

21. Callaway CW, Coppler PJ, Faro J, et al. Association of initial illness severity and outcomes after cardiac arrest with targeted temperature management at 36 °C or 33 °C. JAMA Netw Open 2020;3(7):e208215.

22. Kuroda Y, Kawakita K. Targeted temperature management for postcardiac arrest syndrome. J Neurocrit Care 2020;13(1):1–18.

23. Lascarrou J-B, Merdji H, Le Gouge A, et al. Targeted temperature management for cardiac arrest with Nonshockable rhythm. N Engl J Med 2019;381(24):2327–37.

24. Bray JE, Stub D, Bloom JE, et al. Changing target temperature from 33°C to 36°C in the ICU management of out-of-hospital cardiac arrest: a before and after study. Resuscitation 2017;113:39–43.

25. Badjatia N, Strongilis E, Gordon E, et al. Metabolic impact of shivering during therapeutic temperature modulation: the Bedside Shivering Assessment Scale. Stroke 2008;39(12):3242–7.

26. Olson DM, Grissom JL, Williamson RA, et al. Interrater reliability of the bedside shivering assessment scale. Am J Crit Care 2013;22(1):70–4.

27. Elmer J, Polderman KH. Emergency neurological life support: resuscitation following cardiac arrest. Neurocrit Care 2017;27(Suppl 1):134–43.

28. Geocadin RG, Wijdicks E, Armstrong MJ, et al. Practice guideline summary: Reducing brain injury following cardiopulmonary resuscitation: report of the guideline development, Dissemination, and Implementation Subcommittee of the American Academy of Neurology. Neurology 2017;88(22):2141–9.

29. Elmer J, He Z, May T, et al. Precision care in cardiac arrest: ICECAP (PRECICE-CAP) study protocol and Informatics approach. Neurocrit Care 2022;37(Suppl 2): 237–47.

30. Rittenberger JC, Popescu A, Brenner RP, et al. Frequency and timing of nonconvulsive status epilepticus in comatose post-cardiac arrest subjects treated with hypothermia. Neurocrit Care 2012;16(1):114–22.

31. Elmer J, Torres C, Aufderheide TP, et al. Association of early withdrawal of life-sustaining therapy for perceived neurological prognosis with mortality after cardiac arrest. Resuscitation 2016;102:127–35.

32. Hirsch KG, Fischbein N, Mlynash M, et al. Prognostic value of diffusion-weighted MRI for post-cardiac arrest coma. Neurology 2020;94(16):e1684–92.

33. Iyer VN, Mandrekar JN, Danielson RD, et al. Validity of the FOUR score coma scale in the medical intensive care unit. Mayo Clin Proc 2009;84(8):694–701.

34. Hassler W, Steinmetz H, Gawlowski J. Transcranial Doppler ultrasonography in raised intracranial pressure and in intracranial circulatory arrest. J Neurosurg 1988;68(5):745–51.

35. Tan H, Feng H, Gao L, et al. Outcome prediction in severe traumatic brain injury with transcranial Doppler ultrasonography. Chin J Traumatol 2001;4(3):156–60.

36. Michaeli D, Rappaport ZH. Tissue resonance analysis; a novel method for noninvasive monitoring of intracranial pressure. Technical note. J Neurosurg 2002; 96(6):1132–7.

37. Moretti R, Pizzi B. Optic nerve ultrasound for detection of intracranial hypertension in intracranial hemorrhage patients: confirmation of previous findings in a different patient population. J Neurosurg Anesthesiol 2009;21(1):16–20.

38. Dubourg J, Javouhey E, Geeraerts T, et al. Ultrasonography of optic nerve sheath diameter for detection of raised intracranial pressure: a systematic review and meta-analysis. Intensive Care Med 2011;37(7):1059–68.

39. Robba C, Cardim D, Tajsic T, et al. Ultrasound non-invasive measurement of intracranial pressure in neurointensive care: a prospective observational study. Plos Med 2017;14(7):e1002356.

40. Hénon H, Lebert F, Durieu I, et al. Confusional state in stroke: relation to preexisting dementia, patient characteristics, and outcome. Stroke 1999;30(4):773–9.

41. Mc Manus J, Pathansali R, Hassan H, et al. The evaluation of delirium post-stroke. Int J Geriatr Psychiatry 2009;24(11):1251–6.

42. Mc Manus JT, Pathansali R, Ouldred E, et al. Association of delirium post-stroke with early and late mortality. Age Ageing 2011;40(2):271–4.

43. McManus J, Pathansali R, Stewart R, et al. Delirium post-stroke. Age Ageing 2007;36(6):613–8.

44. Devlin JW, Skrobik Y, Gélinas C, et al. Clinical practice guidelines for the prevention and management of pain, agitation/sedation, delirium, immobility, and sleep disruption in adult patients in the ICU. Crit Care Med 2018;46(9):e825–73.

45. Rollo E, Callea A, Brunetti V, et al. Delirium in acute stroke: a prospective, cross-sectional, cohort study. Eur J Neurol 2021;28(5):1590–600.

46. Roberson SW, Patel MB, Dabrowski W, et al. Challenges of delirium management in patients with traumatic brain injury: from pathophysiology to clinical practice. Curr Neuropharmacol 2021;19(9):1519–44.

47. Shaw RC, Walker G, Elliott E, et al. Occurrence rate of delirium in acute stroke settings: systematic review and meta-analysis. Stroke 2019;50(11):3028–36.

48. Patel MB, Bednarik J, Lee P, et al. Delirium monitoring in neurocritically ill patients: a systematic review. Crit Care Med 2018;46(11):1832–41.

49. Reznik ME, Drake J, Margolis SA, et al. Deconstructing Poststroke delirium in a prospective cohort of patients with Intracerebral hemorrhage. Crit Care Med 2020;48(1):111–8.

50. Hilbert MT, Henkel ND, Spetz SL, et al. The rising status of phenobarbital: A case for use in severe refractory hyperactive Poststroke delirium. Neurologist 2022;(May 9). https://doi.org/10.1097/NRL.0000000000000441. Epub ahead of print.

51. Tidwell WP, Thomas TL, Pouliot JD, et al. Treatment of alcohol withdrawal syndrome: phenobarbital vs CIWA-Ar protocol. Am J Crit Care 2018;27(6):454–60.

52. Romero-Gómez M, Boza F, García-Valdecasas MS, et al. Subclinical hepatic encephalopathy predicts the development of overt hepatic encephalopathy. Am J Gastroenterol 2001;96(9):2718–23.

53. Boyer TD, Haskal ZJ. The role of transjugular intrahepatic portosystemic shunt in the management of portal hypertension. Hepatology 2005;41(2):386–400.

54. Ferenci P, Lockwood A, Mullen K, et al. Hepatic encephalopathy–definition, nomenclature, diagnosis, and quantification: final report of the working party at the 11th World Congresses of Gastroenterology, Vienna, 1998. Hepatology 2002;35(3):716–21.

55. Khungar V, Poordad F. Hepatic encephalopathy. Clin Liver Dis 2012;16(2): 301–20.

56. Bustamante J, Rimola A, Ventura PJ, et al. Prognostic significance of hepatic encephalopathy in patients with cirrhosis. J Hepatol 1999;30(5):890–5.

57. Vilstrup H, Amodio P, Bajaj J, et al. Hepatic encephalopathy in chronic liver disease: 2014 practice guideline by the American association for the study of liver diseases and the European association for the study of the liver. Hepatology 2014;60(2):715–35.

58. Mumtaz K, Ahmed US, Abid S, et al. Precipitating factors and the outcome of hepatic encephalopathy in liver cirrhosis. J Coll Physicians Surg Pak 2010;20(8):514–8.

59. Hadjihambi A, Arias N, Sheikh M, et al. Hepatic encephalopathy: a critical current review. Hepatol Int 2018;12(Suppl 1):135–47.

60. Prakash R, Mullen KD. Mechanisms, diagnosis and management of hepatic encephalopathy. Nat Rev Gastroenterol Hepatol 2010;7(9):515–25.

61. Kircheis G, Nilius R, Held C, et al. Therapeutic efficacy of L-ornithine-L-aspartate infusions in patients with cirrhosis and hepatic encephalopathy: results of a placebo-controlled, double-blind study. Hepatology 1997;25(6):1351–60.

62. Takuma Y, Nouso K, Makino Y, et al. Clinical trial: oral zinc in hepatic encephalopathy. Aliment Pharmacol Ther 2010;32(9):1080–90.

63. Neill L, Rees J, Roddie C. Neurotoxicity-CAR T-cell therapy: what the neurologist needs to know. Pract Neurol 2020;20(4):285–93.

64. Lin YJ, Mashouf LA, Lim M. CAR T cell therapy in primary brain tumors: current investigations and the future. Front Immunol 2022;13:817296.

65. Maggs L, Cattaneo G, Dal AE, et al. CAR T cell-based Immunotherapy for the treatment of Glioblastoma. Front Neurosci 2021;15:662064.

66. Castaneda-Puglianini O, Chavez JC. Assessing and management of neurotoxicity after CAR-T therapy in diffuse large B-cell Lymphoma. J Blood Med 2021; 12:775–83.
67. Lee DW, Santomasso BD, Locke FL, et al. ASTCT Consensus grading for cytokine Release syndrome and neurologic toxicity associated with immune effector cells. Biol Blood Marrow Transpl 2019;25(4):625–38.
68. Roger C, Louart B. Beta-lactams toxicity in the intensive care Unit: an Underestimated Collateral damage? Microorganisms 2021;9(7):1505.
69. Boschung-Pasquier L, Atkinson A, Kastner LK, et al. Cefepime neurotoxicity: thresholds and risk factors. A retrospective cohort study. Clin Microbiol Infect 2020;26(3):333–9.
70. Paulson OB, Strandgaard S, Edvinsson L. Cerebral autoregulation. *Cerebrovasc Brain Metab Rev* Summer 1990;2(2):161–92.
71. Hinchey J, Chaves C, Appignani B, et al. A reversible posterior leukoencephalopathy syndrome. N Engl J Med 1996;334(8):494–500.
72. Ay H, Buonanno FS, Schaefer PW, et al. Posterior leukoencephalopathy without severe hypertension: utility of diffusion-weighted MRI. Neurology 1998;51(5):1369–76.
73. Rabinstein AA, Mandrekar J, Merrell R, et al. Blood pressure fluctuations in posterior reversible encephalopathy syndrome. J Stroke Cerebrovasc Dis 2012; 21(4):254–8.
74. Brightman MW, Klatzo I, Olsson Y, et al. The blood-brain barrier to proteins under normal and pathological conditions. J Neurol Sci 1970;10(3):215–39.
75. Vaughan CJ, Delanty N. Hypertensive emergencies. Lancet 2000;356(9227): 411–7.
76. Arnoldus EP, Van Laar T. A reversible posterior leukoencephalopathy syndrome. N Engl J Med 1996;334(26):1745, author reply 1746.
77. Bakshi R, Bates VE, Mechtler LL, et al. Occipital lobe seizures as the major clinical manifestation of reversible posterior leukoencephalopathy syndrome: magnetic resonance imaging findings. Epilepsia 1998;39(3):295–9.
78. Hayes D Jr, Adler B, Turner TL, et al. Alternative tacrolimus and sirolimus regimen associated with rapid resolution of posterior reversible encephalopathy syndrome after lung transplantation. Pediatr Neurol 2014;50(3):272–5.
79. Tunkel AR, Hartman BJ, Kaplan SL, et al. Practice guidelines for the management of bacterial meningitis. Clin Infect Dis 2004;39(9):1267–84.
80. Gaieski DF, O'Brien NF, Hernandez R. Emergency neurologic life support: meningitis and encephalitis. Neurocrit Care 2017;27(Suppl 1):124–33.
81. Chou SH, Beghi E, Helbok R, et al. Global incidence of neurological manifestations among patients Hospitalized with COVID-19-A report for the GCS-NeuroCOVID Consortium and the ENERGY Consortium. JAMA Netw Open 2021;4(5):e2112131.
82. Michael BD, Walton D, Westenberg E, et al. Consensus clinical guidance for diagnosis and management of adult COVID-19 encephalopathy patients. J Neuropsychiatry Clin Neurosci 2022;(Jul 25). https://doi.org/10.1176/appi.neuropsych.22010002. Epub ahead of print.
83. Illum B, Odish M, Minokadeh A, et al. Evaluation, treatment, and impact of neurologic injury in adult patients on Extracorporeal membrane oxygenation: a review. Curr Treat Options Neurol 2021;23(5):15.
84. Cadena R, Shoykhet M, Ratcliff JJ. Emergency neurological life support: intracranial hypertension and Herniation. Neurocrit Care 2017;27(Suppl 1):82–8.

Neuropharmacology in the Intensive Care Unit

Abdalla Ammar, PharmD, FCCM, BCCCP, BCPS[a],
Mahmoud A. Ammar, PharmD, FCCM, BCCCP, BCPS[b],
Eljim P. Tesoro, PharmD, FNCS, FCCM, BCCCP[c],*

KEYWORDS

- Osmotherapy • Analgesia • Sedation • Anticoagulants • Vasopressors
- Antiseizure drugs

KEY POINTS

- Selection of analgesic and sedative agents should be based on clinical goals and patients' renal and hepatic functions.
- Vasoactive medications can be selected based on clinical goals as well as side-effect profiles.
- Several targeted neuroimmunomodulatory therapies are now available to treat various neuroinflammatory disorders.

ANALGESIA

Neurologically injured patients commonly experience pain and distress because of their underlying injury and invasive procedures, such as endotracheal intubation, extraventricular drain placement, and emergent decompressive craniotomy.[1] Opioids are the mainstay therapy for severe pain management in the acute care setting, which often helps control elevated intracranial pressure (ICP). Commonly used intravenous (IV) formulations in the neurocritical care setting include fentanyl, morphine, and hydromorphone, which can be given either as continuous infusions or as intermittent IV push. Continuous infusions are most appropriate for mechanically intubated patients. Oral agents may be used for maintenance therapy once acute pain is controlled.

Fentanyl, a synthetic opioid, is a commonly used analgesic because of its distinctive pharmacokinetic properties and quick onset of action. However, because of its

[a] Neurocritical Care, New York-Presbyterian/Weill Cornell Medical Center, 525 East 68th Street, New York City, NY 10065, USA; [b] Trauma-Surgical Critical Care, Yale New Haven Hospital, 20 York Street, New Haven, CT 06510, USA; [c] Department of Pharmacy Practice (MC 886), College of Pharmacy, University of Illinois at Chicago, 833 South Wood Street, Room 164, Chicago, IL 60612, USA
* Corresponding author.
E-mail address: etesoro@uic.edu

Crit Care Clin 39 (2023) 171–213
https://doi.org/10.1016/j.ccc.2022.07.007
0749-0704/23/© 2022 Elsevier Inc. All rights reserved.

criticalcare.theclinics.com

lipophilicity, high volume of distribution, and 3-compartmental model, continuous in-fusions of fentanyl may result in a prolonged and unpredictable effect extending beyond infusion discontinuation and hinder liberation from mechanical ventilation. Rapid bolus doses of fentanyl have been associated with chest wall rigidity and can result in inadequate spontaneous ventilation.[2–4] Morphine and hydromorphone are commonly used as alternatives to fentanyl in neurologically injured patients. However, caution should be taken when using morphine in hemodynamically unstable patients, as it can cause systemic histamine release that can lead to hypotension.[1,5] In addition, it is recommended to avoid morphine in status epilepticus patients because of accu-mulation of an active metabolite (morphine-6-glucuronide) that can cause seizures.[1,5] Similarly, hydromorphone is metabolized to hydromorphone-3-glucuronide, a poten-tially neuroexcitatory metabolite. Fentanyl is the preferred agent in patients with renal dysfunction, as it does not have active metabolites that can accumulate like morphine and hydromorphone.[1,5] Common side effects include sedation, hypotension, and con-stipation.[1,5] **Table 1** describes commonly used analgesics in the neurocritical care setting with therapeutic considerations.

SEDATIVES

In mechanically ventilated patients, light sedation is preferred over deep sedation along with daily awakening trials.[1] This strategy is supported with positive short-term outcomes, such as reduced intensive care unit (ICU) length of stay and shorter duration of mechanical ventilation.[12,13] Large studies suggest that using a nonbenzo-diazepine sedative, such as dexmedetomidine or propofol, rather than a benzodiazepine-based regimen in critically ill adults may reduce delirium, ICU length of stay, and duration of mechanical ventilation.[1,14] These outcomes are often extrap-olated to the neurocritical care settings because most published studies excluded pa-tients with neurological injuries since sedatives can interfere with frequent clinical neurologic assessments.[15] In addition, in the neurocritical care setting, sedative agents are often used for other therapeutic indications, such as treatment or preven-tion of elevated ICP, achieved through reduction in cerebral metabolic rate for oxygen, which regulates cerebral blood flow and cerebral perfusion pressure (CPP).[16] Contin-uous anesthetic agents are also used as rescue therapy for patients with refractory status epilepticus on continuous electroencephalogram (EEG) monitoring.[17,18] **Table 2** describes commonly used sedatives in the neurocritical care setting and ther-apeutic considerations.

HYPEROSMOLAR THERAPY

Hyperosmolar therapies, such as mannitol and hypertonic saline (HTS), are used to treat elevated ICP and cerebral edema in the setting of traumatic brain injury (TBI), ischemic and hemorrhagic strokes, and hepatic encephalopathy. HTS is also often used in patients with symptomatic hyponatremia, cerebral salt wasting, and syndrome of inappropriate secretion of antidiuretic hormone. The focus in the following section is on the use of hyperosmolar agents to treat intracranial hypertension and cerebral edema.

Mannitol is a sugar alcohol osmotic diuretic that decreases water and sodium reab-sorption in the renal tubule. Mannitol lowers ICP through 2 distinct mechanisms of ac-tion. The first, mannitol's rheological effect, reduces blood viscosity and promotes plasma expansion and cerebral oxygen delivery. This may eventually potentiate cere-bral vasoconstriction secondary to cerebral autoregulation leading to a reduction in cerebral blood perfusion.[30,31] The second effect occurs through fluid shifts by creating

Table 1
Common analgesics in neurocritical care setting

	Mechanism of Action	Dosing	Pharmacokinetics	Patient Care Considerations
Opioid				
Fentanyl[2-4]	Mu-opioid receptor agonist	Intermittent dosing: 0.35–1.5 μg/kg IV every 30–60 min Infusion: 0.7–10 μg/kg/h IV (most patients require 1-3 μg/kg/h or 50–200 μg/h) titrate by 25 μg every 30 to 60 min to clinical effect	Onset: Immediate Duration: 30–60 min Volume of distribution: 4–6 L/ kg Context-sensitive half-life: >100 min Elimination half-life: 2–4 h Three-compartment distribution model Hepatically metabolized, primarily via CYP3A4 Renally eliminated	Prolonged and unpredictable effects may extend beyond infusion discontinuation and may hinder liberation from mechanical ventilation Chest wall rigidity with rapid administration Accumulation in hepatic dysfunction
Morphine[1,5]		Intermittent dosing: 2–4 mg IV every 1–2 h Infusion: 2–30 mg/h IV titrate by 1 mg/h every 30 to 60 min to clinical effect Enteral: 10–30 mg every 4 h PRN	Onset: 5–10 min Duration: 3–5 h Elimination half-life: 3–4 h Hepatically metabolized to active metabolite morphine-6-glucuronide and inactive metabolite morphine-3-glucuronide Renally eliminated, primarily as morphine-3-glucuronide	Can cause hypotension, bradycardia Metabolite can accumulate in kidney dysfunction (avoid use) Accumulation of morphine-6-glucuronide can cause sedation and morphine-3-glucuronide can cause neurotoxicity (e.g., seizures)

(continued on next page)

Table 1
(continued)

	Mechanism of Action	Dosing	Pharmacokinetics	Patient Care Considerations
Hydromorphone[6,7]		Intermittent dosing: 0.2–0.6 mg IV every 1–2 h Infusion: 0.5–3 mg/h IV titrate by 0.2 mg/h every 30 to 60 min to clinical effect Enteral: 2–4 mg every 4 to 6 h PRN	Onset: 15–30 min Duration: 3–4 h Elimination half-life: 2–3 h Hepatically metabolized to inactive metabolite hydromorphone-3-glucuronide Renally eliminated, primarily as hydromorphone-3-glucuronide	Can cause hypotension 5–7 times more potent than morphine Accumulation of hydromorphone-3-glucuronide in kidney dysfunction can cause neurotoxicity (avoid use)
Oxycodone[5]		Enteral: 5–20 mg every 4 to 6 h	Onset: 10–15 min Duration: 3–6 h Half-life: 4 h Hepatically metabolized via CYP3A4 Renally eliminated	Can cause hypotension (rare) CrCl ≤ 60 mL/min; 50% increase in serum concentration
Methadone[8,9]	Mu-opioid receptor agonist and NMDA receptor antagonist	Enteral: 10–40 mg every 6–12 h Intermittent dosing: 2.5–10 mg IV every 8–12 h	Onset: enteral; 0.5–1 h, IV; 10–20 min Duration: 12–48 h Half-life: 8–59 h Steady state in 3–5 d Hepatic via CYP3A4, CYP2B6, CYP2C19, CYP2C9, and CYP2D6 to inactive metabolites Renally eliminated	QTc prolongation, caution with coadministration with other QTc prolonging drugs Long half-life Prolonged effect in hepatic and renal dysfunction Can cause serotonin syndrome with concomitant use of serotonergic agents

Nonopioid

Drug	Mechanism	Dosing	Pharmacokinetics	Notes
Acetaminophen	Central prostaglandin inhibitor (COX-2 inhibitor)	Enteral: 325–1000 mg q4–6h (maximum 4000 mg/d) IV: 650 mg IV q4h PRN pain OR 1 g IV q6h PRN pain	Onset: 3 min (IV), 11 min (PO) Duration: 3–4 h Half-life: 2–4 h Metabolized hepatically via CYP 2E1 to NAPQI, which is toxic Renally excreted <5% unchanged	Hepatotoxic metabolite (NAPQI) accumulates in renal dysfunction
Gabapentin[10]	Modulated calcium-channel	Enteral: 900–3600 mg/d divided q6–8h	Slow onset of action Half-life: 6 h Renally eliminated	Dizziness, somnolence, ataxia; can rarely cause peripheral edema Dose reduction warranted in renal dysfunction
Carbamazepine[1,11]	Sodium channel inhibitor	Enteral: 200–1200 mg/d divided q8–12h	Peak effect: 4–8 h Hepatic metabolism to active metabolite carbamazepine-10,11-epoxide Half-life: 24 h Major CYP3A4 substrate Major CYP2C19/3A4 inducer Renally eliminated	Dose-dependent hyponatremia Transient elevation of hepatic transaminases Associated with Stevens-Johnson syndrome/toxic epidermal necrolysis and agranulocytosis Consider dose reduction in both severe renal and hepatic impairment
Pregabalin[1]	Calcium-channel modulation (GABA analogue)	Enteral: 150–600 mg/d divided q6–8h	Slow onset of action Half-life: 6 h Renally eliminated (dialyzable)	Rarely peripheral edema Dose reduction warranted in renal dysfunction
Ketorolac[1]	Reversible inhibition of COX 1 and 2 enzymes	Intermittent dosing: 15–30 mg IV/IM q6h up to 5 d	Onset: 30 min Half-life: 2–9 h Renally eliminated	Associated with kidney injury and bleeding Avoid NSAIDs in renal dysfunction, postneurosurgical patients, gastrointestinal bleeding, and platelet dysfunction
Ibuprofen[1]		Enteral: 400 mg q4h (max: 2400 mg/d) Intermittent dosing: 400–800 mg IV every 6 h (max: 3200 mg/d)	Onset: 30 min (PO) Half-life; PO/IV: 2–3 h Renally eliminated	

Abbreviations: COX, cyclooxygenase; CrCl, creatinine clearance; CYP, cytochrome P450; GABA, gamma-aminobutyric acid; IBW, ideal body weight; IM, intramuscular; max, maximum; NAPQI, N-acetyl-*p*-benzoquinone imine; NMDA, N-methyl-D-aspartate; NSAIDs, nonsteroidal anti-inflammatory drugs; PO, per os; PRN, as needed; QTc, corrected QT interval.

Table 2
Common sedatives in neurocritical care setting

	Mechanism of Action	Dosing	Pharmacokinetics	Patient Care Considerations
Nonbenzodiazepines				
Propofol[1,19]	Enhances neurotransmission of GABA neurotransmitter at the GABA$_A$ receptor, increasing the frequency of chloride ion channel opening in response to GABA	Infusion: 5–100 μg/kg/min; titrate by 5 to 10 μg/kg/min every 2 min until goal sedation level is achieved. Doses higher than 80 μg/kg/min may increase risk of PRIS	Onset of action: 30 s. Half-life: initially 3–12 h, but extends to 30–70 h with long-term use. Duration: 3–10 min. Large volume of distribution. Highly lipophilic. Extensively metabolized by liver; also has extrahepatic and extrarenal clearance	May cause respiratory depression, hypotension, hypertriglyceridemia, pancreatitis, and PRIS. Monitor patients for PRIS signs and symptoms of metabolic acidosis, bradycardia, cardiac arrest, rhabdomyolysis, renal failure. Contraindicated in patients with hypersensitivity to egg or soy products. Source of calories (1.1 kcal/mL); adjust nutrition requirements accordingly. Monitor pH, bicarbonate, triglycerides, creatine kinase, lipase with prolonged therapy (>48 h), or high doses (>80 μg/kg/min or 5 mg/kg/h)
Dexmedetomidine[20]	α_2-adrenoreceptor agonist at the brain stem mediating sedation through the locus coeruleus	Loading dose 1 μg/kg over 10 min (not recommended due to cardiovascular side effects). Infusion: 0.2–1.5 μg/kg/h, titrate by 0.2 μg/kg/h every 30 min to sedation goal	Onset: 5–10 min after loading doses, 18–30 min with no loading dose. Half-life: 2–3 h. Accumulates in hepatic failure. Duration: 60–120 min	Can cause bradycardia, negative inotropy, hypotension. Can cause hypertension (with bolus dosing or high infusion rates). No added benefit with doses >1.5 μg/kg/h

Agent	Mechanism	Dose	Pharmacokinetics	Comments / Adverse effects
				Does not provide deep sedation Not associated with respiratory depression compared with other sedatives Has analgesic properties, can be beneficial for opioid-sparing strategies
Ketamine[21-24]	NMDA antagonist	Light sedation, or analgesia: 0.1–1 mg/kg/h Deep sedation: 1–10 mg/kg/h titrate by 0.1 mg/kg/h every 15–30 min to sedation goal	Onset: 30 min Half-life; alpha, 5–17 min; beta, 2.5 h can extend in critically ill patients (~5 h) Volume of distribution increases ~3-fold in the critically ill Duration: Dose and duration-dependent, 15 min to 1 h (prolonged in renal or hepatic dysfunction) Metabolized to active metabolite norketamine	Preserves pharyngeal and laryngeal protective reflexes Lowers airway resistance, increases lung compliance May have sympathomimetic properties, but can also cause hypotension when HR/SBP > 0.9 Has analgesic properties, can be beneficial for opioid-sparing strategies May cause increased pulmonary secretions
Pentobarbital[25]	Barbiturate; enhances neurotransmission of GABA at the GABA$_A$ receptor. Resulting in an increase in the frequency of chloride ion channel opening in response to GABA neurotransmitters	Medically induced coma: Loading dose: 5–15 mg/kg Sedation infusion: 0.5–5 mg/kg/h (not often used due to safety profile)	Onset: 3–5 min Half-life: 15–50 h Duration: 15–45 min Accumulation in severe hepatic failure	Decreases ICP Prolonged half-life (up to 50 h; dose-dependent) May cause hypotension, ileus, myocardial and pulmonary suppression, immunosuppression, and thrombocytopenia IV formulation contains 40% propylene glycol; may cause metabolic acidosis

(continued on next page)

Table 2
(continued)

	Mechanism of Action	Dosing	Pharmacokinetics	Patient Care Considerations
Clonidine[26,27]	α_2-adrenoreceptor agonist at the brain stem mediating sedation through the locus coeruleus	Enteral (sedation): 0.3–1.6 mg/d divided into 3–4 doses	Onset; enteral: 0.5–1 h Half-life: ~12 h in healthy patients, prolonged to ~40 h in patients with renal dysfunction Hepatic metabolism through CYP2D6	Can cause hypotension, bradycardia, and xerostomia Rebound effect may occur; taper off if used for prolonged periods Dexmedetomidine weaning strategy: 0.2–0.5 mg every 6 h, taper clonidine every 24–48 h by increasing dosing frequency, reduce dexmedetomidine infusion by 25% within 6 h of each clonidine dose Has analgesic properties, can be beneficial for opioid-sparing strategies
Benzodiazepines				
Midazolam[28]	Enhances neurotransmission of GABA neurotransmitter at the GABA$_A$ receptor, increasing the frequency of chloride ion channel opening in response to GABA neurotransmitter	Infusion: 0.02–0.1 mg/kg/h (1–10 mg/h) titrate infusion rate to clinical effect Intermittent dosing: 0.5–4 mg IV bolus doses every 15 min to 1 h as needed	Onset: 3–5 min Large volume of distribution Half-life: 3–11 h, prolonged half-life in obese patients Active metabolites (1-hydroxy-midazolam [or	Caution with use in obese patients and patients with renal dysfunction, as it may result in drug accumulation Can cause respiratory depression

Lorazepam[29]	Infusion: 0.01–0.1 mg/kg/h (1–10 mg/h) titrate infusion rate to clinical effect Intermittent dosing: 0.5–4 mg every 2–6 h as needed (oral or IV bolus)	alpha-hydroxymidazolam]) that is renally eliminated Onset: 3 min Half-life: 8–15 h Hepatically metabolized to inactive metabolites Duration: 6–8 h	Preferred to midazolam in morbidly obese patients and patients with renal dysfunction IV formulation contains propylene glycol; may cause metabolic acidosis Monitor for development of propylene glycol toxicity Can cause respiratory depression

Abbreviations: HR, heart rate; SBP, systolic blood pressure.

an osmotic gradient across the blood-brain barrier, resulting in a decrease in cerebral blood volume and ICP.[30,31] Mannitol is available in concentrations ranging from 5% to 25%, with 20% commonly used in acute ICP management with a dose range of 0.5 to 1.5 g/kg/dose over 5 to 15 minutes administered through an in-line filter. Rapid infusion (<5 minutes) of mannitol can cause hypotension, which can be detrimental in hemodynamically unstable patients; slower infusion rates (15–30 minutes) can alleviate this side effect.[32] Mannitol administration should be avoided when the osmolar gap is greater than 20 mOsm/kg to prevent acute renal injury. In general, it is not recommended to use serum osmolality of greater than 320 mOsm/L as a threshold to withhold mannitol therapy, as plasma osmolality is not a valid measure of excess mannitol and can be elevated in other common conditions, such as hyperglycemia.[33–35]

HTS affects ICP and brain edema by creating an osmotic gradient across the blood-brain barrier, leading to the movement of water from the brain tissue into the intravascular space.[36] Other proposed mechanisms of action of HTS include fluid expansion, direct vasodilation, increased cardiac output (CO), and neurochemical and immune-modulating effects.[35,37] HTS can be administered as a continuous infusion or as a series of bolus doses. It is prudent to note that concentration of HTS therapies beyond 3% is recommended to be administered through a central IV line, but there is evidence supporting administration of 3% NaCl and 23.4% NaCl through a peripheral IV line via at least 20-gauge catheters.[38–40] Because of the high sodium content of HTS, ranging from 257 to 4004 mEq/L (1.5%–23.4%), there are concerns for electrolyte imbalances (such as hypernatremia, hyperchloremia, hypokalemia). As such, clinicians should weigh the risk versus benefit of using HTS in patients with decompensated heart failure. Chronic hyponatremia should be excluded before administering HTS to decrease the risk of osmotic demyelinating syndrome (ODS).[39] In the setting of elevated ICP and chronic hyponatremia, consideration should be given to lower serum sodium targets, smaller HTS boluses, or some permissive mild edema in order to avoid sudden overcorrection. Changes in serum sodium should not exceed 12 mEq/L over the first 24 hours to further prevent the risk of ODS.[41]

The current Neurocritical Care Guidelines recommend either HTS or mannitol for acute management of cerebral edema with a higher preference for HTS over mannitol (conditional recommendation, very-low-quality evidence) in TBI and intracranial hemorrhages because of presumed advantages of HTS over mannitol for fluid resuscitation and cerebral perfusion.[42] It is essential to tailor the choice of hyperosmolar therapies based on serum sodium levels, plasma osmolar gap, fluid status, and patient's renal function. Mannitol is associated with profound hypotension secondary to osmotic diuresis, whereas HTS bolus is associated with transient hypotension because of a direct vasodilatory effect.[32] Mannitol could potentially be deleterious in hemodynamically unstable patients. In addition, chronic use of mannitol is associated with an increased incidence of rebound ICP elevation owing to disruption of the blood-brain barrier.[43] **Table 3** summarizes the characteristics of hyperosmolar therapies.

ANTICOAGULANT/ANTIPLATELET REVERSAL AND HEMOSTATIC AGENTS

Anticoagulants, antiplatelet agents, and thrombolytics are the cornerstone for treating and preventing thrombotic or embolic events in various medical conditions. The use of oral anticoagulants, specifically, direct oral anticoagulants (DOACs), is increasing and will continue to grow as the prevalence of atrial fibrillation increases, driven by advances in early detection, prevention, and treatment in an aging population.[44,45] The selection of an anticoagulant must consider both drug-specific and patient-specific

Table 3
Hyperosmolar therapies for intracranial pressure

	Mannitol	Hypertonic Saline
US products	20% mannitol (1100 mOsmol/L) 25% mannitol (1375 mOsm/L)	1.5% (513.5 mOsm/L) 2% (685 mOsm/L) 3% (1027 mOsmol/L) 5% (1711 mOsmol/L) 7.5% (2566 mOsmol/L) 23.4% (8008 mOsmol/L)
Bolus dosing	0.5–1.5 g/kg (average, 1 g/kg) over 5–15 min, can be redosed every 4–6 h	3%: 2.5–5 mL/kg over 5–20 min 5%: 2.5–5 mL/kg over 5–20 min 7.5%: 1.5–2.5 mL/kg over 5–20 min 23.4%: 30 mL over 10–20 min
Pharmacokinetics	Onset: 15 min Duration: 2–6 h Elimination half-life: 0.5–2.5 h Metabolism: Hepatic Excretion: Renal	Onset: ~15 min Duration: ~1.5–10 h Excretion: Renal
Adverse effects	Rebound increased ICP Acute kidney injury Dehydration Hypotension Electrolyte imbalances	Pulmonary edema Heart failure Acute kidney injury Coagulopathy Hypernatremia Metabolic acidosis Thrombophlebitis ODS
Monitoring	Patient's intake and output to maintain adequate intravascular volume Systemic blood pressure to prevent hypotension due to rapid diuresis Trough osmolar gap with threshold goal of <20 to prevent nephrotoxicity	Serum electrolytes, including trough serum sodium level with a holding threshold of 160 mEq/L Avoid increase in sodium by 12 mEq/L/d to further reduce the risk of ODS

factors. **Table 4** describes commonly used anticoagulants in neurosciences. With knowledge of drug-specific properties, clinicians can guide the appropriate application of these agents in the neurocritical care setting. Despite high effectiveness of these treatment modalities, they have been associated with significant bleeding risks.[46,47] In general, the DOACs have a lower risk of bleeding side effects compared with warfarin. **Table 5** lists recommendations for reversal of agents in the setting of intracranial hemorrhages.

ANTISEIZURE MEDICATIONS

The primary goal of managing status epilepticus (clinical and subclinical) focuses on preventing secondary brain injury and systemic complications associated with continuous seizure activity.[64] The first step of treatment, before giving antiseizure medications, is ensuring that the patient's airway is secure and that the patient is hemodynamically stable.[65] A detailed discussion of primary systemic treatment considerations when managing status epilepticus in a stepwise approach is found in later discussion, Status Epilepticus: A Neurological Emergency.

Table 4
Common anticoagulants in neurosciences

Agents	Mechanism of Action	Dosing	Pharmacokinetics	Special Considerations
Argatroban	*Direct thrombin inhibitors* A direct competitive inhibitor of thrombin, thus inhibiting production of fibrin inhibit production of fibrin	IV: 2–10 µg/kg/min Titrate to ACT and aPTT goals	Metabolism: Hepatic Elimination: Biliary excretion Onset of action: Immediate Half-life: 45 min Dose adjustments Hepatic failure: 0.5 mg/kg/min Severe hepatic failure: Avoid use	Lowest affinity to thrombin compared with other direct thrombin inhibitors PT/INR will falsely increase during administration of argatroban Preferred anticoagulant for patients with HITTS
Bivalirudin		IV bolus dose: 0.75 mg/kg, followed by a continuous infusion of 1.75 mg/kg/h Titrate to ACT and aPTT goals	Metabolism: Proteolysis and hepatic Elimination: 20% of the dose is renally eliminated Onset of action: Immediate Half-life: 25 min Dose adjustments: CrCl 15–60 mL/min: 15–50% dose reduction CrCl < 15 mL/min: Avoid use	Intermediate affinity to thrombin compared with other direct thrombin inhibitors Therapeutic option for anticoagulant during endovascular procedures in patients with HIT/HITTS
Dabigatran		NVAF and VTE treatment/ prophylaxis: 150 mg PO twice daily Hip DVT prophylaxis: 110 mg PO on day 1, followed by 220 mg PO once daily × 35 d	Metabolism: Hepatocytes and enterocytes; 20% metabolized to active metabolite Elimination: Biliary 20%; renally 80% Onset of action: 1 h Half-life 12–17 h Dose adjustments: NVAF: CrCl 15–30 mL/min: 75 mg twice daily VTE treatment and hip DVT prophylaxis: CrCl 15–30 mL/min: Avoid use CrCl < 15 mL/min: Avoid use Clinically significant drug-drug interactions: Quinidine, verapamil, amiodarone, rifampicin, St John's wort, strong P-glycoprotein inhibitors	Delayed absorption with food Avoid opening, crushing, or chewing capsule, as it increases its oral bioavailability (must keep in original packaging)
Apixaban	Factor-Xa inhibitors Bind and inhibit factor Xa, which converts	Stroke prophylaxis in NVAF: 5 mg PO twice daily	Metabolism: Hepatic Elimination: Renally (~27%)	Consider in patients with renal insufficiency, as it is the least renally cleared oral Factor-Xa inhibitor

prothrombin to thrombin	VTE prophylaxis: 2.5 mg PO twice daily VTE treatment: 10 mg PO twice daily × 7 d, then 5 mg PO twice daily	Feces (biliary and direct intestinal excretion) Onset of action: 3–4 h Half-life ~12 h Dose adjustments NVAF: If 2 of the following 3: SCr ≥ 1.5, weight ≤60 kg, age ≥80 y/o, 2.5 mg twice daily VTE treatment: None Clinically significant drug-drug interactions: CYP inhibitors ketoconazole and ritonavir CYP inducers Phenytoin, carbamazepine, rifampin, St. John's wort	May be crushed for administration via enteral feeding tube
Dalteparin	VTE prophylaxis: 5000 units SC daily VTE treatment: 100 units/kg SC every 12 h or 200 units/kg SC daily	Metabolism: Hepatic (desulfation) Elimination: Renally Onset of action: 1–2 h Half life IV: 2.21–5.7 h SQ: 3–5 h Dose adjustments CrCl < 30 mL/min: monitor anti-factor Xa level or use alternative	
Edoxaban	Stroke prophylaxis in NVAF: 60 mg PO daily VTE treatment: 60 mg PO daily (30 mg if <60 kg)	Metabolism: Hepatic Elimination: Renally Onset of action: 1–2 h Half-life 10–14 h Dose adjustments NVAF: CrCl > 95 mL/min: Not recommended CrCl 15–50 mL/min: 30 mg daily CrCl < 15 mL/min: not recommend VTE treatment: CrCl ≥ 51 mL/min: none CrCl 15–50 mL/min: 30 mg daily CrCl < 15 mL/min: Not recommend Clinically significant drug-drug interactions: Rifampin, strong P-glycoprotein inhibitors	Least drug-drug interactions of oral Factor-Xa inhibitors NVAF: Should not be used in patients with CrCl > 95 mL/min due to increased drug clearance and elevated risk of ischemic stroke

(continued on next page)

Table 4
(continued)

Agents	Mechanism of Action	Dosing	Pharmacokinetics	Special Considerations
Enoxaparin		VTE prophylaxis: 40 mg SC daily (q12h if BMI > 40 kg/m^2) VTE treatment: 1 mg/kg every 12 h or 1.5 mg/kg daily (based on indication)	Metabolism: Hepatic Elimination: Renally Onset of action: 3–5 h Half-life: 4.5–7 h Dose adjustments VTE prophylaxis: CrCl < 30 mL/min: 30 mg daily VTE treatment: CrCl < 30 mL/min: 1 mg/kg daily	
Fondaparinux		DVT prophylaxis: 2.5 mg SC daily VTE treatment: <50 kg: 5 mg SC daily 50–100 kg: 7.5 mg SC daily >100 kg: 10 mg SC daily	Metabolism: Not metabolized Elimination: Renally Onset of action: 2–3 min Half-life 17–21 h Dose adjustments VTE prophylaxis CrCl 30–50 mL/min: Consider 1.25 mg daily; avoid use if CrCl < 30 mL/min	Option for patients with HIT/HITTS
Rivaroxaban		Stroke prophylaxis in NVAF: 20 mg PO daily VTE prophylaxis: 10 mg PO daily VTE treatment: 15 mg PO twice daily × 21 d, then 20 mg PO daily	Metabolism: Hepatic Elimination: Renally (66%) Onset of action: 2–4 h Half-life 5–9 h Dose adjustments NVAF: CrCl 15–50 mL/min: 15 mg daily CrCl < 15 mL/min: Not recommend VTE treatment: CrCl ≥ 51 mL/min: None CrCl 15–50 mL/min: 30 mg daily CrCl < 15 mL/min: Not recommended Clinically significant drug-drug interactions CYP inhibitors ketoconazole, itraconazole, ritonavir CYP inducers phenytoin, carbamazepine, rifampin, St. John's wort	May be crushed for administration via enteral feeding tube

| Unfractionated heparin | Thrombin inhibitor Binds and activates antithrombin (inhibiting coagulation factors Xa and IIa), resulting in inhibition of fibrin formation | Varies depending on therapeutic indication and targeted aPTT (usually 1.5–2 times baseline aPTT) | Metabolism: Hepatic and splenic Elimination: Renally Onset of action: IV: Immediate SC: 3 h Half-life varies depending on dose (30–150 min) | |
| Warfarin | Vitamin K antagonist Inhibits VKOR and the production of the reduced vitamin K—a cofactor for the carboxylation of intrinsic clotting factors II, VII, IX, and X, and intrinsic anticoagulants protein C and protein S | Dose and targeted INR range (2–3.5) varies depending on therapeutic indication | Metabolism: Hepatic Elimination: Renally Onset of action: Variable Clinical half-life 20–60 h Dose adjustments Consider dose adjustment in renal and hepatic impairment Clinically significant drug-drug interactions: Vitamin K, foods rich with vitamin K (e.g., green leafy vegetables) Significant interactions with drugs that inhibit or induce CYP 2C9, 1A2, and 3A4 isoenzymes | Genetic mutations in the 2C9 isoenzymes and VKOR1 have been associated with variability in dosing requirements |

Abbreviations: ACT, activated clotting time; aPTT, activated partial thromboplastin time; BMI, body mass index; DDI, drug-drug interactions; HIT/HITTS, heparin-induced thrombocytopenia/heparin-induced thrombocytopenia with thrombotic syndrome; INR, international normalized ratio; NVAF, nonvalvular atrial fibrillation; PT, prothrombin time; PTT, partial thromboplastin time; SC, subcutaneous; SCr, serum creatinine; VKOR, vitamin K oxide reductase; VTE, venous thromboembolism. *Data from* Refs.[48-59]

Table 5
Reversal of anticoagulants

Agents	Dialyzable	Reversal Agent (IV)
Direct Thrombin Inhibitors		
Argatroban	20% over 4 h	• aPCC (50 units/kg) OR
Bivalirudin	25% over 4 h	• 4-factor PCC (50 units/kg) OR
		• FFP 15–20 mL/kg OR
		• rFVIIa 20 µg/kg and may repeat
		• Monitor aPTT to confirm reversal
Dabigatran	57%–68% over 4 h	• If patient presents within 2–3 h from ingestion, administer enteral activated charcoal 50 g (caution, aspiration risk)
		• Idarucizumab 5 g (2.5 g × 2 doses)
Factor-Xa Inhibitors		
Apixaban	Minimal	• If patient presents within 2–3 h from ingestion, administer enteral activated charcoal 50 g (caution, aspiration risk)
Rivaroxaban	No	• Andexanet alpha (refer to **Table 6** for recommended dosing) OR
		• 4-Factor PCC 25–50 units/kg OR
		• rFVIIa 40 µg/kg OR
		• aPCC 50 units/kg
Edoxaban	No	• If patient presents within 2–3 h from ingestion, administer enteral activated charcoal 50 g (caution, high aspiration risk)
		• 4-Factor PCC 25–50 units/kg OR
		• rFVIIa 40 µg /kg OR
		• aPCC 50 units/kg
Enoxaparin	No	• Protamine partially reverses the anticoagulant effect of LMWHs (~60%)
Dalteparin	No	○ If <8 h since last dose: 1 mg protamine:1 mg enoxaparin OR 100 units dalteparin (max: 50 mg)
		○ If 8–12 h since last dose: 0.5 mg protamine:1 mg enoxaparin OR 100 units dalteparin (max: 25 mg)
		○ If >12 h since last dose: unlikely to be of benefit; may consider in patients with renal dysfunction (max: 25 mg)
		• Monitor Factor Xa activity to confirm reversal
Fondaparinux	Yes, 20%	• Weak data for reversal effect with the following but may consider:
		○ 4F-PCC 50 units/kg OR
		○ rFVIIa 20 µg/kg and may repeat × 1
		• Protamine not effective
Thrombin Inhibitor		
Unfractionated heparin	No	• Protamine neutralizes heparin
		○ 1 mg per 100 units of heparin administered if stopped immediately

(continued on next page)

Table 5 (continued)		
Agents	**Dialyzable**	**Reversal Agent (IV)**
		○ 0.5 mg per 100 units of heparin administered if stopped 30 min ago ○ 0.25 mg per 100 units of heparin administered if stopped >2 h ago
Vitamin K Antagonist		
Warfarin	No	• Vitamin K 2.5–10 mg IV (onset 4–12 h) or 1–5 mg PO (onset 12–24 h) • 4-Factor PCC (in addition to vitamin K) ○ INR 2–3.9: 25 units/kg (max: 2500 units) ○ INR 4–6: 35 units/kg (max: 3500 units) ○ INR >6: 50 units/kg (max: 5000 units) Recheck INR 30 minutes after 4-Factor PCC administered • Additional 500 units may be given for clinically significant bleeding, repeat INR ≥1.4 OR • FFP 20–30 mL/kg (in addition to vitamin K)

Abbreviations: aPCC, activated prothrombin complex concentrate; FFP, fresh frozen plasma; FXa, Factor Xa; PCC, prothrombin complex concentrate; rFVIIa, recombinant factor VIIa.
   Data from Refs.[60–63]

Benzodiazepines are considered the first-line treatment for status epilepticus followed immediately by antiseizure medications, preferably administered through the IV route; otherwise, intramuscular, intraosseous, nasal, or buccal administration routes are acceptable alternatives.[64,66] Treatment should not be delayed while awaiting IV access. If seizures are refractory to parenteral benzodiazepines and antiseizure medications, then continuous infusions of anesthetic agents are indicated.[66] It is prudent to treat status and refractory status epilepticus rapidly and aggressively to abort seizures. Hence, higher weight-based doses of injectable anesthetics are commonly used compared with standard doses used for sedation. A comprehensive list with pharmacologic considerations for antiseizure medications is provided in **Table 7**.

Table 6 Andexanet-alpha dosing recommendation					
	Factor Xa Inhibitor	**Time Since Last Dose of FXa Inhibitor**		**Low Dose**	**High Dose**
Factor Xa Inhibitor	**Last Dose**	**<8 h or Unknown**	**≥8 h**		
Rivaroxaban	≤10 mg	Low dose	Low dose	*Bolus:* 400 mg over 15 min	*Bolus:* 800 mg over 30 min
	>10 mg/ unknown	High dose		*Infusion:*	*Infusion:*
Apixaban	≤5 mg	Low dose		480 mg over 2 h (4 mg/min)	960 mg over 2 h (8 mg/min)
	>5 mg/ unknown	High dose			

Data from Refs.[60–63]

Table 7
Antiseizure medications

Drug	Dosing	Half-Life in Noncritically Ill Patients	Protein Binding	Clinically Relevant Drug-Drug Interactions	Consideration for Dose Adjustments in Renal Impairment	Consideration for Dose Adjustment in Hepatic Impairment	Special Considerations
Injectable Anesthetic Agents							
Ketamine	LD: 1.5 mg/kg IV push over 3–5 min (max: 150 mg); repeat until seizures suppression; max total load of 4.5 mg/kg MD: initial 1.0 mg/kg/h, range 0.3–7.5 mg/kg/h; titrate to EEG target	2.5 h	27%		None	Consider dose reduction	NMDA antagonist; provides an infusion with a different mechanism of action (non-GABA) May have sympathomimetic properties, but can also cause hypotension when HR/SBP > 0.9
Midazolam	10 mg IM × 1 Alternate: LD: 0.2 mg/kg IV (push over 1–2 min); max 20 mg. Repeat 0.2–0.4 mg/kg boluses (max: 40 mg per bolus) every 5 min until seizures suppression; max total load of 2 mg/kg Continuous infusion: 0.05–3 mg/kg/h; titrate to EEG target	7 h	97%		Consider dose reduction: Risk of active metabolite accumulation (1-hydroxymidazolam)	Consider dose reduction	Enhances neurotransmission of GABA neurotransmitter at the GABA$_A$ receptor, increasing the frequency of chloride ion channel opening in response to GABA neurotransmitter Rapid redistribution Active metabolites (1-hydroxy-midazolam [or alpha-hydroxymidazolam]) May be administered via alternate routes: 0.2 mg/kg (up to 10 mg) IM, intranasal, or buccal routes; all well absorbed rapidly
Pentobarbital	LD: 5 mg/kg IVP (up to 50 mg/min); max 500 mg. Repeat until seizures suppression; max total load of 25 mg/kg MD: 0.5–10 mg/kg/h; titrate to EEG target	22 h	45%–75%		None	Consider dose reduction	Barbiturate; enhances neurotransmission of GABA neurotransmitter at the GABA$_A$ receptor, increasing the duration of chloride ion channel opening in response to GABA neurotransmitter; at higher doses, may activate GABA$_A$ receptor directly Prolonged half-life (up to 50 h; dose-dependent) May cause hypotension, ileus, myocardial, and pulmonary suppression, immunosuppression, and thrombocytopenia IV formulation contains 40% propylene glycol; may cause metabolic acidosis

Propofol	LD: 1–2 mg/kg IV over 5 min; max: 200 mg. Repeat until seizures cessation up to total LD of 10 mg/kg MD: 30–200 µg/kg/min (1.8–12 mg/kg/h); titrate to EEG target	Initially 3–12 h, but extends to 30–70 h with long-term use	90%	None	None	Enhances neurotransmission of GABA neurotransmitter at the GABA$_A$ receptor, increasing the frequency of chloride ion channel opening in response to GABA neurotransmitter May cause respiratory depression, hypotension, hypertriglyceridemia, pancreatitis, and PRIS Monitor patients for PRIS sign and symptoms of metabolic acidosis, bradycardia, cardiac arrest, rhabdomyolysis, renal failure Contraindicated in patients with hypersensitivity to egg or soy products Provides 1.1 kcal/mL, adjust nutritional support accordingly Monitor pH, bicarbonate, triglycerides, creatine kinase, lipase with prolonged therapy (>48 h), or high doses (>80µg/kg/ min or 5 mg/kg/h)
Injectable nonanesthetic agents						
Brivaracetam	LD: 100–400 mg MD: 50–600 mg/d divided every 8–12 h	9 h	<20%	Increase concentrations of carbamazepine active metabolite (carbamazepine epoxide) and phenytoin[67]	None	Binds to synaptic vesicle glycoprotein SV2A, inhibiting pre synaptic calcium channels, thereby reducing neurotransmitter release No added therapeutic benefit when coadministered with levetiracetam
Diazepam	LD: 0.25 mg/kg IV push over 1–2 min (max: 10 mg per dose); repeat every 5 min until seizures stop up to 3 doses or 30 mg MD: not applicable	40 h	98%	Not applicable	Not applicable	Enhances neurotransmission of GABA neurotransmitter at the GABA$_A$ receptor. Resulting in an increase in the frequency of chloride ion channel opening in response to GABA neurotransmitter Has rapid redistribution IV formulation contains propylene glycol IV solution may be administered rectally if no IV access Rectal gel formulation available

(continued on next page)

Table 7
(continued)

Drug	Dosing	Half-Life in Noncritically Ill Patients	Protein Binding	Clinically Relevant Drug-Drug Interactions	Consideration for Dose Adjustments in Renal Impairment	Consideration for Dose Adjustment in Hepatic Impairment	Special Considerations
Fosphenytoin	LD: 20 mg PE/kg IV (up to 150 mg/min); max: 2000 mg. If still seizing, give additional 5 mg/kg IV (max: 500 mg) MD: use phenytoin Note: Fosphenytoin is dosed in PE	IV: 0.25 h IM: 0.5 h	95%–99%	Induces CYP1A2, 2B6, 2C, 3A3/4 Avoid use with most CYP3A4 substrates Coadministration with valproate displaces phenytoin from protein binding site and induces metabolism of valproate	None	Consider dose reduction	Hydantoin-derivative that blocks voltage-gated sodium channels. It is also a class 1b antiarrhythmic medication Conversion half-life to phenytoin ~15 to 30 min May be administered IM if no IV access (up to 99% absorption after IM administration) Compatible with saline, dextrose, and lactated Ringer solution Diluent is nontoxic; decrease cutaneous reactions with extravasation May cause hypotension, arrhythmias Consider obtaining peak phenytoin level 2 h post-IV dose or 4 h post-IM dose (see phenytoin section later)
Lacosamide	LD: 10 mg/kg IV over 5–10 min (max: 500 mg). If still seizing, give an additional 5 mg/kg over 5 min (max: 250 mg IV) MD: 200–600 mg/d divided every 6–12 h Note: Maximum IV push dose is 400 mg administered at a rate of 80 mg/min	13 h	<15%		Reduce dose in severe renal impairment (CrCl < 30 mL/min); max 300 mg/d HD: 50% removed; lower dose based on CrCl, divide every 12 h and add 50% of morning dose to evening dose post-HD CRRT: Lower dose based on CrCl, then increase total daily dose by 50% and divide every 8 h	Consider dose reduction	Functionalized amino acid that enhances slow inactivation of voltage-gated sodium channels. May prolong PR interval or induce tachyarrhythmia, including atrial fibrillation

Drug	Dosing	Half-life	Protein binding	Renal/CRRT adjustment		Mechanism/Notes
Levetiracetam	LD: 60 mg/kg over 15 min (max: 4,500 mg) MD: 1500–4500 mg/d divided every 6–12 h Note: Maximum IV push dose is 1500 mg administered at a rate of 500 mg/min	6 h	<10%	Reduce dose based on CrCl HD: 50% removed; lower dose based on CrCl, divide every 12 h, and add 50% of morning dose to the evening dose post-HD CRRT: lower dose based on CrCl, then increase total daily dose by 50%, and divide every 6 h		Binds to synaptic vesicle glycoprotein SV2A, inhibiting pre synaptic calcium channels, thereby reducing neurotransmitter release. May cause behavioral disturbances (eg, agitation, aggression); consider switching to brivaracetam No added therapeutic benefit when coadministered with brivaracetam
Lorazepam	LD: 4 mg IVP over 2 min; repeat every 5 min until seizures stop up to 3 doses or 12 mg MD: Not applicable	12 h	85%–90%	Not applicable	Not applicable	Enhances neurotransmission of GABA neurotransmitter at the GABA$_A$ receptor. Resulting in an increase in the frequency of chloride ion channel opening in response to GABA neurotransmitter Rapid redistribution IV formulation contains 80% propylene glycol; may cause metabolic acidosis Do not administer IM or SC (IM midazolam preferred if IV access not available)

(continued on next page)

Table 7
(continued)

Drug	Dosing	Half-Life in Noncritically Ill Patients	Protein Binding	Clinically Relevant Drug-Drug Interactions	Consideration for Dose Adjustments in Renal Impairment	Consideration for Dose Adjustment in Hepatic Impairment	Special Considerations
Phenytoin	LD: 20 mg/kg IVP (up to 50 mg/min; 25 mg/min in elderly and patients with preexisting cardiovascular conditions) MD: 200–600 mg/d divided every 8–12 h	7–42 h (nonlinear kinetics)	95%–99%	Induces CYP1A2, 2B6, 2C, 3A3/4 Generally, avoid use with most CYP3A4 substrates Coadministration with valproate displaces phenytoin from protein binding site and induces metabolism of valproate	None	Consider dose reduction	Hydantoin-derivative that blocks voltage-gated sodium channels. It is also a class 1b antiarrhythmic medication May cause rash, fever, hypotension, or arrhythmias IV formulation contains 40% propylene glycol; may cause metabolic acidosis Only compatible in saline (unlike fosphenytoin) Incompatibilities include dextrose solution, potassium, insulin, heparin, norepinephrine, cephalosporin, and dobutamine Severe tissue injury may occur with extravasation, including rare purple glove syndrome Consider obtaining peak phenytoin (free and total) level 2 h post-IV loading dose Therapeutic range: 10–20 μg/mL (total) or 1–2 μg/mL (free)
Phenobarbital	LD: 20 mg/kg IV (up to 60 mg/min); max dose 1500 mg. If still seizing, give an additional 5–10 mg/kg MD: 1–3 mg/kg given every day or divided every 8–12 h	80 h	50%–60%	Strong inducer of UGT, CYP 3A4, 2B6, 2C9, 2A6, 1A2. Dose adjustments of drugs including phenytoin and valproate might be necessary	Consider dose reduction HD: give full daily dose in evening after hemodialysis	Consider dose reduction	Barbiturate; enhances neurotransmission of GABA neurotransmitter at the GABA_A receptor, increasing the frequency of chloride ion channel opening in response to GABA neurotransmitter Prolonged half-life (up to 140 h) May cause hypotension. IV formulation contains 70% propylene glycol; may cause metabolic acidosis Therapeutic range: 15–40 μg/mL

	Dosing	Half-life	Protein binding	Drug interactions	Renal	Hepatic	Comments
Valproate	LD: 40 mg/kg IV (over 5–10 min); max 4000 mg. If still seizing, give additional 20 mg/kg IV (max: 2000 mg) over 5 min. MD: 2000–6000 mg divided every 6–8 h	12 h	90%	Phenytoin and valproate may displace each other from protein binding sites. Valproate markedly inhibits lamotrigine metabolism resulting in increase in lamotrigine levels and risk of side effects including severe rash. Concurrent use with carbapenems may result in markedly decreased valproic acid plasma concentrations	None	Caution in hepatic impairment	Organic acid compound that prolongs sodium channel inactivation, attenuates calcium mediated transient currents and augments GABA. Highly plasma protein-bound (up to 90%). May cause hyperammonemia encephalopathy (treated with L-carnitine supplementation), hepatotoxicity, thrombocytopenia, and platelet dysfunction. Consider obtaining total valproate level 2 h post-IV loading dose. Highly teratogenic and associated with other adverse fetal effects. Therapeutic range: 50–125 µg/mL
Enteral agents							
Cannabidiol	MD: 2.5–20 mg/kg/d divided q12h	58 h	>94%	CYP3A4 and CYP2C19 substrate. Phenytoin and other CYP3A4 inducers decrease levels. Valproic acid and other CYP3A4 inhibitors increase levels	None	Consider dose reduction.	Concomitant use of higher doses of cannabidiol and valproate increases the risk of transaminase elevations and hepatocellular injury. Consider discontinuation or dose adjustment of cannabidiol and/or valproate if liver enzyme elevations occur. If AST and/or ALT >3 times ULN and total bilirubin >2 times ULN, discontinue treatment. If sustained AST and/or ALT >5 times ULN, discontinue treatment
Carbamazepine	LD: 400–800 mg. MD: 400–600 mg/d divided every 12 h	24 h. 8 h (with prolonged use due to autoinduction; 2–4 wk)	75%–90%	Major CYP3A4 substrate; major CYP2C19/3A4 inducer. Phenytoin and other CYP3A4 inducers decrease carbamazepine levels. Valproic acid and other CYP3A4 inhibitors increase carbamazepine levels	Consider dose reduction in severe renal impairment (CrCl < 10 mL/min): reduce dose by 25%	Consider dose reduction undergoes extensive hepatic metabolism	Strong association between the risk of developing Stevens-Johnson syndrome/TEN and the presence of HLA-B*1502 allele (documented mostly in Asian descent). Dose-dependent hyponatremia; decreased incidence compared with oxcarbazepine. Therapeutic range: 4–12 µg/mL

(continued on next page)

Table 7
(continued)

Drug	Dosing	Half-Life in Noncritically Ill Patients	Protein Binding	Clinically Relevant Drug-Drug Interactions	Consideration for Dose Adjustments in Renal Impairment	Consideration for Dose Adjustment in Hepatic Impairment	Special Considerations
Clobazam	LD: 20–40 mg MD: 20–80 mg/d divided q12h	Clobazam: 16 h, N-desmethyl-clobazam: 39 h	80%–90%	Felbamate: Increase plasma concentrations of N-desmethylclobazam	Caution in severe renal impairment (CrCl < 30 mL/min)	Consider dose reduction undergoes extensive hepatic metabolism	Enhances neurotransmission of GABA neurotransmitter at the GABA_A receptor, increasing the frequency of chloride ion channel opening in response to GABA neurotransmitter Decreased sedation compared with other benzodiazepines When ordering drug levels, consider ordering clobazam and active metabolite (N-desmethylclobazam) drug level
Oxcarbazepine	LD: 600–1200 mg MD: 600–2400 mg/d divided q6–12h	5	67%	Increase concentrations of phenobarbital and phenytoin	Consider 50% dose reduction in severe renal impairment HD: IR formulations preferred	ER formulation not recommended	Dose-dependent hyponatremia; more common in elderly
Perampanel	LD: 6–12 mg MD: 4–12 mg/d	105 h	95%		Use not recommended in severe renal impairment (CrCl < 30 mL/min)	Consider dose reduction in mild to moderate hepatic impairment Use not recommended in severe hepatic impairment	A noncompetitive AMPA-receptor antagonist, theoretically effective at regulating the glutamate overload May cause behavioral issues/agitation
Pregabalin	LD: 150–300 mg MD: 150–600 mg/d divided q6–8h	6 h	None		Reduce dose HD: Dose based on CrCl, administer supplemental dose post-HD	None	Occasional peripheral edema

Drug	Dose	Half-life	Protein binding	Notes	Renal impairment/Dialysis	Hepatic impairment	Comments
Topiramate	LD: 200–400 mg MD: 200–600 (reports up to 1600) mg/d divided every 6–12 h	21 h	15%–41%	Use with zonisamide and other carbonic anhydrase inhibitors may worsen metabolic acidosis	Reduce dose by ~50% HD: Supplemental dose may be necessary	Consider dose reduction	Potent broad-spectrum ASM that blocks ionotropic glutamatergic AMPA receptors. May cause metabolic acidosis; caution with propofol, acetazolamide, zonisamide, and metformin. May cause renal stones. May be associated with oligohidrosis, with risk of hyperthermia, mainly in pediatric patients
Vigabatrin	LD: 1500 mg MD: 1000–3000 mg/d divided every 12 h	10 h (but sustained effect for several days)	None		Reduce dose based on CrCl	None	Potential progressive, permanent peripheral vision loss after months to years of use; regular ophthalmology examinations recommended with prolonged use. May markedly reduce liver function test (ALT/AST) in patients with documented liver disease. It is not recommended to use plasma liver function test activity as an index of liver cell damage

Abbreviations: ALT, alanine transaminase; ASM, antiseizure medication; AST, aspartate transaminase; DSW, dextrose 5% in water; ER, extended release; HD, hemodialysis; IM, intramuscular; IR, immediate release; LD, loading dose; MD, maintenance dose; PE, phenytoin equivalent; TEN, toxic epidermal necrolysis; UGT, uridine 5′-diphospho-glucuronosyltransferase; ULN, upper limit of normal.
Adapted from the Yale New Haven Hospital status epilepticus protocol.[68]

ANTISHIVERING AGENTS

Shivering is encountered in neurologically injured patients undergoing targeted temperature management to achieve hypothermia or normothermia. This therapeutic intervention is used in comatose post–cardiac arrest patients and also in patients with acute brain injury with refractory intracranial hypertension or fever, albeit with limited evidence.[69–71] Shivering is an involuntary thermoregulatory response that is centrally mediated and can have detrimental impact on systemic oxygen consumption, brain tissue oxygenation, and ICP. Therefore, it is prudent to evaluate and treat shivering in neurologically injured patients.[72–74] Several antishivering protocols based on Bedside Shivering Assessment Scale (BSAS), to achieve minimal shivering or a BSAS score of 1 (**Table 8**), have been implemented and evaluated in clinical practice. An example of such a protocol is highlighted in **Table 9** along with recommended drug therapies for each BSAS score.

VASOACTIVE AGENTS

Vasoactive agents can be categorized into vasopressors, inotropes, and antihypertensives (**Tables 10** and **11**). Vasopressor agents induce vasoconstriction and are commonly used in neurologically injured patients to augment mean arterial pressure in various scenarios, such as shock or vasospasm, or to improve cerebral or spinal perfusion pressures.[76] Vasopressors exert their effect by augmenting systemic vascular resistance (SVR) and/or increasing CO.[76,77] Catecholamine vasopressors primarily increase blood pressure by increasing SVR through their actions at adrenergic (alpha and/or beta receptors), dopamine, and vasopressin receptors.[76,77] Vasopressin is a unique vasopressor that increases SVR by affecting V_1R/V_2R activity. Selective sparing V_1R in some vascular beds or V_2R-mediated vasodilation leads to decreased vasoconstrictive effects of vasopressin in the coronary, cerebral, and pulmonary circulation.[76,77] Inotropes exert their pharmacologic effect through increasing CO. Dobutamine is a β-agonist that improves cardiac function by augmenting SVR and CO. Milrinone, on the other hand, is a phosphodiesterase type 3 (PDE3) inhibitor. PDE3 inhibition potentiates cyclic adenosine monophosphate, leading to increased inotropy and vasodilation.[76,77] **Table 10** highlights the receptors and pharmacology of various vasopressors agents.

Table 8	
Bedside shivering assessment scale	
Score	**Description**
0	No shivering noted on palpation of the masseter, neck, or chest wall and no electrophysiological evidence of shivering (using electrocardiography)
1	Electrophysiological evidence of shivering (using electrocardiography), without clinical evidence of shivering
2	Shivering localized to the neck and/or thorax only
3	Shivering involves gross movement of the upper extremities (in addition to neck and thorax)
4	Shivering involves gross movements of the trunk, upper, and lower extremities

Adapted from Badjatia N, Strongilis E, Gordon E, et al. Metabolic impact of shivering during therapeutic temperature modulation: the Bedside Shivering Assessment Scale. Stroke. 2008;39(12):3242-3247; with permission.

Table 9
Antishivering medications

Agent	Mechanism of Action in Thermoregulation	Dosing	Key Pharmacology	Clinical Consideration
Score 0: Shivering Prophylaxis (includes skin counter warming at a maximum temperature of 43°C)				
Acetaminophen	Lowers hypothalamic thermoregulatory set point through inhibiting cyclooxygenase-mediated prostaglandin synthesis	Enteral/IV: 650–1000 mg q4–6h	Elimination half-life: 2–3 h (prolonged in hepatic injury) Metabolism: Hepatic with toxic metabolite; NAPQI Excretion: Renal	Increased risk for hepatic injury, dose-dependent hepatic cell necrosis Contraindicated in severe hepatic impairment
Ibuprofen	Lowers hypothalamic thermoregulatory set point through inhibiting cyclooxygenase-mediated prostaglandin synthesis	Enteral: 400–600 mg q4–6h	Elimination half-life: 2 h Metabolism: Hepatic Excretion: Renal	Caution with renal dysfunction or recent gastrointestinal bleed
Buspirone	5-HT1A partial agonist, lowering shivering threshold	Enteral: 20–30 mg q8h	Elimination half-life: 2–3 h (prolonged in severe hepatic or renal impairment) Metabolism: Hepatic into active metabolite Excretion: Renal	Can cause sedation Dose reduction might be needed in severe hepatic or renal impairment
Magnesium sulfate	Direct vasodilator, which counteracts normal adaptive response of vasoconstriction during surface cooling process Antagonist activity at NMDA receptor Impairs thermoregulatory control, reducing time to target temperature	IV bolus: 2–4 g IV q4h to maintain goal serum magnesium level of 2–4 mg/dL	Excretion: Renal	Electrolyte imbalances (calcium, potassium, phosphate levels), flushing, hyporeflexia, respiratory and muscle paralysis, cardiac arrest Dose adjustment might be needed in severe renal failure

(continued on next page)

Table 9
(continued)

Agent	Mechanism of Action in Thermoregulation	Dosing	Key Pharmacology	Clinical Consideration
Score 1 (mild sedation): Select an opioid or dexmedetomidine and maximize therapy				
Score 2 (moderate sedation): Select an opioid and dexmedetomidine if inadequate control with mild sedation and maximize therapy				
Meperidine	Lowers the shivering threshold through agonist effect on α_{2B}-receptor Impair thermoregulatory control through agonist activity at opioid receptors (μ, κ) and antagonist activity at NMDA receptor	25–100 mg IV q4–6h as needed	Meperidine elimination half-life: 3 h (prolonged in hepatic dysfunction) Normeperidine elimination half-life: 15–20 h for (prolonged in hepatic dysfunction) Metabolism: Hepatic to active neurotoxic metabolite; normeperidine Excretion: Renal	CNS stimulation, including tremors, muscle twitches, seizures (accumulation of normeperidine that can lower seizure threshold), hypotension, respiratory depression sedation, constipation Avoid in severe hepatic or renal impairment due to risk of neurotoxicity
Fentanyl	Impair thermoregulatory control through agonist activity at μ-opioid receptor	Infusion: 0.7–10 μg/kg/h IV (most patients require 1–3 μg/kg/h or 50–200 μg/h)	Elimination half-life: 2–4 h (prolonged with continuous infusion due to third-compartment model) Metabolism: Hepatic Excretion: Renal	Respiratory depression sedation, constipation Dose reduction might be needed in severe renal impairment and moderate hepatic impairment Avoid in severe hepatic impairment
Dexmedetomidine	Vasoconstriction and lowers the shivering threshold through agonist effect on α_{2A}-receptor	Infusion 0.2–1.5 μg/kg/h	Elimination half-life: 2–3 h Metabolism: Hepatic Excretion: Renal	Bradycardia, hypotension, sedation

Score 3: Deep sedation				
Propofol	Peripheral vasodilatory effects reduce primarily vasoconstriction, but also shivering thresholds	Infusion: 5–100 μg/kg/min (doses higher than 80 μg/kg/min may increase risk of PRIS)	Elimination half-life: 4–7 h (prolonged with continuous infusion) Metabolism: Hepatic Excretion: Renal	Bradycardia, hypotension, respiratory depression PRIS: risk of PRIS increases at high doses (>80 μg/kg/min) for 48 h. Monitor for metabolic acidosis and creatinine kinase Due to high lipid load, monitor triglycerides and caloric intake (1.1 kcal/mL) Contraindicated in patients with severe allergy to egg and soy proteins
Score 4: Neuromuscular blockade (MUST BE DEEPLY SEDATED PRIOR TO INITIATION)				
Vecuronium	Control involuntary muscle contractions involved in shivering	Bolus: 0.05–0.1 mg/kg (duration 30–45 min) Infusion: 0.05–1.5 μg/kg/min IV titrate to TOF	Elimination half-life: 60–80 min Metabolism: Hepatic Excretion: Renal, fecal	Muscle atrophy and weakness. Loss of neurologic examination (masks insufficient sedation and seizure activity)
Cisatracurium		Bolus: 0.1–0.2 mg/kg (duration 45–60 min) Infusion: 2–10 μg/kg/min	Elimination half-life: 22–29 min Metabolism: Nonenzymatic degradation in the bloodstream (Hofmann elimination) Excretion: Renal (85%), fecal (4%)	Prolonged paralysis may occur in severe hepatic or renal failure Cisatracurium is metabolized to laudanosine that is associated with CNS stimulation, including seizures

Abbreviations: 5-HT1A, serotonin 1A receptor; CNS, central nervous system; TOF, train-of-four; κ, kappa; μ, delta.
Data from Refs.[62,72,75]

Table 10
Common parenteral vasoactive agents

	Adrenergic Receptor Activation	Mechanism of Action	Dose	Common Indications	Clinical Considerations
Vasopressors					
Norepinephrine	α_1 β_1	Potent α-adrenergic agonist with less pronounced β-adrenergic agonist effects	Typical dose 2–40 µg/min or 0.025–1 µg/kg/min (max dose for refractory shock 3 µg/kg/min)	Septic shock with low SVR	First line for septic shock Risk of dysrhythmias and myocardial ischemia, decrease renal, splanchnic, or peripheral blood flow
Dopamine	α_1 β_1 DA	Natural precursor of norepinephrine and epinephrine, with distinct dose-dependent pharmacologic effects	Dopa: 1–3 µg/kg/min α: 3–10 µg/kg/min β: 10–20 µg/kg/min	Septic shock with low SVR and/or low CO	Highest risk of dysrhythmias (especially at higher doses)
Epinephrine	α_1 β_1 β_2	Potent α- and β-adrenergic agent; increases mean arterial pressure by increasing both the cardiac index and peripheral vascular tone	Typical dose 1–40 µg/min or 0.01-2 µg/kg/min	Septic shock with low SVR and/or low CO Anaphylactic shock	Risk of dysrhythmias, myocardial ischemia, and hypoglycemia Tachyarrhythmias, hyperglycemia, lactic acidosis
Phenylephrine	α_1	Selective α_1-adrenergic agonist; increases MAP by vasoconstriction increasing SVR	Typical dose 40–400 µg/min or 0.25–5 µg/kg/min	Septic shock with low SVR or tachyarrhythmia CPP augmentation	May cause reflex bradycardia No β effects, therefore less arrhythmogenic Can be added or used as an alternative agent when tachyarrhythmias limit therapy

Drug	Receptor	Mechanism	Dose	Indication	Comments
Vasopressin	V_1R V_2R	Constricts vascular smooth muscle directly via V_1R and increases responsiveness of the vasculature to catecholamines	0.04 units/min	Refractory hypotension in septic shock; Central diabetes insipidus	Refractory shock for vasopressors sparing effect; May decrease splanchnic perfusion and increase gut ischemia
Inotropes					
Dobutamine	α_1 β_1 β_2	A racemic mixture of 2 isomers; D-isomer with β_1- and β_2-adrenergic affinity and an L-isomer with β_1- and a1-adrenergic affinity; Predominant inotropic effect via stimulation of β_1 receptors	Typical dose 2–10 µg/kg/min (max dose for refractory shock is 20 µg/kg/min)	Acute decompensated heart failure, cardiogenic shock, septic shock with depressed cardiac function	Tolerance may occur with prolonged administration
Milrinone	PDE3	PDE3 inhibitor; PDE3 inhibition potentiates cyclic adenosine monophosphate, leading to increased inotropy and vasodilation	0.25–0.75 µg/kg/min (doses up to 2 µg/kg/min have been reported for refractory cerebral vasospasm); Reduce dose if CrCl < 50 mL/min	Acute decompensated heart failure cardiogenic shock, septic shock with depressed cardiac function	Dose adjustment might be needed in renal dysfunction; Can cause hypotension and arrhythmias

Abbreviations: α, alpha; β, beta; V_1A, vasopressin V_1A; V_2A, vasopressin V_2A.
Data from Refs.[62,76,77]

Table 11
Common parenteral antihypertensive agents

	Mechanism of Action	Dosing	Pharmacokinetics	Patient Care Considerations
Vasodilators				
Hydralazine	Potent arterial vasodilator decreasing afterload	IV bolus 10–20 mg every 30 min as needed IM: 10–40 mg every 30 min as needed	Onset: IV: 10 min, IM: 20 min Duration: IV: 1–4 h, IM: 2–6 h Half-life: 2–8 h	Can cause reflex tachycardia, headache, flushing
Sodium nitroprusside	Potent arterial and venous vasodilator decreasing both afterload and preload	IV 0.3–10 μg/kg/min Increase rate by 0.1–0.2 μg/kg/min IV every 5 min	Onset: seconds Duration: 1–2 min Half-life: 3–4 min	Concerns for coronary steal through shunting of oxygenated blood from diseased coronary arteries to nondiseased coronary artery Theoretical concerns regarding increasing ICP through cerebral arteries vasodilation potentially decreasing CPP Risk for cyanide toxicity, especially in patients with chronic liver disease, alcoholism, prolonged use (>3 d), and malnutrition; concern for thiocyanate neurotoxicity in patients with renal dysfunction

Calcium Channel Blockers

Drug	Mechanism	Dosing	Pharmacokinetics	Comments
Nicardipine	Dihydropyridine; peripherally selective to L-type calcium channel blockers. Inhibit calcium influx through calcium channels along the vascular smooth muscle leading to vasodilation	IV 5–15 mg/h; Increase rate by 2.5 mg/h every 5–15 min	Onset: 5–15 min; Duration: 0.5–2 h; Half-life: 2 h	Can cause reflex tachycardia, headache, nausea, flushing. Contraindicated in patients with severe aortic stenosis
Clevidipine		IV 1–2 mg/h; Increase rate by 1–2 mg/h every 90 s to maximum dose of 21 mg/24 h (for more aggressive dosing, may double rate every 90 s up to a dose of 16 mg/h, then increase by 2 mg/h once within 10 mmHg of goal blood pressure to a typical max of 24 mg/h)	Onset: 1–4 min; Duration: 90 s; Half-life: 1 min	Contraindication in patients with soy or egg product allergy (as it is formulated in a lipid compound) and severe aortic stenosis. Provides 2 kcal/mL, adjust nutritional support as needed. Monitor triglycerides, lipase, and amylase. Discard vials within 12 h due to the risk of bacterial growth. Can cause reflex tachycardia
Nimodipine		Enteral: 60 mg q4h (or 30 mg q2h) for 21 consecutive days	Onset: 0.25–1 h; Half-life: 1–2 h	Indicated for use in aneurysmal subarachnoid hemorrhage to decrease delayed cerebral ischemia (no indication for hypertension)

Beta-blockers

Drug	Mechanism	Dosing	Pharmacokinetics	Comments
Esmolol	Beta selective antagonist	IV 25–300 µg/kg/min; Increase rate by 25 µg/kg/min every 3–5 min	Onset: 1–2 min; Duration: 10–20 min; Half-life: 9 min	Avoid in patient with systolic heart failure
Labetalol	Combined alpha and beta antagonist	IV bolus: 10–20 mg; may repeat escalating doses by 20–80 mg every 5–10 min as needed; IV 0.5–10 mg/min; increase dose by 1–2 mg/min every 2 h	Onset: 2–5 min; Peak effect: 5–15 min; Duration: 2–18 h; Half-life: 4–8 h	Avoid in patient with systolic heart failure

(continued on next page)

Table 11
(continued)

	Mechanism of Action	Dosing	Pharmacokinetics	Patient Care Considerations
Metoprolol	Beta selective antagonist	IV bolus: 5–15 mg every 5–15 min as needed	Onset: 5–20 min Duration 2–6 h Half-life: 3–4 h	Avoid in patient with systolic heart failure Due to long duration of activity, less titratable, can cause extended, unintentional correction of blood pressure
Angiotensin-Converting Enzyme Inhibitor				
Enalaprilat	Inhibits ACE preventing the conversion of angiotensin I to angiotensin II, a potent vasoconstrictor	IV bolus: 1.25 mg over 5 min every 6 h. Maximum dose: 5 mg/dose every 6 h	Onset: 15 min Duration: 6 h Half-life: 35 h	Can cause angioedema, cough, hyperkalemia Due to long duration of activity, less titratable, can cause extended, unintentional correction of blood pressure Use in pregnancy is contraindicated

Abbreviation: ACE, angiotensin-converting enzyme.
Data from Refs.[62,78,79]

Table 12
Immunomodulatory therapies

Drug	Mechanism of Action	Dosing	Adverse Effects	Patient Care Consideration
Glucocorticoids (methylprednisolone, prednisone, dexamethasone)	Cytokine modulation	(Varies by specific condition) Methylprednisolone 1 g IV daily for 3–5 d Prednisone 1 mg/kg/d to start Dexamethasone 1–40 mg IV every 6 h	Hyperglycemia, psychosis, infection, adrenal suppression, osteoporosis, myopathy	Ensure proper GI prophylaxis Monitor blood glucose, lipid panel
IV immunoglobulins	Autoantibodies; modulates complement, cytokines	Chronic inflammatory demyelinating polyneuropathy/Guillain-Barré syndrome/ myasthenia gravis/ multifocal motor neuropathy/ encephalomyelitis: 2 g/kg IV divided over 3–5 d	Hypersensitivity/infusion reactions, thromboembolism, renal failure, aseptic meningitis, hemolytic anemia, neutropenia	May premedicate with acetaminophen, diphenhydramine Monitor vital signs during infusion, renal function
Cyclophosphamide (CYC)	DNA alkylation/crosslinking; suppresses T- and B-cell mediated immunity; decreases secretion of IL-12, Th-1-cytokine LFNγ	Various Multiple sclerosis: 1. IV induction therapy with MP: 600 mg/m² IV CYC given on days 1, 2, 4, 6, 8 plus IV MP given daily for 8 d 2. IV pulse therapy with CYC/ MP after MP induction (1 g daily for 5 d): IV CYC pulses begun at 800 mg/ m² with dose escalation designed to produce leukopenia of 2000/mm³;	Nausea/vomiting, cytopenias, infections, hemorrhagic cystitis, alopecia, myelosuppression	Provide IV hydration, Mesna (to reduce hemorrhagic cystitis), antiemetics Monitor CBC w/diff, BUN/ creatinine Maximum lifetime dose: 80–100 g

(continued on next page)

Table 12
(continued)

Drug	Mechanism of Action	Dosing	Adverse Effects	Patient Care Consideration
		every 4 wk for 12 wk, every 6 wk for 12, every 2 mo for 12 mo; 1 g IV MP given with CYC (maximum dose 1600 mg/m^2) 3. IV pulse therapy with CYC at a fixed dose: IV CYC pulses given at 800–1000 mg/m^2 every 4–8 wk for 12–24 mo; given with or without IV MP		
Rituximab	Anti-CD20 antibody, depletes B cells and plasmablasts	Myasthenia gravis: 1000 mg IV every 2 weeks for 2 doses or 375 mg/m^2 IV weekly × 4 (usually every 6 mo) Multiple sclerosis: 1000 mg IV every 2 wk for 2 doses. Consider repeating 1000 mg once every 6 mo Neuromyelitis optica: 1000 mg every 2 wk for 2 doses or 375 mg/m^2 weekly for 4 wk	Hypersensitivity reactions, hypogammaglobulinemia, infections, PML	Monitor vital signs, telemetry during infusion, CBC w/ diff, CD19/20 counts, IgG/IgM levels Hepatitis B reactivation can occur following rituximab administration in patients who are hepatitis B core antibody positive regardless of surface antigen positivity. Screening and monitoring for HBV reactivation is recommended
Infliximab, Adalimumab	TNFα inhibitor, inhibits macrophage activation via decrease in TNFR1/2 stimulation	Infliximab 5 mg/kg IV at 0, 2, 6 wk, then every 4–8 wk Adalimumab 40 mg SC every 2 wk	Hypersensitivity reactions, hepatotoxicity, demyelination/optic neuritis, TB reactivation	Monitor vital signs during infusion, CBC w/diff, LFTs

Drug	Mechanism	Dosing	Adverse effects	Monitoring
Azathioprine	DNA intercalation, inhibits purine synthesis	Myasthenia gravis: PO: 25–50 mg once daily; increase by 50 mg every 1–4 wk to maximum 2 to 3 mg/kg or 200 mg/d once daily	Hepatotoxicity, cytopenias, infections, nausea, diarrhea	Monitor CBC w/diff, LFTs
Methotrexate	Inhibits thymidylate and purine synthesis	Multiple sclerosis: PO/SC: start 7.5 mg weekly, then increase to 15–25 mg weekly	Nausea, diarrhea, mucositis, cytopenias, hepatotoxicity, pneumonitis	Consider folic acid supplementation Monitor CBC w/diff, LFTs
Mycophenolate mofetil	Inhibits guanosine synthesis	Myasthenia gravis: Start 250 or 500 mg twice daily, then increase by 500 mg/d every 1–2 weeks to 1000–1500 mg twice daily	Nausea, diarrhea, abdominal pain, hepatotoxicity, cytopenias, hypertension, nephrotoxicity, cough, dyspnea, infections, headache, tremor	Monitor CBC w/diff, LFTs, BUN/creatinine
Eculizumab	Anti-C5 antibody	Myasthenia gravis/ neuromyelitis optica spectrum disorder: Induction: 900 mg IV weekly for 4 doses Maintenance: 1200 mg IV weekly for 1 dose, then 1200 mg IV every 2 weeks	Hypersensitivity reactions, hypertension, anemia	May premedicate with acetaminophen, diphenhydramine Meningococcal vaccines at least 2 wk before treatment initiation is recommended. CDC recommends both MenACWY vaccine and the full series of MenB vaccine (2–3 doses depending on brand) for eculizumab recipients. Patients should be administered a booster dose of MenACWY vaccine every 5 y, for the duration of eculizumab therapy.

(continued on next page)

Table 12
(continued)

Drug	Mechanism of Action	Dosing	Adverse Effects	Patient Care Consideration
Tocilizumab	Anti-IL-6R antibody	Giant cell arteritis: 4–8 mg/kg IV every 4 wk OR 162 mg SC every wk	Hypersensitivity reactions, GI perforation, hepatotoxicity, neutropenia, thrombocytopenia, TB reactivation	May premedicate with acetaminophen, diphenhydramine Monitor CBC, LFTs
Natalizumab	Anti-α4-integrin antibody	Multiple sclerosis: 300 mg infusion every 4 wk	PML, hypersensitivity reactions	May premedicate with acetaminophen, diphenhydramine Monitor vital signs during infusion, CBC, LFTs

Abbreviations: BUN, blood urea nitrogen; CBC, complete blood count; GI, gastrointestinal; LFTs, liver function tests; MP, methylprednisolone; PML, progressive multifocal leukoencephalopathy.

Data from Refs.[80–90]

IMMUNOSUPPRESSANT THERAPIES

Immunosuppressive medications and selective immunomodulatory agents acting on specific immune system components have been increasingly used due to improved understanding of the pathophysiology of immune-mediated neurologic conditions and the recent development of new immunosuppressant and selective immunomodulatory therapeutic agents. **Table 12** lists the most common medications used for immune-mediated neurologic disorders.

SUMMARY

Pharmacologic management of patients with neurological injury is challenging. Therapy choices and doses should be tailored to each patient based on patient's comorbidities and medications' pharmacokinetic and pharmacodynamic properties. Using this knowledge, clinicians should optimize appropriate therapies while minimizing further cognitive dysfunction and adverse events.

CLINICS CARE POINTS

- Osmotherapy can be guided by intracranial pressures (when available) as well as laboratory criteria (i.e., osmolar gap for mannitol, serum sodium for hypertonic saline).
- Proper reversal of anticoagulant therapy in the setting of severe bleeding requires evaluation of the anticoagulant half-life, time of last known ingestion, and patient's renal and hepatic function.
- Benzodiazepines are the first-line agents in status epilepticus followed by an antiseizure medication, which may be selected based on formulation, side-effect profile, drug interactions, and onset of action.

REFERENCES

1. Devlin JW, Skrobik Y, Gelinas C, et al. Clinical practice guidelines for the prevention and management of pain, agitation/sedation, delirium, immobility, and sleep disruption in adult patients in the ICU. Crit Care Med 2018;46:e825–73.
2. Peng PW, Sandler AN. A review of the use of fentanyl analgesia in the management of acute pain in adults. Anesthesiology 1999;90:576–99.
3. Roan JP, Bajaj N, Davis FA, et al. Opioids and chest wall rigidity during mechanical ventilation. Ann Intern Med 2018;168:678.
4. Coruh B, Tonelli MR, Park DR. Fentanyl-induced chest wall rigidity. Chest 2013; 143:1145–6.
5. Dowell D, Haegerich TM, Chou R. CDC guideline for prescribing opioids for chronic pain - United States, 2016. MMWR Recomm Rep 2016;65:1–49.
6. Vallner JJ, Stewart JT, Kotzan JA, et al. Pharmacokinetics and bioavailability of hydromorphone following intravenous and oral administration to human subjects. J Clin Pharmacol 1981;21:152–6.
7. Sarhill N, Walsh D, Nelson KA. Hydromorphone: pharmacology and clinical applications in cancer patients. Support Care Cancer 2001;9:84–96.
8. Fishman SM, Wilsey B, Mahajan G, et al. Methadone reincarnated: novel clinical applications with related concerns. Pain Med 2002;3:339–48.
9. Gazelle G, Fine PG. Methadone for pain: No. 75. J Palliat Med 2004;7:303–4.

10. Attal N, Cruccu G, Baron R, et al. EFNS guidelines on the pharmacological treatment of neuropathic pain: 2010 revision. Eur J Neurol 2010;17:1113-e88.

11. Pandey CK, Raza M, Tripathi M, et al. The comparative evaluation of gabapentin and carbamazepine for pain management in Guillain-Barre syndrome patients in the intensive care unit. Anesth Analg 2005;101:220–5, table of contents.

12. Girard TD, Kress JP, Fuchs BD, et al. Efficacy and safety of a paired sedation and ventilator weaning protocol for mechanically ventilated patients in intensive care (Awakening and Breathing Controlled trial): a randomised controlled trial. Lancet 2008;371:126–34.

13. Strom T, Martinussen T, Toft P. A protocol of no sedation for critically ill patients receiving mechanical ventilation: a randomised trial. Lancet 2010;375:475–80.

14. Fraser GL, Devlin JW, Worby CP, et al. Benzodiazepine versus nonbenzodiazepine-based sedation for mechanically ventilated, critically ill adults: a systematic review and meta-analysis of randomized trials. Crit Care Med 2013;41:S30–8.

15. Sharshar T, Citerio G, Andrews PJ, et al. Neurological examination of critically ill patients: a pragmatic approach. Report of an ESICM expert panel. Intensive Care Med 2014;40:484–95.

16. Oddo M, Crippa IA, Mehta S, et al. Optimizing sedation in patients with acute brain injury. Crit Care 2016;20:128.

17. Betjemann JP, Lowenstein DH. Status epilepticus in adults. Lancet Neurol 2015; 14:615–24.

18. Glauser T, Shinnar S, Gloss D, et al. Evidence-based guideline: treatment of convulsive status epilepticus in children and adults: report of the guideline committee of the American Epilepsy Society. Epilepsy Curr 2016;16:48–61.

19. DIPRIVAN (propofol injection epiLZ. IL: Fresenius Kabi USA, LLC; 2020.

20. Naaz S, Ozair E. Dexmedetomidine in current anaesthesia practice- a review. J Clin Diagn Res 2014;8:GE01–4.

21. Patanwala AE, Martin JR, Erstad BL. Ketamine for analgosedation in the intensive care unit: a systematic review. J Intensive Care Med 2017;32:387–95.

22. Lippmann M, Appel PL, Mok MS, et al. Sequential cardiorespiratory patterns of anesthetic induction with ketamine in critically ill patients. Crit Care Med 1983;11:730–4.

23. Erstad BL, Patanwala AE. Ketamine for analgosedation in critically ill patients. J Crit Care 2016;35:145–9.

24. Christ G, Mundigler G, Merhaut C, et al. Adverse cardiovascular effects of ketamine infusion in patients with catecholamine-dependent heart failure. Anaesth Intensive Care 1997;25:255–9.

25. Tobias JD, Deshpande JK, Pietsch JB, et al. Pentobarbital sedation for patients in the pediatric intensive care unit. South Med J 1995;88:290–4.

26. Gagnon DJ, Fontaine GV, Riker RR, et al. Repurposing valproate, enteral clonidine, and phenobarbital for comfort in adult ICU patients: a literature review with practical considerations. Pharmacotherapy 2017;37:1309–21.

27. Sakamoto H, Fukuda S, Minakawa Y, et al. Clonidine induces sedation through acting on the perifornical area and the locus coeruleus in rats. J Neurosurg Anesthesiol 2013;25:399–407.

28. Midazolam injection. USP [prescribing information]. Lake Zurich, IL: Hospira, Inc; 2019.

29. Lorazepam injection. USP [prescribing information]. Eatontown, NJ: West-Ward Pharmaceuticals Corp; 2008.

30. Smith QR, Rapoport SI. Cerebrovascular permeability coefficients to sodium, potassium, and chloride. J Neurochem 1986;46:1732–42.

31. Messeter K, Nordstrom CH, Sundbarg G, et al. Cerebral hemodynamics in patients with acute severe head trauma. J Neurosurg 1986;64:231–7.

32. Rosner MJ, Coley I. Cerebral perfusion pressure: a hemodynamic mechanism of mannitol and the postmannitol hemogram. Neurosurgery 1987;21:147–56.
33. Garcia-Morales EJ, Cariappa R, Parvin CA, et al. Osmole gap in neurologic-neurosurgical intensive care unit: its normal value, calculation, and relationship with mannitol serum concentrations. Crit Care Med 2004;32:986–91.
34. Fink ME. Osmotherapy for intracranial hypertension: mannitol versus hypertonic saline. Continuum (Minneap Minn) 2012;18:640–54.
35. Brophy GM, Human T. Pharmacotherapy pearls for emergency neurological life support. Neurocrit Care 2017;27:51–73.
36. Rangel-Castilla L, Gopinath S, Robertson CS. Management of intracranial hypertension. Neurol Clin 2008;26:521–41, x.
37. Strandvik GF. Hypertonic saline in critical care: a review of the literature and guidelines for use in hypotensive states and raised intracranial pressure. Anaesthesia 2009;64:990–1003.
38. Dillon RC, Merchan C, Altshuler D, et al. Incidence of adverse events during peripheral administration of sodium chloride 3. J Intensive Care Med 2018;33:48–53.
39. Faiver L, Hensler D, Rush SC, et al. Safety and efficacy of 23.4% sodium chloride administered via peripheral venous access for the treatment of cerebral herniation and intracranial pressure elevation. Neurocrit Care 2021;35:845–52.
40. Meng L, Nguyen CM, Patel S, et al. Association between continuous peripheral i.v. infusion of 3% sodium chloride injection and phlebitis in adults. Am J Health Syst Pharm 2018;75:284–91.
41. Ennis KM, Brophy GM. Management of intracranial hypertension: focus on pharmacologic strategies. AACN Adv Crit Care 2011;22:177–82 [quiz: 83-4].
42. Cook AM, Morgan Jones G, Hawryluk GWJ, et al. Guidelines for the acute treatment of cerebral edema in neurocritical care patients. Neurocrit Care 2020;32:647–66.
43. Dunn IFKA, Gormley WB. Brain trauma. In: Squire LR, editor. Encyclopedia of neuroscience. Oxford: Academic Press; 2009. p. 407–16.
44. Huttner HB, Schellinger PD, Hartmann M, et al. Hematoma growth and outcome in treated neurocritical care patients with intracerebral hemorrhage related to oral anticoagulant therapy: comparison of acute treatment strategies using vitamin K, fresh frozen plasma, and prothrombin complex concentrates. Stroke 2006;37:1465–70.
45. Alotaibi GS, Wu C, Senthilselvan A, et al. Secular trends in incidence and mortality of acute venous thromboembolism: the AB-VTE population-based study. Am J Med 2016;129:879.e19-25.
46. Shoeb M, Fang MC. Assessing bleeding risk in patients taking anticoagulants. J Thromb Thrombolysis 2013;35:312–9.
47. Melkonian M, Jarzebowski W, Pautas E, et al. Bleeding risk of antiplatelet drugs compared with oral anticoagulants in older patients with atrial fibrillation: a systematic review and meta-analysis. J Thromb Haemost 2017;15:1500–10.
48. Tulinsky A. Molecular interactions of thrombin. Semin Thromb Hemost 1996;22:117–24.
49. Schindewolf M, Steindl J, Beyer-Westendorf J, et al. Use of fondaparinux off-label or approved anticoagulants for management of heparin-induced thrombocytopenia. J Am Coll Cardiol 2017;70:2636–48.
50. Robson R, White H, Aylward P, et al. Bivalirudin pharmacokinetics and pharmacodynamics: effect of renal function, dose, and gender. Clin Pharmacol Ther 2002;71:433–9.
51. Reed MD, Bell D. Clinical pharmacology of bivalirudin. Pharmacotherapy 2002;22:105S-11S.

52. Hirsh J, Fuster V, Ansell J, et al. American Heart A, American College of Cardiology f. American Heart Association/American College of Cardiology Foundation guide to warfarin therapy. Circulation 2003;107:1692–711.
53. Garcia DA, Baglin TP, Weitz JI, et al. Parenteral anticoagulants: antithrombotic therapy and prevention of thrombosis, 9th ed: American College of Chest Physicians evidence-based clinical practice guidelines. Chest 2012;141:e24S–43S.
54. Cuker A, Arepally GM, Chong BH, et al. American Society of Hematology 2018 guidelines for management of venous thromboembolism: heparin-induced thrombocytopenia. Blood Adv 2018;2:3360–92.
55. Chan KE, Edelman ER, Wenger JB, et al. Dabigatran and rivaroxaban use in atrial fibrillation patients on hemodialysis. Circulation 2015;131:972–9.
56. Blech S, Ebner T, Ludwig-Schwellinger E, et al. The metabolism and disposition of the oral direct thrombin inhibitor, dabigatran, in humans. Drug Metab Dispos 2008;36:386–99.
57. Bates SM, Weitz JI. The mechanism of action of thrombin inhibitors. J Invasive Cardiol 2000;12(Suppl F):27F–32F.
58. Alban S. Pharmacological strategies for inhibition of thrombin activity. Curr Pharm Des 2008;14:1152–75.
59. COUMADIN(R) oral tablets ii, warfarin sodium oral tablets, intravenous injection. Princeton, NJ: Bristol-Myers Squibb Company; 2010.
60. Frontera JA, Lewin JJ 3rd, Rabinstein AA, et al. Guideline for reversal of antithrombotics in intracranial hemorrhage: a statement for healthcare professionals from the neurocritical care society and society of critical care medicine. Neurocrit Care 2016;24:6–46.
61. Bower MM, Sweidan AJ, Shafie M, et al. Contemporary reversal of oral anticoagulation in intracerebral hemorrhage. Stroke 2019;50:529–36.
62. Brophy GM, Human T, Shutter L. Emergency neurological life support: pharmacotherapy. Neurocrit Care 2015;23(Suppl 2):S48–68.
63. Writing Group M, January CT, Wann LS, et al. 2019 AHA/ACC/HRS focused update of the 2014 AHA/ACC/HRS guideline for the management of patients with atrial fibrillation: a report of the American College of Cardiology/American Heart Association task force on clinical practice guidelines and the Heart Rhythm Society. Heart Rhythm 2019;16:e66–93.
64. Tesoro EP, Brophy GM. Pharmacological management of seizures and status epilepticus in critically ill patients. J Pharm Pract 2010;23:441–54.
65. Claassen J, Goldstein JN. Emergency neurological life support: status epilepticus. Neurocrit Care 2017;27:152–8.
66. Brophy GM, Bell R, Claassen J, et al. Guidelines for the evaluation and management of status epilepticus. Neurocrit Care 2012;17:3–23.
67. Klein P, Diaz A, Gasalla T, et al. A review of the pharmacology and clinical efficacy of brivaracetam. Clin Pharmacol 2018;10:1–22.
68. Ameli PA, Ammar AA, Owusu KA, et al. Evaluation and management of seizures and status epilepticus. Neurol Clin 2021;39:513–44.
69. Nolan JP, Morley PT, Vanden Hoek TL, et al. Therapeutic hypothermia after cardiac arrest: an advisory statement by the advanced life support task force of the International Liaison Committee on Resuscitation. Circulation 2003;108:118–21.
70. Sadaka F, Veremakis C. Therapeutic hypothermia for the management of intracranial hypertension in severe traumatic brain injury: a systematic review. Brain Inj 2012;26:899–908.

71. Lewis SR, Evans DJ, Butler AR, et al. Hypothermia for traumatic brain injury. Cochrane Database Syst Rev 2017;9:CD001048.
72. Choi HA, Ko SB, Presciutti M, et al. Prevention of shivering during therapeutic temperature modulation: the Columbia anti-shivering protocol. Neurocrit Care 2011;14:389–94.
73. Oddo M, Frangos S, Maloney-Wilensky E, et al. Effect of shivering on brain tissue oxygenation during induced normothermia in patients with severe brain injury. Neurocrit Care 2010;12:10–6.
74. Badjatia N, Strongilis E, Gordon E, et al. Metabolic impact of shivering during therapeutic temperature modulation: the Bedside Shivering Assessment Scale. Stroke 2008;39:3242–7.
75. Jain A, Gray M, Slisz S, et al. Shivering treatments for targeted temperature management: a review. J Neurosci Nurs 2018;50:63–7.
76. Bangash MN, Kong ML, Pearse RM. Use of inotropes and vasopressor agents in critically ill patients. Br J Pharmacol 2012;165:2015–33.
77. Hollenberg SM. Vasoactive drugs in circulatory shock. Am J Respir Crit Care Med 2011;183:847–55.
78. Rhoney D, Peacock WF. Intravenous therapy for hypertensive emergencies, part 2. Am J Health Syst Pharm 2009;66:1448–57.
79. Aggarwal M, Khan IA. Hypertensive crisis: hypertensive emergencies and urgencies. Cardiol Clin 2006;24:135–46.
80. Awad A, Stüve O. Cyclophosphamide in multiple sclerosis: scientific rationale, history and novel treatment paradigms. Ther Adv Neurol Disord 2009;2(6):50–61.
81. Cree BA, Lamb S, Morgan K, et al. An open label study of the effects of rituximab in neuromyelitis optica. Neurology 2005;64(7):1270–2.
82. Ciron J, Audoin B, Bourre B, et al. Recommendations for the use of Rituximab in neuromyelitis optica spectrum disorders. Rev Neurol (Paris) 2018;174(4):255–64.
83. Salzer J, Svenningsson R, Alping P, et al. Rituximab in multiple sclerosis: a retrospective observational study on safety and efficacy. Neurology 2016;87(20):2074–81.
84. Zebardast N, Patwa HS, Novella SP, et al. Rituximab in the management of refractory myasthenia gravis. Muscle Nerve 2010;41(3):375–8.
85. Sharshar T, Porcher R, Demeret S, et al. Comparison of corticosteroid tapering regimens in myasthenia gravis: a randomized clinical trial. JAMA Neurol 2021;78(4):426–33.
86. Farrugia ME, Goodfellow JA. A practical approach to managing patients with myasthenia gravis-opinions and a review of the literature. Front Neurol 2020;11:604.
87. Goodkin DE, Rudick RA, VanderBrug Medendorp S, et al. Low-dose (7.5 mg) oral methotrexate reduces the rate of progression in chronic progressive multiple sclerosis. Ann Neurol 1995;37(1):30–40.
88. Howard JF Jr, Utsugisawa K, Benatar M, et al. Safety and efficacy of eculizumab in anti-acetylcholine receptor antibody-positive refractory generalised myasthenia gravis (REGAIN): a phase 3, randomised, double-blind, placebo-controlled, multicentre study. Lancet Neurol 2017;16(12):976–86.
89. Villiger PM, Adler S, Kuchen S, et al. Tocilizumab for induction and maintenance of remission in giant cell arteritis: a phase 2, randomised, double-blind, placebo-controlled trial. Lancet 2016;387(10031):1921–7.
90. Clerico M, De Mercanti SF, Signori A, et al. Extending the interval of natalizumab dosing: is efficacy preserved? Neurotherapeutics 2020;17(1):200–7.

Brain Death/Death by Neurological Criteria

International Standardization and the World Brain Death Project

Gene Sung, MD, MPH

KEYWORDS

• Death • Brain death • End of life

KEY POINTS

- One legal definition of death in most of the world is brain death.
- The method for determining brain death is to follow local policies for determining death by neurologic criteria.
- Difficulties in brain death determination can be lessened by developing a protocol based on national or regional guidelines.
- The World Brain Death Project was an attempt to develop a resource for the current understanding and determination of brain death.

INTRODUCTION

From the moment humans developed self-awareness, attempts at understanding the concepts of life and death inevitably followed and are debated to this day. As science developed, clinical definitions of death and determining death formed and were continually refined. Over time, cardiorespiratory death was the clinical standard used to determine death, although with no standard criteria, and sometimes cases of misdiagnosis were reported. As medical care advanced, resuscitation techniques and mechanical ventilation methods were developed, and newer definitions of death were needed.

Eventually it became clear that even after resuscitation and ventilation, many patients could not be saved and in fact never recovered, never woke, and often continued to deteriorate. In 1959, the 2 French neurologists Mollaret and Goulon presented a paper describing the condition as "coma de depassé"[1]; which subsequently became known as "brain death." In 1968, formal criteria for the clinical definition of

University of Southern California, LAC+USC Medical Center, 2051 Marengo Street, Inpatient Tower A4E111, Los Angeles, CA 90033, USA
E-mail address: gsung@usc.edu

Crit Care Clin 39 (2023) 215–219
https://doi.org/10.1016/j.ccc.2022.08.005
0749-0704/23/© 2022 Elsevier Inc. All rights reserved.

brain death were developed and published; this became known as the Harvard Brain Death Criteria.[2] Many other guidelines and protocols for the determination of brain death have been developed, published, adopted, and revised in numerous countries. The general concept of brain death, also known as death by neurologic criteria (BD/DNC), has been accepted by medical groups, major religious groups, and governments worldwide.[3,]

DEVELOPMENT OF THE WORLD BRAIN DEATH PROJECT

Despite this general acceptance, there remains confusion and dilemmas that arise around BD/DNC. An issue that promotes more confusion is the widespread inconsistency and variance in the practice of BD/DNC determination between and even within countries.[3] Certainly, the fact that it is difficult to perform large-scale or randomized controlled clinical trials on issues of BD/DNC leads to an inability to have evidence-based recommendations and guidelines. In addition, challenges occasionally arise to the validity of different facets of BD/DNC determination. For all these reasons and more, the World Brain Death Project was undertaken to improve the rigor and harmonize the practice of BD/DNC determination.

Initially, this project was conceived by the author when he was in the leadership track of the Neurocritical Care Society (NCS). However, it became known that there was a similar concurrent effort by the World Health Organization (WHO). The NCS effort was set aside until it became clear that the eventual goals and product of the WHO were insufficient for the perceived needs of the global medical community. The World Brain Death Project initiative was revived in 2014 with the premise that BD/DNC determination is a medical practice issue and should be addressed by medical societies.

As a leader of the NCS, a member society of the World Federation of Intensive and Critical Care (WFICC—formerly known as World Federation of Societies of Intensive and Critical Care Medicine), the author approached the leadership of WFICC to support the initiative and consider endorsement when the document was completed. In turn, the leadership of the other world federations whose practitioners are involved in the determination of BD/DNC were approached, including the World Federation of Pediatric Intensive and Critical Care Societies, World Federation of Neurology, World Federation of Neurosurgery, and the World Federation of Critical Care Nurses. Following successfully obtaining support for this initiative, a steering committee was formed in 2015. Subsequently, an authorship committee totaling 44 members was established and included those nominated from the world federations as well as other topic experts.

It was recognized from the outset that the lack of high-quality data from randomized clinical trials or large studies available to be assessed by GRADE, AGREE, or other analyses would mean that recommendations would have to be formulated based on consensus of contributors and medical societies that represented all relevant disciplines, including critical care, neurology, and neurosurgery.

A topic list of the issues to be addressed was created:

1. Worldwide Variance in Brain Death/Death by Neurologic Criteria
2. The Science of Brain Death/Death by Neurologic Criteria
3. The Concept of Brain Death/Death by Neurologic Criteria
4. Minimum Clinical Criteria for Determination of Brain Death/Death by Neurologic Criteria
5. Beyond Minimum Clinical Determination of Brain Death/Death by Neurologic Criteria

6. Pediatric and Neonatal Brain Death/Death by Neurologic Criteria
7. Determination of Brain Death/Death by Neurologic Criteria in Patients on Extra-corporeal Support: ECMO
8. Determination of Brain Death/Death by Neurologic Criteria after Treatment with Targeted Temperature Management
9. Documentation of Brain Death/Death by Neurologic Criteria
10. Qualification for and Education on Determination of Brain Death/Death by Neuro-logic Criteria
11. Somatic Support after Brain Death/Death by Neurologic Criteria for Organ Dona-tion and Other Special Circumstances
12. Religion and Brain Death/Death by Neurologic Criteria: Managing Requests to Forego a Brain Death/Death by Neurologic Criteria Evaluation or Continue So-matic Support after Brain Death/Death by Neurologic Criteria
13. Brain Death/Death by Neurologic Criteria and the Law

The evidence was reviewed, and recommendations were generated according to the following criteria. Recommendations were strong *(It is recommended that)* based on expert consensus that clinicians should follow the recommendation unless a clear and compelling rationale for an alternative approach was present, and where actions could be adopted as policy. Strong recommendations were made as a precautionary, conservative approach to prevent premature or erroneous determinations of death (false positives). Recommendations were conditional or weak *(It is suggested that)* when there were potentially different options and the best action may differ depending on circumstances, patients, resources, societal values, or where there is a need for further evidence or discussion among clinicians and stakeholders. No recommenda-tions were made when there was insufficient evidence and the balance of benefits versus harms was neutral.

In addition to the recommendations and suggestions for each of the topics, a list of research questions was generated to understand some of the unresolved issues for each topic. Finally, a flow chart and a checklist were also included to ease the process of incorporating the recommendations into practice.

The findings of the literature review and preliminary recommendations were pre-sented and discussed at an open preconference forum of the World Federation of Intensive and Critical Care 2017 meeting in Brazil and then again at a plenary session of that conference. The text and recommendations for all sections were then reviewed by the Steering Committee who provided the primary investigators with comments and recommended revisions and then distributed to the entire writing/review commit-tee for comments and content consensus. The final draft was sent to international so-cieties for final review and endorsement before publication. The summary of the final draft was published in JAMA, and the entire publication including all 15 appendices are available online.[4]

POSSIBLE AMBIGUITIES AND COMPLICATIONS IN BRAIN DEATH DETERMINATION

This project attempted to be as thorough as possible, but there will always be issues that may not be specifically addressed. The clinical brain death examination, when properly done and under the proper circumstances, is sufficient to accurately deter-mine brain death. There is no absolute proper order in which the clinical examination needs to be performed. General medical care of critically ill patients by nurses and res-piratory therapists will include regular assessments of level of consciousness, pupil-lary function, and cough reflex (for respiratory care of mechanical ventilation), so there should already be clinical suspicion of brain death before a complete evaluation.

Generally, in the performance of the examination, 2 considerations in the order of the examination are that (1) because the apnea test is more involved and presents potential risk of instability, it is best to perform it as the last component of the clinical examination and, if needed, ancillary testing should be performed last and (2) in the vestibular ocular examination (cold water caloric) the stimulus is a temperature differential causing current of the endolymph in the semicircular canal, so one should examine one side and then wait for a few (3 or more) minutes (perhaps check motor and peripheral reflexes on the same side) before performing the vestibular ocular examination on the other side. As an aside, doing the vestibular ocular examination in the setting of perforated or ruptured tympanic membranes is likely to be accurate, although there may be an infection risk that may cause harm if it is determined that the patient does not meet criteria for brain death.

However, there are times when the clinical examination alone is not sufficient, a clear example being when physical ocular trauma precludes being able to complete a pupillary examination. A little more complicated is the situation when the confounder to the clinical brain death examination is the presence or use of pharmacologic agents that depress central nervous system activity. In general, the goal of identifying confounders is to avoid situations where the patient examination may falsely lead to the apparent absence of clinical brain function. Specifically with certain pharmacologic agents, one must determine whether the agent is capable of, and at a level high enough, to suppress all brain function including brainstem reflexes before evaluating for brain death. A case where this is true is the setting of pentobarbital coma, sometimes used for refractory intracranial hypertension or super-refractory status epilepticus.

The principles and process of brain death determination remain the same in these situations. First, one must know that the patient has a disease process that can lead to brain death. Second, a clinical examination must be consistent with brain death. If the clinical examination was incomplete or unreliable because of possible toxicologic interference or another confounder, only then should one proceed to an ancillary test. In the case of toxicologic interference, the ancillary test should probably be a cerebral blood flow study. Each test has specific parameters that should be carefully followed as noted in the section "Beyond Minimal Clinical Determination of Brain Death," particularly if transcranial Doppler ultrasound is to be used as an ancillary test. In this way, knowing the pathology, having an examination and an ancillary test all together helps reduce the potential for error in determining brain death. Finally, perhaps the most important principle in brain death determination is to err on the conservative side; if there is some doubt or question, it is better to avoid a "false-positive declaration," declaring a patient to be brain dead when they are not.

Brain death determination protocols in some countries have mandatory ancillary testing. Certainly, one's national protocols or laws need to be followed; however, the authors of the World Brain Death Project felt that the clinical examination alone is sufficient. The case against requiring ancillary tests is that (1) there have been no documented cases where a patient determined to be brain dead in a properly done clinical brain death examination was later found not to be brain dead and (2) doing ancillary tests when unnecessary can be prohibitive in situations with limited resources.

Once brain death is determined, another complication can occur when families either do not accept the determination or want to wait days for family members to come from long distances to see the family member in the hospital before removal of medical ventilation. In most countries that have brain death laws and protocols, brain death is an accepted means of determining death, and patients who have died do not stay longer in the hospital, so all medical support is discontinued and removed. Having said that, the body of the patient who has reached brain death can be maintained for some time with good critical care. Continuing somatic support for a finite period for families to pay respects is reasonable, but the length of time that is appropriate is always a question; this should be determined in a hospital policy that can be applied to all patients and should be a finite time period of at most the same day; in the author's hospitals' policies, it is measured in hours. One consideration to be made when establishing policies is the potential for abuse of a corpse if prolonged somatic support is maintained.

SUMMARY

The World Brain Death project represents the first step toward harmonization of the differences that exist in determining brain death/death based on neurologic criteria throughout the world, understanding that given long-standing practice and understanding, there will likely be some continued variances in practice. The Neurocritical Care Society has developed a sample brain death policy that can be modified for any hospital to use here: https://higherlogicdownload.s3.amazonaws.com/NEUROCRITICALCARE/9359e17f-978d-4f0e-a978-2dbaa842daad/UploadedImages/Brain_Death_Toolkit_Docs/Brain_Death_Policy.pdf. The presence of a policy can minimize variation in practice and also help families understand that there is a standard process of brain death determination.

CLINICS CARE POINTS

- There can be controversies in the determination of brain death that development of protocols can minimize. These protocols should be based on science and follow national or regional laws and guidelines.

- Brain death determination is a clinical evaluation, but occasionally ancillary testing is required.

- Good family communication is always recommended, especially when discussing end-of-life issues; this is particularly important in notification of impending brain death, evaluation of the same, and explanation of the need for a finite time of continued somatic support after brain death determination.

DISCLOSURE

No conflicts of interest to disclose.

REFERENCES

1. Mollaret P, Goulon M. Le coma depasse. Rev Neurol (Paris) 1959;101:3–15.
2. A definition of irreversible coma. Report of the Ad Hoc committee of the Harvard medical School to examine the definition of brain death. JAMA 1968;205(6):337–40.
3. Wijdicks EF. Brain death worldwide: accepted fact but no global consensus in diagnostic criteria. Neurology 2002;58(1):20–5.
4. Greer DM, Shemie SD, Lewis A, et al. Determination of brain death/death by neurologic criteria: the world brain death project. JAMA 2020;324(11):1078–97.

Physiological Monitoring in Patients with Acute Brain Injury: A Multimodal Approach

Tracey H. Fan, DO[a,b], Eric S. Rosenthal, MD[a,c],*

KEYWORDS

- Neuromonitoring • Multimodal monitoring • Acute brain injury
- Traumatic brain injury • Subarachnoid hemorrhage • Secondary brain injury

KEY POINTS

- Integration of multimodality monitoring with clinical neurologic examination enhances the detection of impending secondary brain injury.
- No one modality has proven sufficient in isolation; monitoring strategies have synergistic value when viewed together and in context of clinical trends in laboratory values, imaging, and neurologic examinations.
- An integration of multiple neuromonitoring tools using multimodal monitoring approach allows for iterative, individualized treatment strategies in real time.

INTRODUCTION

Neuromonitoring is increasingly used in acute brain injury (ABI). Patient outcomes are determined by secondary brain injury (SBI) resulting from a complex cascade of pathophysiologic sequelae in addition to severity of preadmission ABI.[1] Goals of neuromonitoring include identifying impending neurologic deterioration, individualizing management, assessing treatment response, and mitigating SBI.[2] The neurologic examination is the standard for neurocritical care (NCC) monitoring, although often limited by the use of sedation and existing neurologic deficits (eg, encephalopathy, coma, aphasia, and neglect). Changes found during examination may provide insufficient time to prevent SBI.[3]

T.H. Fan is a Lead author.
^a Department of Neurology, Division of Neurocritical Care, Massachusetts General Hospital, 55 Fruit Street, Boston, MA 02493, USA; ^b Department of Neurology, Division of Neurocritical Care, Brigham and Women's Hospital, 55 Fruit Street, Boston, MA 02493, USA; ^c Department of Neurology, Division of Clinical Neurophysiology, Massachusetts General Hospital, 55 Fruit Street, Boston, MA 02493, USA
* Corresponding author. 55 Fruit Street, Lunder 644, Boston, MA 02114.
E-mail address: erosenthal@mgh.harvard.edu

Crit Care Clin 39 (2023) 221–233
https://doi.org/10.1016/j.ccc.2022.06.006
0749-0704/23/© 2022 Elsevier Inc. All rights reserved.
criticalcare.theclinics.com

Multimodal monitoring (MMM) augments the clinical examination by acquiring and synchronizing data, including blood pressure (BP), heart rate, end tidal carbon dioxide, intracranial pressure (ICP), cerebral perfusion pressure (CPP), brain tissue oxygenation (BTO), cerebral blood flow (CBF), cerebral autoregulation (CA), cerebral electrical activity, and cerebral metabolism.[4] Here, we review the physiology and principles of MMM in ABI.

Pathophysiology of Secondary Brain Injury

Primary ABI triggers a complex cascade of pathologic changes in the central nervous system (CNS) physiology. These include biochemical, cellular and physiologic changes such as glutamate-related excitotoxicity, mitochondrial dysfunction, oxidative stress, neuroinflammation, and vascular changes including CA dysfunction and vasospasm.[5] The resulting imbalance of cerebral oxygen delivery (cDO$_2$) and consumption can lead to brain tissue hypoxia, cerebral metabolic crisis, and epileptiform activity.[5] When metabolic crisis persists, cell death and cerebral edema may ensue, further propagating SBI.

Impaired brain tissue oxygenation
When severe, ABI may result in an imbalance between cDO$_2$ and oxygen consumption.[6] Brain parenchyma has limited emergency reserves, a high metabolic demand, and critical dependence on continuous substrate supply. cDO$_2$ is dominated by hemoglobin (Hgb) concentration, saturation of arterial oxygen (SaO$_2$), and cardiac output (CO): cDO$_2$ = CO $\times$ (1.34 $\times$ Hgb $\times$ SaO$_2$) + (Pao$_2$ $\times$ 0.03).[7] Thus, systemic factors, such as CO, Hgb, SaO$_2$, metabolic rate (fever, agitation, or shivering), and cerebral vasospasm, adversely affect BTO, aggravating SBI. Low BTO has been associated with poor outcomes in patients with ABI especially during the acute period.[8] CPP has been used to estimate CBF and monitor for cerebral ischemia. However, oxygen deprivation can occur despite normal CPP and ICP.[9] Thus, direct monitoring of BTO and oxygen utilization has shown promise over monitoring CPP alone.[10]

Cerebral metabolic dysfunction
Reduced CBF following ABI promotes a switch from aerobic to anaerobic metabolism causing lactate accumulation.[11] This dysregulation limits glucose entry into the brain promoting the breakdown of lactate instead of glucose, resulting in an energy production deficit.[11] Reduced metabolic consumption following traumatic brain injury is thought to be an independent risk factor for worse outcome.[12] Brain tissue hypoxia and metabolic crisis lead to a massive release of excitatory amino acid neurotransmitters, particularly glutamate.[13] Excess glutamate overstimulates neurons and astrocytes, triggering blood–brain barrier (BBB) breakdown, and ultimately cell apoptosis and necrosis.[11] Increased brain extracellular glycerol levels are seen with cell membrane or BBB breakdown and may be associated with unfavorable outcome.[14]

Impaired cerebrovascular autoregulation
The brain tightly autoregulates blood flow and any perturbance affects its normal metabolic landscape. Cerebral ischemia and hyperemia result from CBF and cerebral metabolism mismatch. One pathogenic mechanism of this mismatch is impaired cerebrovascular autoregulation, which can be transient or persistent.[15] Failure to maintain CPP within the range of optimal autoregulation is associated with a worse outcome in various acute neurologic diseases.[16]

Development of cerebral edema

ABI induces a release of proinflammatory cytokines, neurotoxic mediators, and activation of glial cells.[5] Vasogenic cerebral edema follows the loss of BBB integrity and uncontrolled ion and protein shifts from the intravascular to extracellular compartment with water accumulation.[5] Cytotoxic edema involves the accumulation of intracellular water in neurons and glial cells. Increased membrane permeability for ions, ion pump failure from energy depletion and cellular reabsorption of osmotically active solutes follows.[5]

Cortical spreading depolarizations

Ischemic brain insults can provoke cortical spreading depolarizations,[17] which result in significant loss of the neuronal gradient, massive energy expenditure to reestablish the gradient, calcium influx, and ensuing hyperemia or oligemia that exacerbate metabolic crisis.[6] A hallmark is the slow 3 to 5 mm/min spreading wave of depolarizing "brain tsunamis" throughout the hemisphere along gyri.[18] Point monitoring via a subdural electrode strip enables whole hemispheric surveillance.[19]

Tools for Brain Physiologic Monitoring

Brain tissue oxygenation

Cerebral oxygen monitoring includes 2 invasive techniques, brain parenchymal oxygen tension ($PbtO_2$, regional) and jugular bulb oxygen saturation ($SjvO_2$, global), or noninvasive cerebral near-infrared spectroscopy (cNIRS, regional).

Intraparenchymal oxygen monitor. An intraparenchymal oxygen monitor (IOM) is a pressure-based measurement that can be used to survey regional BTO in normal-appearing brain tissue, typically at 2.5 to 3.5 cm below the skull's inner table. Controversy exists on whether monitoring should occur peri-injury to monitor vulnerable tissue at risk or contralateral to the injury. The rate of potential complications including hemorrhage, migration, and infection are low.[20] Measures of BTO represent a composite of cerebral arteriovenous oxygen tension, relating to arterial oxygen content, CBF, and tissue oxygen extraction. Normal $PbtO_2$ is 23 to 35 mm Hg. A $PbtO_2$ less than 20 mm Hg represents compromised BTO correlating with insufficient brain oxygen delivery on positron emission tomography and reduced focal and global CBF on computed tomography (CT) perfusion.[21] Low parenchymal oxygenation occurs with periods of poor blood flow or oxygen delivery: high ICP, low cerebral perfusion, anemia, and systemic hypoxia.[22] However, IOM is subject not only to variation in oxygen delivery but also to increased oxygen extraction and cerebral metabolic demands.[23] BTO also decreases in the setting of fever,[23] seizure and high-frequency periodic sharp waves or spikes on ictal-interictal continuum.[24] The depth and proximity of the probe to the region at risk for ischemia affects results. Interpretation should consider probe location per postinsertion CT.[2] $PbtO_2$ monitoring provides accurate data for up to 10 days, with measured responses to interventions (eg, CPP augmentation, ventilator adjustment, pharmacologic sedation, and red blood cell transfusion) and can be used to guide therapy.[25] Observational studies suggest close correlation between reduced $PbtO_2$ and worse outcome in subarachnoid hemorrhage (SAH) and traumatic brain injury (TBI) populations in which $PbtO_2$ monitoring has been most studied.[26] A multicenter phase 2 trial, Brain Oxygen Optimization in Severe TBI, compared ICP and $PbtO_2$-guided treatment protocol with one using ICP alone for severe TBI patients. The approach combining ICP and $PbtO_2$ had a lower burden of brain tissue hypoxia, decreased mortality, and more favorable outcome prompting an ongoing phase 3 trial.

Jugular bulb oximetry

$SjvO_2$ assesses the balance between global brain oxygen supply and consumption when the dominant jugular bulb is cannulated. An oxygen saturation fiber-optic probe is inserted, under ultrasound guidance, above the facial vein and into the dominant jugular vein, allowing for sampling from the intracranial venous circulation.[27] Placement confirmation posterior to the mastoid and above the first vertebra via skull radiographs or CT is advised. Brain oxygen extraction is calculated by arterial oxygen content subtract $SjvO_2$ recorded by the probe.[27] Normal $SjvO_2$ ranges from 60% to 75%, and the recognized threshold for ischemia and need for intervention is less than 55%. Low $SjvO_2$ is an indication for increased oxygen demands such as fever, seizure, or reduced oxygen delivery such as anemia, vasospasm, or reduced CPP. Brain oxygen extraction was found to increase greater than 24 hours before symptomatic cerebral vasospasm. Aside from early vasospasm detection, this technique also presents a potential early therapeutic target.[28] However, positioning, catheter surface clot formation, and poor sampling technique can influence $SjvO_2$ accuracy. Errors are common, thus monitoring of $SjvO_2$ is more challenging and less reliable than $PbtO_2$.[29] The International Multidisciplinary Consensus Conference on MMM guidelines recommended that jugular bulb oximetry should be used in conjunction with other MMM techniques.[2] Although BTO monitoring with $PbtO_2$ is preferable, jugular bulb oximetry may resolve questions of whether brain tissue hypoxia may be a late result of sustained hyperemia, suggested by a discordant elevation in jugular oximetry.

Cerebral Near-infrared Spectroscopy

cNIRS is a noninvasive technique that can continuously detect real-time changes in regional cortical oxygenation (rSO_2) through the skull via 2 photoelectrodes that measure attenuation of reflected light back from human tissues. The amount of absorbed light depends on tissue oxygenation or metabolism.[30] Different cNIRS techniques are available. Continuous-wave NIRS systems are readily available and reflect dynamic changes in rSO_2 but may be subject to drift. In general, rSO_2 values between 60% and 80% are considered within normal.[31] Although low cost and high sampling rate is an advantage of cNIRS, low penetration depth, measuring approximately 2.5 cm beneath the skin of the frontal bone is a limitation, which is exacerbated by the presence of frontal pneumocephalus, contusion, hematoma, and skin pigmentation as early validation work was in Caucasians.[30] Lower rSO_2 in cNIRS may be associated with brain injury[32,33] and has been linked with worse neurologic outcomes after cardiac surgery[34] and cardiopulmonary resuscitation.[35] However, accuracy of cerebral rSO_2, its hypoxic/ischemic threshold, and evidence of improved outcomes in ABI with its use have yet to be established. For these reasons, cNIRS is not validated for routine use in ABI, although a new study suggests a role in CA evaluation along with systemic BP and ICP monitors. Newer optical methods include frequency-domain or time-domain systems, as well as paired optodes in each sensor, controlling for superficial oxygenation yielding more accurate parenchymal oximetry.

Cerebral metabolism

Cerebral microdialysis (CMD) estimates cerebral metabolism by measuring metabolic intermediates (glucose, lactate, and pyruvate), a marker of cellular membrane damage (glycerol) and glutamate level, a marker of postinjury parenchymal excitotoxicity.[20] These analytes are measured from small amounts of extracellular fluid, obtained via insertion of a flexible catheter with a 10 mm semipermeable membrane into the white matter via an intracranial bolt. This catheter is then constantly infused with a dialysate approximating composition of cerebral spinal fluid (CSF). This allows neuronal metabolites with a specific size range (20–100 kDa) to equilibrate across the semipermeable membrane such that frequent sampling of dialysate is possible.[36] In SAH, increased levels of glutamate, lactate, and glucose were associated with worse neurologic outcomes[37] and increased lactate pyruvate ratio (LPR) and glutamate may detect delayed cerebral ischemia (DCI) 11 to 13 hours before symptom onset.[38] In TBI, an increased LPR and decreased glucose were associated with poor neurologic outcome.[39] Elevated glycerol levels indicate cerebral ischemia that has progressed to cell damage.[40] Moreover, the trend of metabolic markers can inform clinical management.[36] Although this technique provides invaluable information on brain metabolism, it has significant limitations. It is labor and time intensive, has low temporal resolution, interpretation depends on catheter and lesion location and type, and poorly defined interpretation for specific clinical contexts. Furthermore, evidence showing improved clinical outcomes with CMD-guided care is lacking. Therefore, guidelines recommend combining CMD is with clinical indicators and other monitoring modalities for prognostication.[2]

Cerebral blood flow
CBF is a direct indicator of the quantity of blood flow delivery. Although not monitoring oxygen content, it can clarify whether brain tissue hypoxia is related to oligemia or hyperemia and can measure effects of cerebral vasospasm. Changes in CA and metabolic, chemical, and neurogenic regulation all affect CBF.[41] Regional CBF can be measured by 2 types of invasive flowmetry: thermal diffusion flowmetry and laser Doppler flowmetry. Both involve probe placement within tissue at risk for DCI and afford continuous, monitoring of CBF. Thermal diffusion flowmetry (TDF) estimates blood flow by deducing dissipation of heat, whereas laser Doppler flowmetry (LDF) directly measures erythrocyte flux.[20] The TDF method is validated using xenon-enhanced CT and has a 90% sensitivity and 75% specificity for vasospasm.[42] In TBI patients, TDF may identify adequate perfusion or optimal CPP. Unfortunately, TDF has several limitations:

- Measures only regional CBF in the immediate vicinity of the probe and cannot represent global CBF.
- Sensitive to positioning, tissue contact.
- Systemic temperature fluctuation causes reduced accuracy and reliability.
- Requires autorecalibration often every 30 minutes with intervening data loss.

LDF remains a research tool for continuous bedside measurements of microvascular perfusion, regional CBF fluctuation, autoregulation, and carbon dioxide reactivity.[43] Limitations relate to incomplete understanding of how reported values translate to clinical practice.[44]

Currently no continuous noninvasive CBF monitoring method exists. Transcranial Doppler (TCD) can be used to measure CBF, monitor for vasospasm, and assess for hypoperfusion and hyperperfusion in TBI. Its specificity for intracranial circulatory arrest in brain death is high, and sensitivity and specificity to predict angiographic vasospasm is good. TCD is limited by operator variability.[45,46] Furthermore, no studies have demonstrated improved outcomes with treatment strategies directed by devices assessing CFBs or ischemic risk.

Cerebral autoregulation
CA ensures constant CBF over a wide range of mean arterial pressure (MAP). Failure of CA is associated with worse outcome after ABI when CA range is smaller than healthy controls (80 to 120 mm Hg vs 50 to 150 mm Hg) and can have substantial

interindividual variability.[16,47] Identifying the correct range of CA and targeting optimal CPP for individual ABI patients is possible by determining the index of CA. Computer software integration of real-time continuous hemodynamic (arterial line) and ICP monitoring yields the index of CA. CA is obtained traditionally by invasive BTO and ICP monitoring and can also be delineated by noninvasive method including NIRS and TCD. Several CA indices have been studied, including pressure reactivity index (PRx), cerebral oximetry index, and mean velocity index.[20] PRx is a linear correlation coefficient (ranging from 1 to −1) between arterial BP and ICP, with negative values reflecting intact and impaired CA, respectively.[47] Multiple observational studies found an associated between both a positive PRx and nonoptimized CPP range with increased mortality and unfavorable outcome in severe TBI, ICH, and aneurysmal SAH.[48–50] These studies suggest the importance of monitoring and preventing hypoperfusion and hyperperfusion when CA is impaired. However, the safety of titrating therapy to target an optimal CPP requires further study and validation.

Intracranial pressure

ICP and CPP-guided management is recommended by a joint statement of the Neurocritical Care Society and European Society of Intensive Care Medicine for patients with ABI at risk for elevated ICP based on clinical or imaging features.[2] The Brain Trauma Foundation recommends monitoring ICP in TBI patients with Glasgow Coma Scale (GCS) lesser than 8 and neuroimaging demonstrating high risk of ICP elevation.[51] The current consensus supports treating when ICP is greater than 22 mm Hg. In addition to ICP, intracranial compliance through ICP waveform analysis, cerebrovascular reactivity, and autoregulation can be obtained via ICP monitoring.[52]

Invasive ICP monitoring. Current methods of invasive ICP monitoring, including external ventricular drain (EVD) and intraparenchymal devices, are comparable in reliability and accuracy.[53] However, EVD has the therapeutic advantage of CSF diversion and intrathecal medication access in patients with patent ventricles. EVDs can also be recalibrated after placement and are not subject to temporal drift. However, EVDs introduce the risk of infection and bleeding.[54] Additionally, only few EVD catheters have a mechanism for continuous ICP monitoring, and these may be of greater expense.[54] Intraparenchymal pressure monitoring involves placing a fiberoptic, strain gauge, or air bladder device in brain parenchyma with less risk than an EVD.[54] Subdural, subarachnoid, and epidural bolts are less accurate, subject to daily drift, and not routinely recommended.[55] Although ICP monitoring has been available for a long time, the only randomized controlled trial assessing their use in TBI reported that ICP monitoring guided care did not improve outcome compared with management based on clinical and examination findings.[56] Several important considerations include the following:

- Barbiturate use only in the ICP-guided group.
- Uncertain generalizability as many centers had no prior experience with ICP monitoring.
- Mortality was higher (38%) than other randomized controlled trials (RCTs) of TBI patients.
- Many patients lacked prehospital emergency care and/or posthospital rehabilitation.
- Treating ICP with a numeric threshold is an oversimplification because hypoxia and cellular dysfunction can occur despite normal ICP.
- Heterogeneity of underlying brain injuries may require management tailored to specific pathophysiology.

Therefore, ICP should be interpreted in the context of ICP waveform morphology, intracranial compliance, and CA.[57]

Noninvasive ICP monitoring. There are many noninvasive ICP monitoring tools including TCD, optic nerve sheath diameter (ONSD) measurement, tympanometry, and pupillometry. None is yet recognized as sufficiently accurate measure of ICP for routine clinical care.

TCD can assess changes of flow velocity pulse waveform and the pulsatility index (PI) to estimate ICP and CPP noninvasively.[58] PI can be calculated by the difference between systolic and diastolic flow velocity and dividing by the mean flow velocity in the middle cerebral artery.[59] PI values between 1.26 and 1.33 are 81% to 100% sensitive and 82% to 97% specific for predicting ICP greater than $20mmH_2O$.[60] However, TCD-based methods currently predict mean ICP with insufficient overall accuracy of ±12 mm Hg. Additional studies are required to systematically compare and validate TCD-based methods across different populations.[58]

ONSD measurement relies on transmission of ICP through CSF in the subarachnoid space translating to optic nerve sheath dilation and can be detected via transocular ultrasonography. It is a useful screening tool for ICP when invasive monitoring is not promptly available.[61]

Tympanic membrane displacement (TMD) is another ICP measurement technique under development based on communication of the perilymph and CSF via the perilymphatic duct. A normal or low ICP produces an outward (positive values), whereas a high ICP causes inward (negative values) displacement of the tympanic membrane.[62] However, clinical feasibility is questionable due to difficulties in achieving an accurate TMD measurement compared with invasive ICP monitoring, with very wide predictive values of $\pm$ 25 mm Hg.[63]

Pupillometry is frequently used in NCC for assessing Neurological Pupil index (NPi), calculated from pupil size, constriction and dilation velocity, and latency. Changes in NPi along with pupillary light reflex may be the first sign of impending clinical deterioration in CNS insults.[64–66]

Cerebral electrical activity

Electroencephalography (EEG) has long been used to (1) detect seizure, (2) assess response to antiseizure treatment, (3) provide prognostic information, and (4) predict DCI. Up to 26% of TBI and ICH patients in the intensive care unit (ICU) develop seizures, of which 5% to 15% are nonconvulsive, exacerbating SBI.[67–70] Similar to convulsive seizures, nonconvulsive seizures can cause toxic spikes in glutamate levels and increase LPR.[69] Although no adequately powered, RCT has demonstrated treating nonconvulsive seizures or nonconvulsive status epilepticus improves outcomes, continuous EEG is recommended in ABI patients with unexplained altered mental status and those with clinical seizure without return to baseline within 60 minutes of antiseizure medication.[70] Although low risk, the cost is considerable and should be weighed against potential benefit.

Neuronal activity and CBF are coupled, so EEG can rapidly reflect a reduction in CBF. EEG first loses faster frequencies, then as CBF reaches approximately 17 mL/100 g/min, slower frequencies gradually increase.[71] Therefore, EEG can detect a window when intervention may prevent irreversible injuries. Quantitative continuous EEG measures are validated in SAH to trend changes in background activity total power, variability of relative alpha, and alpha/delta ratio overtime to detect DCI.[72] A drop in alpha/delta ratio or percent of alpha variability occurs up to 3 days before clinical or radiographic evidence of DCI.[73] Although epileptiform activity is associated with

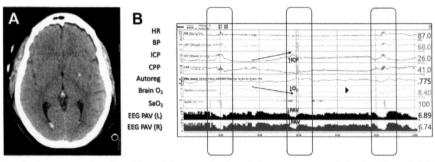

Fig. 1. Case example of multimodality monitoring following traumatic brain injury. Initial CT imaging (*A*) of a patient with potential diffuse axonal injury. Boxes (*B*) show 3 episodes of ICP crisis during a 6-hour period. Figure 1B shows an increase in ICP commensurate with a drop in CPP and PbtO$_2$, punctuated by drop out of EEG PAV at peak severity. Arrowhead (*B*) shows a 2-minute trial of Fio$_2$ 1.0 confirming the brain tissue oximetry probe was functional. Values reported on the right legend correspond to the ICP crisis episode marked by the second box. CPP, cerebral perfusion pressure; EEG, electroencephalography; ICP, intracranial pressure; PAV; percent alpha variability; PbtO$_2$, partial pressure of brain tissue oxygen.

impending ischemia, predicting DCI, and long-term outcome, changes in background activity are associated only with DCI and not long-term outcome, potentially due to treatment response.[74]

Some limitations of EEG in ICU relate to cost, labor intensiveness, and technical challenges (electrical artifacts in noisy neuro ICU; altered cranial anatomy).

Case Example

A 26-year-old woman (GCS 3) presented as a multivehicle crash victim. Initial CT imaging (**Fig. 1**A) revealed potential diffuse axonal injury. Through a multilumen bolt, ICP and PbtO$_2$ monitors, with and a 2-cm, 8-contact depth electrode were placed. Monitoring revealed multiple episodes of ICP crisis, each with concordant brain tissue hypoxia and decrement of EEG Percent Alpha Variability (**Fig. 1**B arrows). A 2-min trial of 100% Fio$_2$ confirmed the brain tissue oximetry probe was functional (see **Fig. 1**B arrowhead). The patient was treated with ventricular drainage, osmotherapy, and sedation.

SUMMARY

The ideal neuromonitoring tool would be cost-effective, quick, safe, easy to use, with the ability to provide continuous real-time monitoring of all brain regions with a high sensitivity and specificity and allow for early detection of subclinical physiologic changes in neurologic status. However, noninvasive monitoring tools are limited by inaccuracy, lack of specificity, and cost. Invasive monitoring tools are limited by the risk of surgical implantation and limited to only regional monitoring ability. No one modality is sufficient. An integration of multiple neuromonitoring tools using the MMM approach can provide real-time information on multiple parameters of brain function supporting individualized therapeutic strategies. Considering trends instead of responding to individual critical thresholds allows for more goal-directed therapy. As such the MMM concept will rapidly evolve bioinformatics and artificial intelligence applications. The biggest barrier to broad adoption of MMM in NCC practice is the lack of a common data management system to link neuromonitoring data to other patient-level data within the medical record. Clinical trials evaluating these strategies are ongoing but results will reflect the treatment protocol used to translate monitoring values into patient care.

CLINICS CARE POINTS

- Integration of MMM with neurologic examination enhances detection of impending SBI.
- Physiologic parameters measured by neuromonitoring are best interpreted in concert and along with clinical data.
- Invasive ICP monitors are standard of care in patients with ABI at risk for elevated ICP. The gold standard ICP monitor is the ventriculostomy catheter.
- Accuracy of noninvasive ICP monitors is yet to be validated.
- Continuous EEG is recommended in persistent or unexplained altered mental status, status epilepticus not promptly returning to baseline, therapeutic hypothermia, and aneurysmal SAH.
- For noninvasive oximetry measures such as NIRS, methods that mitigate scalp contributions and drift should be considered. For invasive focal measures of oximetry, consideration of probe placement relative to surrounding injury is necessary. Monitoring from perilesional tissue is likely more dynamic and treatment-responsive than from the core infarction, contusion, or hemorrhage.
- CA monitoring provides data to calculate optimal individualized MAP and CPP targets.

DISCLOSURE

Dr T.H. Fan has nothing to disclose. Dr E. Rosenthal reports consulting fees from UCB Inc.; consulting fees from Ceribell, Inc.; and grant funding from the Department of Defense (as subcontract from Moberg Analytics; W81XWH-18-DMRDP-PTCRA) as well as from NIH/NIINDS (1R01NS117904, 1R01NS113541 1K23NS105950, and U54NS100064).

REFERENCES

1. Chesnut RM, Marshall LF, Klauber MR, et al. The role of secondary brain injury in determining outcome from severe head injury. J Trauma 1993;34(2):216.
2. le Roux P, Menon DK, Citerio G, et al. Consensus summary statement of the international multidisciplinary consensus conference on multimodality monitoring in neurocritical care: a statement for healthcare professionals from the neurocritical care Society and the European Society of intensive care medicine. Neurocrit Care 2014;21(Suppl 2):1–26.
3. Vespa P, Menon DK, le Roux P, et al. The international multi-disciplinary consensus conference on multimodality monitoring: future directions and emerging technologies. Neurocrit Care 2014;21(Suppl 2):270–81.
4. Le Roux P, Menon DK, Citerio G, et al. The international multidisciplinary consensus conference on multimodality monitoring in neurocritical care: Evidentiary Tables: a statement for healthcare professionals from the neurocritical care Society and the European Society of intensive care medicin. Neurocrit Care 2014; 21(2):297–361.
5. Ng SY, Lee AYW. Traumatic brain injuries: pathophysiology and potential therapeutic targets. Front Cell Neurosci 2019;13:528.

6. von Bornstädt D, Houben T, Seidel JL, et al. Supply-demand mismatch transients in susceptible peri-infarct hot zones explain the origin of spreading injury depolarizations. Neuron 2015;85(5):1117.

7. Schneeweiss B, Druml W, Graninger W, et al. Assessment of oxygen-consumption by use of reverse Fick-principle and indirect calorimetry in critically ill patients. Clin Nutr (Edinburgh, Scotland) 1989;8(2):89–93.

8. de Georgia MA. Brain tissue oxygen monitoring in neurocritical care. J Intensive Care Med 2015;30(8):473–83.

9. Stiefel MF, Udoetuk JD, Spiotta AM, et al. Conventional neurocritical care and cerebral oxygenation after traumatic brain injury. J Neurosurg 2006;105(4):568–75.

10. Okonkwo DO, Shutter LA, Moore C, et al. Brain tissue oxygen monitoring and management in severe traumatic brain injury (BOOST-II): a phase II randomized trial. Crit Care Med 2017;45(11):1907.

11. Algattas H, Huang JH. Traumatic Brain Injury pathophysiology and treatments: early, intermediate, and late phases post-injury. Int J Mol Sci 2013;15(1):309–41.

12. Matsushima K, Peng M, Velasco C, et al. Glucose variability negatively impacts long-term functional outcome in patients with traumatic brain injury. J Crit Care 2012;27(2):125–31.

13. Hinzman JM, Thomas TC, Quintero JE, et al. Disruptions in the regulation of extracellular glutamate by neurons and glia in the rat striatum two days after diffuse brain injury. J Neurotrauma 2012;29(6):1197–208.

14. Peerdeman SM, Girbes ARJ, Polderman KH, et al. Changes in cerebral interstitial glycerol concentration in head-injured patients; correlation with secondary events. Intensive Care Med 2003;29(10):1825–8.

15. Dewitt DS, Prough DS. Traumatic cerebral vascular injury: the effects of concussive brain injury on the cerebral vasculature. J Neurotrauma 2003;20(9):795–825.

16. Czosnyka M, Smielewski P, Kirkpatrick P, et al. Continuous assessment of the cerebral vasomotor reactivity in head injury. Neurosurgery 1997;41(1):11–9.

17. Hinzman JM, Andaluz N, Shutter LA, et al. Inverse neurovascular coupling to cortical spreading depolarizations in severe brain trauma. Brain 2014;137(11):2960–72.

18. Hartings JA, Shuttleworth CW, Kirov SA, et al. The continuum of spreading depolarizations in acute cortical lesion development: Examining Leão's legacy. J Cereb Blood Flow Metab 2017;37(5):1571.

19. Dreier JP, Major S, Lemale CL, et al. Correlates of spreading depolarization, spreading depression, and negative ultraslow potential in epidural versus subdural Electrocorticography. Front Neurosci 2019;13:373.

20. Lara LR, Püttgen HA. Multimodality monitoring in the neurocritical care unit. Contin Lifelong Learn Neurol 2018;24(6):1776–88.

21. Pennings FA, Schuurman PR, van den Munckhof P, et al. Brain tissue oxygen pressure monitoring in awake patients during functional neurosurgery: the assessment of normal values. J Neurotrauma 2008;25(10):1173–7.

22. Sarrafzadeh AS, Sakowitz OW, Kiening KL, et al. Bedside microdialysis: a tool to monitor cerebral metabolism in subarachnoid hemorrhage patients? Crit Care Med 2002;30(5):1062–70.

23. Rose JC, Neill TA, Hemphill JC. Continuous monitoring of the microcirculation in neurocritical care: an update on brain tissue oxygenation. Curr Opin Crit Care 2006;12(2):97–102.

24. Witsch J, Frey HP, Schmidt JM, et al. Electroencephalographic periodic discharges and frequency-dependent brain tissue hypoxia in acute brain injury. JAMA Neurol 2017;74(3):301–9.

25. Pascual JL, Georgoff P, Maloney-Wilensky E, et al. Reduced brain tissue oxygen in traumatic brain injury: are most commonly used interventions successful? J Trauma 2011;70(3):535–46.

26. Oddo M, Bösel J, le Roux P, et al. Monitoring of brain and systemic oxygenation in neurocritical care patients. Neurocrit Care 2014;21(Suppl 2):103–20.

27. Kistka H, Dewan MC, Mocco J. Evidence-based cerebral vasospasm surveillance. Neurol Res Int 2013;2013:256713.

28. Heran NS, Hentschel SJ, Toyota BD. Jugular bulb oximetry for prediction of vasospasm following subarachnoid hemorrhage. Can J Neurol Sci 2004;31(1):80–6.

29. Coplin WM, O'Keefe GE, Sean Grady M, et al. Thrombotic, infectious, and procedural complications of the jugular bulb catheter in the intensive care unit. Neurosurgery 1997;41(1):101–9.

30. Scheeren TW, Schober P, Schwarte LA. Monitoring tissue oxygenation by near infrared spectroscopy (NIRS): background and current applications. J Clin Monit Comput 2012;26(4):279–87.

31. Misra M, Stark J, Dujovny M, et al. Transcranial cerebral oximetry in random normal subjects. Neurol Res 1998;20(2):137–41.

32. M Oddo FT. How to monitor the brain in septic patients? Minerva Anestesiol 2015; 81(7):776–88.

33. Chock VY, Chock SH, Kwon N, et al. Cerebral oxygenation and autoregulation in preterm infants (early NIRS study). J Pediatr 2020;227:94–100.e1.

34. Colak Z, Borojevic M, Ivancan V, et al. The relationship between prolonged cerebral oxygen desaturation and postoperative outcome in patients undergoing coronary artery bypass grafting. Coll Antropol June 2012;381–8.

35. Storm C, Leithner C, Krannich A, et al. Regional cerebral oxygen saturation after cardiac arrest in 60 patients–a prospective outcome study. Resuscitation 2014; 85(8):1037–41.

36. Bellander BM, Cantais E, Enblad P, et al. Consensus meeting on microdialysis in neurointensive care. Intensive Care Med 2004;30(12):2166–9.

37. Staub F, Graf R, Gabel P, et al. Multiple interstitial substances measured by microdialysis in patients with subarachnoid hemorrhage. Neurosurgery 2000;47(5): 1106–16.

38. Skjøth-Rasmussen J, Schulz M, Kristensen SR, et al. Delayed neurological deficits detected by an ischemic pattern in the extracellular cerebral metabolites in patients with aneurysmal subarachnoid hemorrhage. J Neurosurg 2004; 100(1):8–15.

39. Nagel A, Graetz D, Schink T, et al. Relevance of intracranial hypertension for cerebral metabolism in aneurysmal subarachnoid hemorrhage. Clinical article. J Neurosurg 2009;111(1):94–101.

40. Hlatky R, Valadka AB, Goodman JC, et al. Patterns of energy substrates during ischemia measured in the brain by microdialysis. J Neurotrauma 2004;21(7): 894–906.

41. Roh DJ, Morris NA, Claassen J. Intracranial multimodality monitoring for delayed cerebral ischemia. J Clin Neurophysiol 2016;33(3):241–9.

42. Vajkoczy P, Horn P, Thome C, et al. Regional cerebral blood flow monitoring in the diagnosis of delayed ischemia following aneurysmal subarachnoid hemorrhage. J Neurosurg 2003;98(6):1227–34.

43. Kirkpatrick PJ, Smielewski P, Czosnyka M, et al. Continuous monitoring of cortical perfusion by laser Doppler flowmetry in ventilated patients with head injury. J Neurol Neurosurg Psychiatry 1994;57(11):1382–8.

44. Miller C, Armonda R, le Roux P, et al. Monitoring of cerebral blood flow and ischemia in the critically ill. Neurocrit Care 2014;21(Suppl 2):121–8.

45. Lysakowski C, Walder B, Costanza MC, et al. Transcranial Doppler versus angiography in patients with vasospasm due to a ruptured cerebral aneurysm: a systematic review. Stroke 2001;32(10):2292–8.

46. Wartenberg KE, Schmidt JM, Mayer SA. Multimodality monitoring in neurocritical care. Crit Care Clin 2007;23(3):507–38.

47. Copplestone S, Welbourne J. A narrative review of the clinical application of pressure reactiviy indices in the neurocritical care unit. Br J Neurosurg 2018; 32(1):4–12.

48. Zweifel C, Lavinio A, Steiner LA, et al. Continuous monitoring of cerebrovascular pressure reactivity in patients with head injury. Neurosurg Cocus 2008;25(4).

49. Aries MJH, Czosnyka M, Budohoski KP, et al. Continuous determination of optimal cerebral perfusion pressure in traumatic brain injury. Crit Care Med 2012;40(8):2456–63.

50. Rivera-Lara L, Zorrilla-Vaca A, Geocadin RG, et al. Cerebral autoregulation-oriented therapy at the bedside: a comprehensive review. Anesthesiology 2017;126(6):1187–99.

51. Carney N, Totten AM, O'Reilly C, et al. Guidelines for the management of severe traumatic brain injury, Fourth Edition. Neurosurgery 2017;80(1):6–15.

52. Steiner LA, Czosnyka M, Piechnik SK, et al. Continuous monitoring of cerebrovascular pressure reactivity allows determination of optimal cerebral perfusion pressure in patients with traumatic brain injury. Crit Care Med 2002;30(4):733–8.

53. Lescot T, Reina V, le Manach Y, et al. In vivo accuracy of two intraparenchymal intracranial pressure monitors. Intensive Care Med 2011;37(5):875–9.

54. Dey M, Stadnik A, Riad F, et al. Bleeding and infection with external ventricular drainage: a systematic review in comparison with adjudicated adverse events in the ongoing Clot Lysis Evaluating Accelerated Resolution of Intraventricular Hemorrhage Phase III (CLEAR-III IHV) trial. Neurosurgery 2015;76(3):291–300.

55. Eide PK, Sorteberg W. Simultaneous measurements of intracranial pressure parameters in the epidural space and in brain parenchyma in patients with hydrocephalus. J Neurosurg 2010;113(6):1317–25.

56. Melhem S, Shutter L, Kaynar AM. A trial of intracranial pressure monitoring in traumatic brain injury. Crit Care (London, England) 2014;18(1):302.

57. le oux P. Physiological monitoring of the severe traumatic brain injury patient in the intensive care unit. Curr Neurol Neurosci Rep 2013;13(3):331.

58. Bratton SL, Chestnut RM, Ghajar J, et al. Guidelines for the management of severe traumatic brain injury. VI. Indications for intracranial pressure monitoring. J Neurotrauma 2007;24(Suppl 1):S37–44.

59. Bellner J, Romner B, Reinstrup P, et al. Transcranial Doppler sonography pulsatility index (PI) reflects intracranial pressure (ICP). Surg Neurol 2004;62(1):45–51.

60. Wakerley BR, Kusuma Y, Yeo LLL, et al. Usefulness of transcranial Doppler-derived cerebral hemodynamic parameters in the noninvasive assessment of intracranial pressure. J Neuroimaging 2015;25(1):111–6.

61. Harary M, Dolmans RGF, Gormley WB. Intracranial pressure monitoring-review and avenues for development. Sensors (Basel) 2018;18(2).

62. Al-Mufti F, Smith B, Lander M, et al. Novel minimally invasive multi-modality monitoring modalities in neurocritical care. J Neurol Sci 2018;390:184–92.

63. Shimbles S, Dodd C, Banister K, et al. Clinical comparison of tympanic membrane displacement with invasive intracranial pressure measurements. Physiol Meas 2005;26(6):1085–92.

64. Traylor TY, El Ahmadieh, Bedros NM, et al. Quantitative pupillometry in patients with traumatic brain injury and loss of consciousness: a prospective pilot study. J Clin Neurosci 2021;91:88–92.
65. Riker RR, Sawyer ME, Fischman VG, et al. Neurological pupil index and pupillary light reflex by pupillometry predict outcome early after cardiac arrest. Neurocrit Care 2020;32(1):152–61.
66. Chen JW, Gombart ZJ, Rogers S, et al. Pupillary reactivity as an early indicator of increased intracranial pressure: the introduction of the Neurological Pupil index. Surg Neurol Int 2011;2(1):82.
67. Vespa PM, Nuwer MR, Nenov V, et al. Increased incidence and impact of nonconvulsive and convulsive seizures after traumatic brain injury as detected by continuous electroencephalographic monitoring. J Neurosurg 1999;91(5):750–60.
68. Vespa PM, O'Phelan K, Shah M, et al. Acute seizures after intracerebral hemorrhage: a factor in progressive midline shift and outcome. Neurology 2003; 60(9):1441–6.
69. Vespa PM, Miller C, McArthur D, et al. Nonconvulsive electrographic seizures after traumatic brain injury result in a delayed, prolonged increase in intracranial pressure and metabolic crisis - PubMed. Crit Care Med 2007;35(12):2830–6.
70. Claassen J, Vespa P, le Roux P, et al. Electrophysiologic monitoring in acute brain injury. Neurocrit Care 2014;21(Suppl 2):129–47.
71. Foreman B, Claassen J. Quantitative EEG for the detection of brain ischemia. Crit Care (London, England) 2012;16(2):216.
72. Rosenthal ES, Biswal S, Zafar SF, et al. Continuous electroencephalography predicts delayed cerebral ischemia after subarachnoid hemorrhage: a prospective study of diagnostic accuracy. Ann Neurol 2018;83(5):958–69.
73. Rots ML, van Putten MJAM, Hoedemaekers CWE, et al. Continuous EEG monitoring for early detection of delayed cerebral ischemia in subarachnoid hemorrhage: a pilot study. Neurocrit Care 2016;24(2):207–16.
74. Lissak IA, Locascio JJ, Zafar SF, et al. Electroencephalography, hospital complications, and longitudinal outcomes after subarachnoid hemorrhage. Neurocrit Care 2021;35(2):1.

Artificial Intelligence and Big Data Science in Neurocritical Care

Shraddha Mainali, MD[a],*, Soojin Park, MD[b]

KEYWORDS

- Artificial intelligence • Big data • Neurocritical care • Machine learning

KEY POINTS

- The digitization of health care has paralleled the development of technology to support efficient and affordable processing of large amounts of complex data.
- There are many areas in neurocritical care that could benefit from big data science including process, diagnostics, and clinical decision-making.
- The future awaits rigorous implementation studies and examination of bias and generalizability of promising big data science in neurocritical care.

INTRODUCTION

Big data refers to the rapidly growing large volumes of digitalized web-based information that utilizes modern computer-based technology for storage, processing, and analysis.[1] Machine learning (ML) is a subfield of artificial intelligence (AI) that uses computerized algorithms to automatically improve performance through an iterative learning process or experience.[2] As a field of study, ML sits at the intersection of a variety of fields including computer science, statistics, psychological study of human learning, study of evolution, adaptive control theory, study of educational practices, neuroscience, organizational behavior, and economics, that relate to automatic augmentation of performance over time with acquired ability to reason and make decisions under uncertainty.[3] In recent years, ML technology has emerged as the method of choice for developing practical software for a wide range of fields including health care, where ML technology can be used to process large volumes of clinical data to derive clinically meaningful output.

[a] Department of Neurology, Virginia Commonwealth University, Richmond, 1101 East Marshall Street, Sanger-6-04, Richmond, VA 23298, USA; [b] Department of Neurology, Department of Biomedical Informatics, Columbia University, 8-Milstein-300 center, 177 Fort, Washington Avenue, New York, NY 10032, USA
* Corresponding author. Virginia Commonwealth University, 1101 East Marshall Street, Sanger 6-004, Richmond, VA 23298.
E-mail address: shraddha.mainali@vcuhealth.org

Crit Care Clin 39 (2023) 235–242
https://doi.org/10.1016/j.ccc.2022.07.008
0749-0704/23/© 2022 Elsevier Inc. All rights reserved.
criticalcare.theclinics.com

The neurocritical care environment is a process-intense one with multiple simultaneous high-frequency data variables being monitored and recorded for clinical decision-making. The increase in adoption of multimodal monitoring and the Health Information Systems such as the Electronic Health Records (EHR), Nursing Information Systems, and the Picture Archiving and Communication Systems have led to "big data." Big data consists of a deluge (volume) of evolving data (variety) collected at a high frequency (velocity) with high degree of uncertainty regarding correlations of variable data streams (veracity). However, studies have shown that the human brain can process no more than 4 variables at any given time for cognitive tasks pertaining to reasoning and decision-making.[4] Sensory overload with a plethora of indiscriminate simultaneous data can therefore lead to cognitive burden and decision errors, especially in the intensive care unit (ICU) setting that demands expeditious decisions.[5,6] In such high-stake environments where clinical decisions greatly impact outcome trajectories, computer-based clinical decision support tools have the potential to streamline and process multivariable data in a clinically meaningful and reliable manner that significantly enhances performance of the treating team. Modern technology and innovation have brought us to a juncture of health information revolution with recent increase in integration of tools for management, assimilation, and exchange of electronic clinical data. This increase in human–computer interface aids clinical decisions and enables data exchange between individual silos within the multiprofessional care team. Utilization of data science in neurocritical care now spans the spectrum of clinical diagnosis, event prediction, and determination of prognostic trajectories. This article provides an overview of applications of AI and big data science in neurocritical care. We will also discuss the challenges and limitations of AI-based technology that needs careful consideration before integrating such automated tools into clinical practice.

BIG DATA SCIENCE FOR EARLY DIAGNOSIS/DETECTION OF PATHOLOGIC CONDITION

Supportive care and prevention of secondary brain injury is the cornerstone of neurocritical care management. Conforming to the maxim, "a stitch in time saves nine," early detection of pathologic condition and timely intervention is key to preventing secondary brain injury and poor clinical outcomes. Given the complexity of decision-making, laden with data-overload from clinical observations as well as abundant monitoring devices, diagnostic error in the ICU tends to be very high. It has been estimated that diagnostic errors in the ICU may lead to more than 40,000 adult deaths annually, with infections and vascular events culminating a vast majority of these errors.[7] This alarming number indicates the dire need to develop and implement innovative strategies to simplify data interpretation and facilitate prompt delivery of critical interventions. Various ways to harness big data in clinical medicine have been attempted. Computerized decision support (CDS) systems have been introduced as tools for automated data interpretation to aid in clinical decision-making. Several early warning systems have been developed to enable clinicians to respond proactively toward potentially detrimental impending clinical events.[8] High-impact areas for CDS include conditions with high stakes for rapid deterioration such as cerebrovascular events, severe traumatic brain injury (TBI), hemodynamic instability, respiratory distress, and sepsis.

Arterial hypotension is a commonly encountered pathologic condition in the ICU with high risk for cerebral hypoperfusion and subsequent secondary brain injury. In a recent multicenter study, Donald and colleagues[9] used the Bayesian artificial neural network (BANN) model to give neurointensive care teams early warning (>15 minutes) of potential hypotensive events before they emerge, with area under the receiver operating characteristic (AUROC) of 0.74, sensitivity of 35% to 40% and specificity of 91%. Investigators have also developed a clinical prediction model using ML algorithms to predict the development of septic shock in ICU patients with the ability to predict an event at a median of 28.2 hours before onset.[10] The score called the Targeted Real-Time Early Warning score (TREWScore) had an AUROC of 0.83 with 85% sensitivity at 67% specificity, indicating better performance than the commonly used Modified Early Warning Score.

In the milieu of acute brain injury, an ML-based model has been developed for adult and pediatric patients with TBI to predict future increase in intracranial pressure (ICP) episodes about 30 minutes in advance, by analyzing the ICP and mean arterial pressure characteristics of the preceding hours.[11] This model demonstrated an AUROC of 0.90 with sensitivity and specificity of 70% and 90%, respectively, for adults and AUROC of 0.79 with sensitivity and specificity of 91% and 48%, respectively, for the pediatric TBI cohort. Another model in pediatric patients used ML technology to identify patients at risk for hemodynamic instability in the hours before the required clinical intervention and was found to have better classification performance results with AUROC of 0.80 (0.70), sensitivity of 0.66 (0.50), and specificity of 0.78 (0.77) at 1 hour (and 12 hours) before the event compared with the systolic blood pressure based and shock-index based models.[12] Although modern day ML technology has the potential to significantly enhance our ability to process big data for clinical use, utilization is often limited by artifactual and incomplete data in the real-time dynamic, and at-times chaotic, ICU environment. Additionally, there is much room for improvement in optimization of user interface and minimization of false alarms to avoid provider burnout and facilitate smooth clinical implementation.

BIG DATA AND ARTIFICIAL INTELLIGENCE FOR PREDICTION OF EVENTS AND OUTCOMES

The availability of big data has enabled future event prediction based on the vast database of historic events, obviating comprehensive understanding of the underlying disease dynamics for an individual patient.[13] Data mining techniques using ML models have been adopted to predict disease-related events using physiological and clinical data.[14] Prognostic models using vital sign (VS) parameters stored in cloud platforms demonstrated the ability to accurately predict significant clinical events by using information learned from changes in VS parameters from a large database of patients.[15] Such models have potential utility in routine clinical settings or as remote monitoring tools for physicians to observe patients at risk for deterioration. Similarly, a recent study has demonstrated successful use of deep learning technology to predict future VSs with greater than 80% accuracy, which was then used for prognostic index calculation with the intent to guide early therapeutic interventions before overt clinical deterioration.[16] Such an ability to predict future clinical events could be highly beneficial in the ICU by providing forewarning of imminent life-threatening events.

Outcome prediction is a critical component of routine patient care in the ICU that influences major clinical decisions surrounding therapeutic strategies and management plans. Conventionally, clinical ordinal severity illness scores such as the Acute Physiological Score (APS),[17] Multiorgan Dysfunction Score,[18] Sequential Organ Failure Assessment (SOFA),[19] and International Mission on Prognosis and Analysis of Clinical Trials[20] scores are used for outcome prediction. Although statistical and algorithmic prediction models have been developed over the years, neither neural networks nor regression models have demonstrated sufficient predictive power for integration into routine clinical care.[21] Johnson and colleagues[22] used gradient boosting ML model on granular patient data (including physiology, laboratories, and demographics but excluding diagnosis or comorbidities) in critically ill patients to derive real-time mortality prediction, and demonstrated superior performance (AUROC = 0.920) compared with conventional scores such as the simplified APS and SOFA. Xu and colleagues[23] proposed recurrent attentive and intensive model to jointly analyze continuous monitoring data (eg, electroencephalography [EEG]) and discrete clinical events (eg, specific diagnosis, laboratory value, or medication use) and applied this architecture to predict physiologic decompensation (AUC-ROC 90.18%) and length of stay (accuracy of 87% in a cohort of adult ICU patients). Casteniera and colleagues[24] introduced a methodology designed to automatically extract information (features) from continuous-real-time VS data collected from bedside monitors to predict patient outcomes using ML technology and noted improved performances of 90% (area under the ROC curve [AUC]) with combination of dynamic VS and static clinical data extracted from EHR. Most recently, Bhattacharyay and colleagues[25] have demonstrated that computational analysis of time series motor activity (from extremities of severe brain injury patients) quantitatively captured by wearable accelerometers can yield clinically important insights regarding underlying neurologic states and short-term clinical outcomes. It is important however, to note that in a critical care environment where patients are often on sedation and pain medications, confounding effects of such medications must be considered. Nevertheless, with the availability of efficient and cost-effective data archival and evolving deep learning techniques such as recurrent neural networks, we now have the infrastructure required to explore ML technology on big data to determine clinical events and outcomes.

BIG DATA AND ARTIFICIAL INTELLIGENCE FOR NEUROPROGNOSTICATION

The task of neurologic prognostication is a major challenge for clinicians given the complexity of disease dynamics and uncertainty of prognostic trajectories especially in the acute setting.[26] Moreover, prognostication has a major impact on the course of patient management as prediction of good prognosis leads to offerings of hope and aggressive therapy, whereas prediction of poor prognosis may lead to withdrawal of life supporting therapy.[27] Therefore, prognostication needs to be objective, accurate, and evidence-based. Accurate neuroprognostication requires consideration of various factors including clinical assessment, review of medical comorbidities, neuroimaging, brain physiology and metabolism, electrophysiology, serum biomarkers, therapeutic intensity, and genetic factors. It is therefore a complex process requiring an objective and scientific approach with integration of multimodal data points for educated judgment about possible prognostic trajectories. Use of data-intensive computational methods with the help of ML technology shows great promise in improving the accuracy of prognostication. What is needed to improve ML performance are large, diverse but harmonized observational patient datasets.

Investigators have applied ML technology in outcome predictions and neuroprognostication models. For example, Stapleton and colleagues[28] used an ML classifier to analyze more than 150 metabolites obtained via mass spectrometry in 137 patients with subarachnoid hemorrhage and noted increased plasma taurine as the leading metabolite associated with 90-day functional outcome ($P < .0001$). Recent studies have also trained ML algorithms on models using continuous electroencephalography (cEEG) data acquired in the ICU. In one of the prospective studies with 864 patients from 5 medical centers (model trained and validated internally with data from 2 centers and externally validated using data from 3 other centers) where cEEG was started within 12 to 24 hours after cardiac arrest (CA) and maintained for up to 72 hours, the convoluted neural network classifier discriminated between favorable and unfavorable outcomes (dichotomized cerebral performance category [CPC] score at 6 months) with AUROC of 0.92 at 12 hours after CA and 0.90 at 24 hours.[29] Similarly, in a retrospective study of 438 CA patients from 4 US centers, investigators used statistical and ML technique in an array of 52 quantitative EEG signal features using single-channel or multichannel cEEG recordings and combined the EEG findings with clinical variables (age, gender, initial cardiac rhythm, and time to return of spontaneous circulation) to predict 6-month outcome (dichotomized CPC score).[30] Investigators noted that compared with a clinical model, the integration of time-sensitive cEEG features with clinical variables had the best performance with AUC of 0.83.

BIG DATA AND ARTIFICIAL INTELLIGENCE FOR PRECISION IN INDIVIDUAL PATIENT OR DISEASE TRAJECTORY

Given the heterogeneity of cause, disease trajectory, and outcomes related to acute brain injury, generalized management framework and treatment approaches are often inadequate to achieve optimum patient outcome. The goal of precision medicine is to provide the right treatment to the right patient at the right time. Classically, precision medicine approaches have been based on genetics and multiomics[31]; however, with the evolution of big data and improved ML techniques to mine and leverage various types of patient-specific *unstructured*, *semistructured*, and *structured data* into clinically relevant parameters, applicability of precision medicine in critical care settings is poised to improve. Patient-specific data in the ICU involve clinical variables that characterize individual chronicles of the temporal course reflecting the disease trajectory and effects of clinical intervention. Utilization of patient-specific genetic and/or clinical data including real-time physiologic data can guide individualized management. In the ICU, the ability to predict potential complications or impending clinical deteriorations in each patient will be extremely valuable in determining timely interventions to prevent bad outcomes. Similarly, the ability to accurately predict patient trajectory will be useful in guiding goals of care discussions with families and surrogate decision makers. One important example of ML in outcome prediction is the recent study by Claassen and colleagues,[32] where investigators used supervised learning algorithms from EEG to demonstrate evidence of covert consciousness in 15% of individuals with absence of behavioral responses to motor commands following an acute brain injury. Similarly, a deep-learning artificial neural network trained on EEG data in comatose patients was able to predict 6-month functional outcome in CA patients.[29] With regards to physiologic data, as previously mentioned, Casteniera and colleagues described a methodology designed to automatically extract information from continuous VS data to predict prolonged length of mechanical ventilation (defined as >4 days) in a pediatric ICU. The ML based model had an AUC of >83% using only VSs and AUC of 90% when vitals were combined with static clinical data (demographics, the pediatric index of mortality, and clinical history).[24] In the field of stroke, the development of U.S. Food and Drug Administration (FDA)-approved automated ML-based technology to detect stroke core and penumbra have significantly improved stroke triage and workflow.[2,33] Although AI and big data have shown significant advancement and promise to improve efficiency in care delivery in the neurocritical care setting, much research is needed before routine implementation of these tools to improve the lives of critically ill neurological and neurosurgical patients.

LIMITATIONS AND CHALLENGES

Dr Isaac Kohane said, "If statistics lie, then Big Data can lie in a very, very big way."[34] The axiom "garbage in, garbage out" holds true for ML-based models as poor feature selection, biased data, or use of inadequately labeled outcomes will inevitably lead to meaningless use of data despite adequate ML performance. The effectiveness of ML predictions, particularly that of supervised models largely depends on human judgment. For example, human input is required for the identification of labels or the ground truth regarding the event, the selection of features or variables to input in the model, the selection of proper statistical methods and ML classifiers used to train models, and finally for the evaluation of ML performance using statistical indices. For reliable performance, it is important to have large and diverse training, validation, and testing sets. A prospective study with a set of carefully selected data points reflective of a real-world scenario is ideal for testing an ML algorithm. In actuality, pseudoprospective validations are more feasible; sample size is often limited and frequently mixed with confounders and missing variables. "Overfitting" can occur when the model is too complex for the sample size and features, and when tested on a disparate dataset, such models may fail to perform adequately.[2] Similarly, "underfitting" can occur when a model is oversimplified with generalization of features in the training set, which then becomes unable to capture the specifics within a complex pattern of a larger test set.[2] ML models should be validated by testing the algorithm on independent unseen data, ideally from a center other than the one of model origin to prove generalizability and as a test of overfitting. The paucity of large, high-quality datasets in the ICU population can limit this quality control measure. Additionally, the logistics including need for data-sharing agreements, patient privacy concerns, high costs of data storage and security, arbitration of quality control of the input data can all limit availability of ideal training, testing, and validation data sets. This is reflected in available ML models where only a minority of studies has been validated in an independent cohort. Federated learning represents a potential solution to some of these barriers (challenges still exist regarding harmonization of data sets).

Although momentum is strong among the scientific community to utilize ML in the clinical setting, certain clinical (effects of sedation, analgesia, paralytics) and ethical limitations (eg, who is liable if there is prognostic error related to ML algorithm?) exist. It is important to consider medications and other clinical confounders while building training and testing models. Further, care must be taken to assess whether societal bias baked into patient data is not inadvertently carried forward (or amplified) in learned models. The cryptic (black-box) nature of ML algorithms make it difficult to produce interpretable outputs that can be engineered to provide clinical decision support while allowing false positives and negatives to remain transparent to good clinical judgment. Other barriers are of a more practical nature, including robustness of implementation at centers distal from the center of model origin. Model stability must be demonstrated to ensure reliability of outputs, especially when large amounts of high-frequency real-time data must be ingested. Models developed on retrospective data and validated in pseudoprospective studies of external datasets must be examined in prospective implementation for accuracy and unintended consequences of clinical adoption.

CLINICS CARE POINTS

- Computer-based technologies are being developed for use in the ICU environment.
- Significant limitations and challenges still exist and must be addressed as clinical applications of this technology advance.

DISCLOSURE

S.M: No disclosure; S.P: Receives funding support from NIH R21NS113055.

REFERENCES

1. Flechet M, Grandas FG, Meyfroidt G. Informatics in neurocritical care: new ideas for Big Data. Curr Opin Crit Care 2016;22(2):87–93.
2. Mainali S, Darsie ME, Smetana KS. Machine learning in action: stroke diagnosis and outcome prediction. Front Neurol 2021;12:734345.
3. Jordan MI, Mitchell TM. Machine learning: trends, perspectives, and prospects. Science 2015;349(6245):255–60.
4. Halford GS, Baker R, McCredden JE, et al. How many variables can humans process? Psychol Sci 2005;16(1):70–6.
5. Rebitzer JB, Rege M, Shepard C. Influence, information overload, and information technology in health care. Bingley, United Kingdom.: Emerald Group Publishing Limited; 2008.
6. Montgomery VL. Effect of fatigue, workload, and environment on patient safety in the pediatric intensive care unit. Pediatr Crit Care Med 2007;8(2 Suppl):S11–6.
7. Winters B, Custer J, Galvagno SM, et al. Diagnostic errors in the intensive care unit: a systematic review of autopsy studies. BMJ Qual Saf 2012;21(11):894–902.
8. Medic G, Kosaner Kließ M, Atallah L, Weichert J, Panda S, Postma M, El-Kerdi A. Evidence-based Clinical Decision Support Systems for the prediction and detection of three disease states in critical care: A systematic literature review. F1000Res 2019 Oct 8;8:1728. https://doi.org/10.12688/f1000research.20498.2. PMID: 31824670; PMCID: PMC6894361.
9. Donald R, Howells T, Piper I, et al. Forewarning of hypotensive events using a Bayesian artificial neural network in neurocritical care. J Clin Monit Comput 2019;33(1):39–51.
10. Henry KE, Hager DN, Pronovost PJ, et al. A targeted real-time early warning score (TREWScore) for septic shock. Sci Translational Med 2015;7(299). 299ra122-299ra122.
11. Güiza F, Depreitere B, Piper I, et al. Early detection of increased intracranial pressure episodes in traumatic brain injury: external validation in an adult and in a pediatric cohort. Crit Care Med 2017;45(3):e316–20.
12. Potes C, Conroy B, Xu-Wilson M, et al. A clinical prediction model to identify patients at high risk of hemodynamic instability in the pediatric intensive care unit. Crit Care 2017;21(1):1–8.
13. Zhao L. Event prediction in the big data era: a systematic survey. ACM Comput Surv (CSUR) 2021;54(5):1–37.
14. Clifton L, Clifton DA, Watkinson PJ, et al: Identification of patient deterioration in vital-sign data using one-class support vector machines. In: 2011 federated conference on computer science and information systems (FedCSIS): September 18-21, 2011: IEEE; 2011: 125-131.

15. Forkan ARM, Khalil I, Atiquzzaman M, et al. A learning model for early discovery and real-time prediction of severe clinical events using vital signs as big data. Computer Networks 2017;113:244–57.
16. da Silva DB, Schmidt D, da Costa CA, et al. DeepSigns: a predictive model based on deep learning for the early detection of patient health deterioration. Expert Syst Appl 2021;165:113905.
17. Knaus WA, Zimmerman JE, Wagner DP, et al. APACHE-acute physiology and chronic health evaluation: a physiologically based classification system. Crit Care Med 1981;9(8):591–7.
18. Marshall JC, Cook DJ, Christou NV, et al. Multiple organ dysfunction score: a reliable descriptor of a complex clinical outcome. Crit Care Med 1995;23(10):1638–52.
19. Vincent J-L, Moreno R, Takala J, et al. The SOFA (Sepsis-related Organ Failure Assessment) score to describe organ dysfunction/failure. Springer-Verlag; 1996.
20. Dijkland SA, Helmrich I, Nieboer D, et al. Outcome prediction after moderate and severe traumatic brain injury: external validation of two established prognostic models in 1742 European patients. J Neurotrauma 2021;38(10):1377–88.
21. Bulgarelli L, Deliberato RO, Johnson AE. Prediction on critically ill patients: the role of "big data". J Crit Care 2020;60:64–8.
22. Johnson AE, Mark RG: Real-time mortality prediction in the Intensive Care Unit. In: AMIA Annual Symposium Proceedings: September 18-21, 2011: American Medical Informatics Association; 2017: 994.
23. Xu Y, Biswal S, Deshpande SR, Maher KO, Sun J: Raim: Recurrent attentive and intensive model of multimodal patient monitoring data. In: Proceedings of the 24th ACM SIGKDD international conference on Knowledge Discovery & Data Mining: September 18-21, 2011; 2018: 2565-2573.
24. Castineira D, Schlosser KR, Geva A, et al. Adding continuous vital sign information to static clinical data improves the prediction of length of stay after intubation: a data-driven machine learning approach. Respir Care 2020;65(9):1367–77.
25. Bhattacharyay S, Rattray J, Wang M, et al. Decoding accelerometry for classification and prediction of critically ill patients with severe brain injury. Scientific Rep 2021;11(1):1–17.
26. Stevens RD, Sutter R. Prognosis in severe brain injury. Crit Care Med 2013;41(4):1104–23.
27. Gill TM. The central role of prognosis in clinical decision making. JAMA 2012;307(2):199–200.
28. Stapleton CJ, Acharjee A, Irvine HJ, et al. High-throughput metabolite profiling: identification of plasma taurine as a potential biomarker of functional outcome after aneurysmal subarachnoid hemorrhage. J Neurosurg 2019;133(6):1842–9.
29. Tjepkema-Cloostermans MC, da Silva Lourenço C, Ruijter BJ, et al. Outcome prediction in postanoxic coma with deep learning. Crit Care Med 2019;47(10):1424–32.
30. Ghassemi MM, Amorim E, Al Hanai T, et al. Quantitative eeg trends predict recovery in hypoxic-ischemic encephalopathy. Crit Care Med 2019;47(10):1416.
31. MacEachern SJ, Forkert ND. Machine learning for precision medicine. Genome 2021;64(4):416–25.
32. Claassen J, Doyle K, Matory A, et al. Detection of brain activation in unresponsive patients with acute brain injury. N Engl J Med 2019;380(26):2497–505.
33. Murray NM, Unberath M, Hager GD, et al. Artificial intelligence to diagnose ischemic stroke and identify large vessel occlusions: a systematic review. J Neurointerventional Surg 2020;12(2):156–64.
34. Ghassemi M, Celi LA, Stone DJ. State of the art review: the data revolution in critical care. Crit Care (London, England) 2015;19(1):118.

Printed and bound by CPI Group (UK) Ltd, Croydon, CR0 4YY

03/10/2024

01040467-0006